Rare Cancers

Editor

GUY ESLICK

HEMATOLOGY/ONCOLOGY CLINICS OF NORTH AMERICA

www.hemonc.theclinics.com

Consulting Editors
GEORGE P. CANELLOS
NANCY BERLINER

December 2012 • Volume 26 • Number 6

ELSEVIER

1600 John F. Kennedy Blvd. • Suite 1800 • Philadelphia, PA 19103-2899

http://www.theclinics.com

HEMATOLOGY/ONCOLOGY CLINICS OF NORTH AMERICA Volume 26, Number 6
December 2012 ISSN 0889-8588, ISBN 13: 978-1-4557-4942-3

Editor: Patrick Manley
Developmental Editor: Donald Mumford

Hematology/Oncology Clinics (ISSN 0889-8588) is published bimonthly by Elsevier Inc., 360 Park Avenue South,
New York, NY 10010-1710. Months of issue are February, April, June, August, October, and December. Business
and Editorial Offices: 1600 John F. Kennedy Blvd., Ste. 1800, Philadelphia, PA 19103–2899. Customer Service
Office; 3251 Riverport Lane, Maryland Heights, MO 63043. Periodicals postage paid at New York, NY and at additional mailing offices. Subscription prices are $353.00 per year (domestic individuals), $576.00 per year (do-
mestic institutions), $173.00 per year (domestic students/residents), $401.00 per year (Canadian individuals),
$705.00 per year (Canadian institutions) $477.00 per year (international individuals), $705.00 per year (interna-
tional institutions), and $233.00 per year (international and Canadian students/residents). International air speed
delivery is included in all *Clinics* subscription prices. All prices are subject to change without notice. **POSTMASTER:**
Send address changes to *Hematology/Oncology Clinics of North America*, Elsevier Health Sciences Division,
Subscription Customer Service, 3251 Riverport Lane, Maryland Heights, MO 63043. Customer Service (orders,
claims, online, change of address): Elsevier Health Sciences Division, Subscription Customer Service, 3251 Riverport Lane, Maryland Heights, MO 63043. Tel: 1-800-654-2452 (U.S. and Canada); 314-447-8871 (outside U.S.
and Canada). Fax: 314-447-8029. E-mail: journalscustomerservice-usa@elsevier.com (for print support); jour-
nalsonlinesupport-usa@elsevier.com (for online support).

Reprints. For copies of 100 or more, of articles in this publication, please contact the Commercial Reprints
Department, Elsevier Inc., 360 Park Avenue South, New York, New York 10010-1710; Tel.: 212-633-3813,
Fax: 212-462-1935, E-mail: reprints@elsevier.com.

Hematology/Oncology Clinics of North America is covered in *MEDLINE/PubMed (Index Medicus), EMBASE/
Excerpta Medica, and BIOSIS.*

Printed and bound by CPI Group (UK) Ltd, Croydon, CR0 4YY

Transferred to digital print 2013

Contributors

CONSULTING EDITORS

GEORGE P. CANELLOS, MD
William Rosenberg Professor of Medicine, Department of Medical Oncology, Dana-Farber Cancer Institute, Boston, Massachusetts

NANCY BERLINER, MD
Chief, Division of Hematology, Brigham and Women's Hospital; Professor of Medicine, Harvard Medical School, Boston, Massachusetts

GUEST EDITOR

GUY D. ESLICK, DrPH, PhD, FACE, FFPH
Co-Director and Associate Professor of Surgery and Cancer Epidemiology, The Whiteley-Martin Research Centre, Discipline of Surgery, Sydney Medical School Nepean, The University of Sydney, Sydney, New South Wales, Australia

AUTHORS

MATTHEW BAK, MD
Assistant Professor, Eastern Virginia Medical School, Norfolk, Virginia

THERESA CANAVAN, BS
Medical Student, Department of Dermatology, University of California, San Francisco, San Francisco, California

RONALD Y. CHIN, Bsc(Med), MBBS, FRACS
Department of Otolaryngology Head and Neck Surgery, Nepean Hospital, Lecturer, The University of Sydney, Sydney, Australia

MATTHEW DAVENPORT, MD
Assistant Professor, Department of Radiology, University of Michigan, Ann Arbor, Michigan

BURTON L. EISENBERG, MD
Professor of Surgery, Surgical Oncology, Geisel School of Medicine at Dartmouth; Deputy Director, Norris Cotton Cancer Center, Dartmouth-Hitchcock Medical Center, Lebanon, New Hampshire

HATEM EL HALABI, MD, FACS
Department of Surgical Oncology, Mercy Medical Center, Baltimore, Maryland

GUY D. ESLICK, DrPH, PhD, FACE, FFPH
Co-Director and Associate Professor of Surgery and Cancer Epidemiology, The Whiteley-Martin Research Centre, Discipline of Surgery, Sydney Medical School Nepean, The University of Sydney, Sydney, New South Wales, Australia

FELIX FENG, MD, PhD
Assistant Professor, Department of Radiation Oncology, University of Michigan, Ann Arbor, Michigan

STEPHEN J. FULLER, MBBS, PhD, FRACP, FRCPA
Senior Lecturer, Department of Medicine, Sydney Medical School Nepean, The University of Sydney, Penrith, New South Wales, Australia

ROB GLYNNE-JONES, FRCP, FRCR
Mount Vernon Centre for Cancer Treatment, Mount Vernon Hospital, Northwood, Middlesex, United Kingdom

PETROS D. GRIVAS, MD, PhD
Fellow, Division of Hematology/Oncology, Department of Internal Medicine, University of Michigan, Ann Arbor, Michigan

VADIM GUSHCHIN, MD, FACS
Department of Surgical Oncology, Institute for Cancer Care, Mercy Medical Center, Baltimore, Maryland

SANDRA Y. HAN, MD
Procedural Dermatology Fellow, Department of Dermatology, University of California, San Francisco, San Francisco, California

SHRUTI JAYACHANDRA, MBBS, BBioMedSc
Department of Otolaryngology Head and Neck Surgery, Nepean Hospital, Sydney, Australia

IVANA K. KIM, MD
Associate Professor of Ophthalmology, Retina Service, Harvard Medical School, Massachusetts Eye and Ear Infirmary, Boston, Massachusetts

NANCY KIM, MD
Attending Physician, Spectrum Dermatology, Scottsdale, Arizona

L. PRIYA KUNJU, MD
Associate Professor, Department of Pathology, University of Michigan, Ann Arbor, Michigan

PANAYOTIS LEDAKIS, MD
Department of Medical Oncology, Institute for Cancer Care, Mercy Medical Center, Baltimore, Maryland

ARASH MOHEBATI, MD
Department of Surgery, Memorial Sloan-Kettering Cancer Center, New York, New York

JAMES E. MONTIE, MD
Vallasis Professor of Urologic Oncology, Department of Urology, University of Michigan, Ann Arbor, Michigan

JEFFREY P. NORTH, MD
Dermatopathology Fellow, Department of Dermatology, University of California, San Francisco, San Francisco, California

J. MARC PIPAS, MD
Associate Professor of Medicine; Director, Gastrointestinal Oncology Program, Norris Cotton Cancer Center, Gastrointestinal Department, Dartmouth-Hitchcock Medical Center, Lebanon, New Hampshire

ANDREW RENEHAN, PhD, FRCS
Department of Surgery, Christie NHS Foundation Trust, Institute of Cancer Sciences, Manchester Academic Health Science Centre, University of Manchester, Manchester, United Kingdom

ARMANDO SARDI, MD, FACS
Department of Surgical Oncology, Institute for Cancer Care, Mercy Medical Center, Baltimore, Maryland

JATIN SHAH, MD
Chief of Head and Neck, Department of Surgery, Memorial Sloan-Kettering Cancer Center, New York, New York

ASHOK SHAHA, MD
Department of Surgery, Memorial Sloan-Kettering Cancer Center, New York, New York

SUVEN SHANKAR, MBBS
Department of Surgical Oncology, Institute for Cancer Care, Mercy Medical Center, Baltimore, Maryland

PETER WALSHE, FRCSI, ORL, MD
Department of Otolaryngology Head and Neck Surgery, Beaumont Hospital, Lecturer, Royal College of Surgeons in Ireland, Dublin, Ireland

RICHARD O. WEIN, MD, FACS
Associate Professor, Tufts Medical Center, Boston, Massachusetts

ALON Z. WEIZER, MD, MS
Associate Professor, Department of Urology, University of Michigan, Ann Arbor, Michigan

YOSHIHIRO YONEKAWA, MD
Retina Service, Department of Ophthalmology, Harvard Medical School, Massachusetts Eye and Ear Infirmary, Boston, Massachusetts

SIEGRID S. YU, MD
Associate Professor of Dermatology, Department of Dermatology, University of California, San Francisco, San Francisco, California

Contents

Many rare cancers are essentially an enigma, with little to no information in the medical literature. Defining a rare cancer is not as easy as it might seem. As a guide, generally an incidence of fewer than 6/100,000 is considered rare. Much of the research regarding rare diseases is in its infancy.

This review describes developments in understanding normal mast cell function and genetic changes that predispose to malignant transformation to mastocytosis. Most mastocytosis cases are associated with somatically acquired activating mutations in the KIT receptor. The role these mutations play in the development of mastocytosis is discussed. Mastocytosis is classified into cutaneous mastocytosis and systemic mastocytosis. The classification of mastocytosis and clinical presentation of each variant is detailed in this report. Progress has been made in developing drugs that target the wild-type and mutated KIT receptor, and these and other new therapeutic strategies for the treatment of mastocytosis are reviewed.

Uveal melanoma is the most common primary intraocular malignancy in adults. The annual incidence is approximately 5 per million in the United States. Risk factors include white race, fair skin, light iris color, ancestry from northern latitudes, and ocular/oculodermal melanocytosis. Historically, enucleation was the definitive treatment for uveal melanoma, but brachytherapy and proton beam irradiation are now the most commonly employed treatments. However, there are no effective therapies against metastatic uveal melanoma. Recent studies suggest that the pathogenesis of uveal melanoma includes activation of the MAPK pathway via GNAQ/11, and that metastatic potential may be modulated by mechanisms involving BAP1.

Esthesioneuroblastoma (ENB) is a rare malignancy, representing only 3% to 6% of all sinonasal malignancies. A wide array of treatment options for ENB have been described in the literature, but prospective clinical trials are absent given the tumor's rarity and natural history. Delay in diagnosis leading to an initial advanced stage of presentation is common secondary to the clinically hidden primary site at the anterior skull base. This article presents data from the current body of literature and reviews the advocated roles for surgery, radiation therapy and chemotherapy.

Synovial cell sarcoma represents a rare group of cancers, particularly in the head and neck region, that typically affects young individuals and has a male preponderance. Prognosis varies with patient age, site and size of the malignancy, degree of necrosis, high level of mitotic activity, and neurovascular invasion. Complete surgical resection of the tumor via partial or total laryngectomy is the first-line treatment in locally invasive disease. CO_2 lasers have been shown to be useful in controlling localized disease. There is also a role for adjuvant radiotherapy. Ifosfamide-based chemotherapy is most useful for malignant disease.

Parathyroid carcinoma is a malignant neoplasm affecting 0.5% to 5.0% of all patients with primary hyperparathyroidism. Since it was first described by De Quervain in 1904 to this day, it continues to defy diagnosis and treatment because of its rarity, overlapping features with benign parathyroid disease, and lack of distinct characteristics. En bloc surgical extirpation of the tumor with clear margins remains the best curative treatment. Although prolonged survival is possible with recurrent or metastatic disease, cure is rarely achievable. Efficacy of adjuvant therapies, such as radiotherapy and chemotherapy, in management of persistent, recurrent, or metastatic disease has been disappointing.

Gastrointestinal stromal tumor (GIST) represents the most common mesechymal tumor of the gastrointestinal tract. Discovery of the relationship between unregulated KIT kinase and GIST transformation has led to diagnostic and therapeutic targeting. Imatinib is the recommended first-line treatment of metastatic GIST. In addition, the combination of surgery and imatinib for primary GIST is indicated in the adjuvant setting of high-risk patients and there may be benefit for this combination in the neoadjuvant setting. The success of molecular targeted therapy in GIST represents an important and exciting advance in solid tumor oncology.

The purpose of this article is to update the medical community on the current management of patients with appendiceal neoplasms. The authors discuss clinical evidence of medical and surgical treatment with emphasis on presentation, diagnosis, pathology, and surgical technique. Current available clinical evidence on the use of systemic chemotherapy is included. The authors describe in detail management of peritoneal carcinomatosis arising from tumors of the appendix with cytoreductive surgery and hyperthermic intraperitoneal therapy as standard of care.

Petros D. Grivas, Matthew Davenport, James E. Montie, L. Priya Kunju, Felix Feng, and Alon Z. Weizer

Urethral carcinoma is a rare tumor with predominantly poor survival. Both the disease and its treatment can affect both sexual and urinary function. The natural history of urethral carcinoma varies, therefore the appropriate application of surgery, radiation, and chemotherapy remain unknown. Management of this disease remains driven by individual clinician experience and data derived from small case series. This article discusses the histology and anatomy of the male and female urethra, as well as their natural history. In addition, the epidemiology, clinical presentation, diagnosis, staging, treatment, and future directions of management of cancer arising in the urethra are addressed.

Rob Glynne-Jones and Andrew Renehan

The primary aim of anal cancer treatment is loco-regional control with preservation of anal function. Phase III trials consistently demonstrate radiotherapy with concurrent 5FU and mitomycin (MMC) chemoradiation is the standard of care for anal cancer. Salvage surgery is associated with considerable morbidity and requires specialised input. With current sophisticated radiological staging and the ability to spare critical normal tissues with intensity-modulated radiotherapy, a "one-size-fits-all" approach is probably inappropriate. Radiotherapy dose-escalation and intensification of the concurrent chemotherapy might improve local control, but may also adversely affect colostomy-free survival. Integration of biologic therapy with conventional chemotherapies looks hopeful in the future.

Sandra Y. Han, Jeffrey P. North, Theresa Canavan, Nancy Kim, and Siegrid S. Yu

Merkel cell carcinoma (MCC) is a rare but aggressive carcinoma of the skin, arising most commonly in sun-exposed sites of elderly patients. The diagnosis is based on characteristic histopathologic features. In 2008, the discovery of the Merkel cell polyomavirus led to intensified research into the viral pathogenesisis of MCC. MCC staging guidelines were established in 2010, and it demonstrated the importance of distinguishing clinical vs. pathologic evaluation of lymph nodes in MCC. Surgery and/or radiation is of the mainstay of therapy for early disease, while chemotherapy is reserved for more advanced disease. Treatments based on immunologic mechanisms are currently in development.

HEMATOLOGY/ONCOLOGY CLINICS OF NORTH AMERICA

DOWNLOAD
Free App!

Review Articles
THE CLINICS

NOW AVAILABLE FOR YOUR iPhone and iPad

Preface

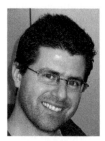

Guy D. Eslick, DrPH, PhD, FACE, FFPH
Guest Editor

The Starfish Story
(Inspired by Loren Eiseley)

One day a man was walking along the beach when he noticed a boy picking something up and gently throwing it into the ocean.
Approaching the boy, he asked, "What are you doing?"
The youth replied, "Throwing starfish back into the ocean. The surf is up and the tide is going out. If I don't throw them back, they'll die."
"Son," the man said, "don't you realize there are miles and miles of beach and hundreds of starfish?
You can't make a difference!"
After listening politely, the boy bent down, picked up another starfish, and threw it back into the surf. Then, smiling at the man, he said…
"I made a difference for that one."

This is one way to think about those with rare cancer; we should view them all as individuals with an uncommon condition that requires special attention so that on an individual level we can make a difference and, if this is done on multiple beaches (hospitals/countries), will affect thousands of lives. It should be remembered that while each individual's cancer type is rare, collectively these can add up to a substantial number of cancer patients worldwide. There are more than one thousand different histological variants of rare cancer, with some being extremely rare and providing a handful of incident cases annually and others reaching into the thousands of cases globally.

Previously, these patients had little if any guidance in their rare cancer journey; physicians had usually only anecdotal evidence with which to provide treatment and management and, for all concerned, patient outcomes were an unknown. However, out of this abyss comes hope! In recent years there has been a growing interest in rare cancers with the development of Rare Cancer Networks, specifically set up to pool resources and cancer cases for inclusion in studies and clinical trials around the world. They offer a multidisciplinary approach to these cancers, which in turn will increase the availability and quality of evidence for treatment studies, thus improving patient outcomes. There have also been a number of workshops conducted by leading health institutes and organizations including the National Cancer Institute in the United States, Rare Cancers

Hematol Oncol Clin N Am 26 (2012) xi–xii
http://dx.doi.org/10.1016/j.hoc.2012.09.003

Europe, Union for International Cancer Control, and the European Society for Medical Oncology.

The Internet has also provided a major source of information on rare cancers with a number of rare cancer/rare diseases Web sites available. Moreover, there are now specific medical peer-reviewed journals dedicated to these conditions (eg, *Rare Tumors*, *Orphanet Journal of Rare Diseases*), which will provide options to publish new data that previously was difficult to publish in mainstream journals. Generally, there is a lack of dedicated literature on rare cancers; there are some books on the topic and these are certainly excellent resources.

This issue of *Hematology/Oncology Clinics of North America* is dedicated to "Rare Cancers." Obviously, this is a select group of cancers due to the constraints of space and the majority if not all are generally adult cancers. Rare cancers in the pediatric population make a substantial contribution (up to 10%) to the overall pediatric cancer burden. I would like to sincerely thank all the authors who contributed their expertise and time to creating such an excellent collection of articles on such a diverse group of rare cancers. I hope this issue fills a gap in the literature and provides up-to-date information that will be useful to physicians, rare cancer patients, and their families.

I would like to thank the editor of *Hematology/Oncology Clinics of North America*, Patrick J. Manley, for his patience and assistance in putting this issue into publication and the consulting editors, Dr George P. Canellos and Dr Nancy Berliner, for inviting me to contribute to *Hematology/Oncology Clinics of North America*. I would also like to give special thanks to my wife, Enid, my daughter, Marielle, and my son, Guillaume, for their love and support.

Guy D. Eslick, DrPH, PhD, FACE, FFPH
The Whiteley-Martin Research Centre
Discipline of Surgery
Sydney Medical School Nepean
The University of Sydney
Level 5, South Block, PO Box 63
Penrith
Sydney, New South Wales 2751
Australia

E-mail address:
guy.eslick@sydney.edu.au

DEDICATION

I would like to dedicate this issue of *Hematology/Oncology Clinics of North America* to my soon-to-be third child (aka Sunrise). Right now, we are wondering, are you a girl or a boy? Enjoy the quiet inside while it lasts. Welcome to the family!

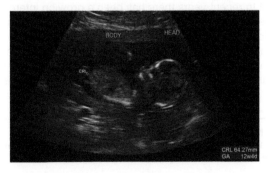

What is a Rare Cancer?

Guy D. Eslick, DrPH, PhD, FFPH

KEYWORDS

- Rare cancer • Rare diseases • Epidemiology • RARECARE

KEY POINTS

- Defining a rare cancer is not as easy as it might seem.
- As a guide, generally an incidence of fewer than 6/100,000 is considered rare.
- Much of the research regarding rare diseases is in its infancy.

Many rare cancers are essentially an enigma. For some there is little to no information in the medical literature.[1,2] Based on a MEDLINE search (1950–2012) using the keyword "rare cancer" in the title, the first published literature occurs in 1953 with 2 articles on rare cancers, and over the years this progressively increases (**Fig. 1**). While this increase is a good start, it is still a long way from what will be required to make substantial improvements in the treatment and quality of life for individuals with a rare cancer. On comparing this with other rare conditions, such as Creutzfeldt-Jakob disease (which affects 1 person in every million individuals), there are disparate differences in the number of publications, and this probably also correlates with levels of funding provided to research these conditions.

DEFINITION OF RARE CANCERS

The Oxford English Dictionary defines "rare" as "of an event, situation, or condition not occurring very often." Defining a rare cancer is not as easy as it might seem, and many organizations have used different definitions, whereas others have simply used definitions applied by other groups or organizations. The following provides examples of differing definitions of rare cancers.

RARECARE. This is the list of tumor entities from which rare tumors are identified as those with an incidence of fewer than 6 per 100,000 persons per year. The list presents the number of cases reported by European cancer registries during the period 1995 to 2002 and the corresponding incidence rates. Both figures are derived from the data of 70 population-based cancer registries adhering to the RARECARE project.

Discipline of Surgery, The Whiteley-Martin Research Centre, Nepean Hospital, The University of Sydney, Level 5, South Block, PO Box 63, Penrith, New South Wales 2751, Australia
E-mail address: guy.eslick@sydney.edu.au

Hematol Oncol Clin N Am 26 (2012) 1137–1141
http://dx.doi.org/10.1016/j.hoc.2012.09.002
0889-8588/12/$ – see front matter Crown Copyright © 2012 Published by Elsevier Inc. All rights reserved.

hemonc.theclinics.com

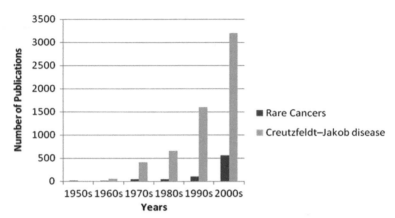

Fig. 1. Number of publications on rare cancers.

Rare Cancers Europe. Rare cancers are generally classified in the group of rare diseases, which is defined in the European Union as diseases with a prevalence of fewer than 5 cases out of a population of 10,000. According to this definition, rare cancers are identified as those with an incidence of fewer than 6 per 100,000 persons per year. Using this definition would help minimize the risk of mistaking a rare cancer (such as testicular cancer), which is frequently cured and thus has a rather high prevalence, for a common cancer, or a frequent cancer (such as small-cell lung cancer), which has a low life expectancy and thus a low prevalence, for a rare cancer.

Office of Rare Diseases. A rare (or orphan) disease is generally considered to have a prevalence of fewer than 200,000 affected individuals in the United States. The Office of Rare Diseases provides a searchable list of almost 7000 rare diseases with links to information from federally supported databases and information sources. The Rare Disease Act of 2002 (HR 4013) and the US Orphan Drug Act define a rare disease or condition as one that "(A) affects fewer than 200,000 persons in the United States, or (B) affects more than 200,000 in the United States and for which there is no reasonable expectation that the cost of developing and making available in the United States a drug for such disease or condition will be recovered from sales in the United States of such drug." Statistically speaking, with a population of 287,400,000, this means roughly 0.07% of the United States population.

The European Commission on Public Health defines rare diseases as "life-threatening or chronically debilitating diseases which are of such low prevalence that special combined efforts are needed to address them. As a guide, low prevalence is taken as prevalence of fewer than 5 per 10,000 in the Community." This would calculate into 0.05% of the overall population.

Rare Cancers US. The definition of "rare" was adopted from a recent National Cancer Institute–sponsored cancer epidemiology workshop: an incidence of fewer than 150 per million per year (ie, 15 per 100,000 per year), roughly corresponding in the United States to 40,000 new cases per year or fewer.

European Action Against Rare Cancers. Rare is defined as fewer than 50 out of 100,000 cases per year.

These are just some of the definitions of rare cancers, and the approximate number per 100,000 to be considered rare is less than 6. However, these are just numbers and like common cancers some attract more media attention, more funding, and more researchers than others. Based on the definition of 6/100,000 cases, Rare Cancers Europe has developed a list of 186 rare cancers (**Fig. 2**). It should be remembered

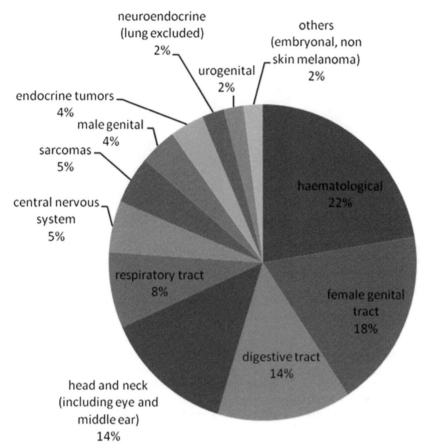

Fig. 2. The categories of rare cancers. (RARECARE (surveillance of rare cancers in Europe www.rarecare.eu). Graph courtesy of Annalisa Trama, Fondazione IRCCS Istituto Nazionale dei Tumori, Milan; with permission.)

that the study of rare cancers is not limited to rare histologic variants, but also includes subgroups that can be difficult to study in common cancers (eg, T4N0 breast cancer). Conversely, rare cancers can be rare episodes of common cancers that present in uncommon hosts (eg, male breast cancer).

RECENT DATA

Recent data using these definitions suggest that in Europe, 1 in 4 patients with cancer have a rare cancer. A recent study using a definition of rare cancer (incidence <6/100,000/yr) reported 108 per 100,000 cases in Europe, which equates to 541,000 new diagnoses annually or 22% of all cancer diagnoses.[3] Thus, it was estimated that approximately 4,300,000 individuals currently living in the European Union have a rare cancer, which accounts for almost one-quarter of the total cancer burden. This study also suggested that survival over 5 years was worse for rare cancers than for common cancer, and that those older than 40 years showed significant differences (**Fig. 3**). Other studies found worse outcomes for rare cancers in some

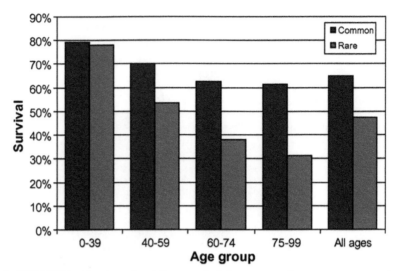

Fig. 3. RARECARE estimates of relative survival for rare and common cancers in the European Union by age group. (*From* Gatta G, van der Zwan JM, Casali PG, et al, RARECARE working group. Rare cancers are not so rare: the rare cancer burden in Europe. Eur J Cancer 2011; 47:2493–511; with permission.)

European countries but not in others.[4] In addition, rare cancers appear to affect children more than adults (**Fig. 4**), but by age 30 this finding changes, with more adults having rare cancers. Recent data from the United States lend support to some of these initial findings, including the important finding that 25% of all cancers can be classified as rare cancers.[5] This study also highlighted that rare cancers were more common among younger individuals and those who were nonwhite. These studies highlight the benefits of using national data sets for analysis, as there are usually few other sources of information available.

Obviously much of this research is in its infancy and there is a lot more to be done, with many other countries yet to contribute to the output. Thus far Europe is leading the way, and it is hoped that others will see the importance and potential benefit of further study to those who have a rare cancer.

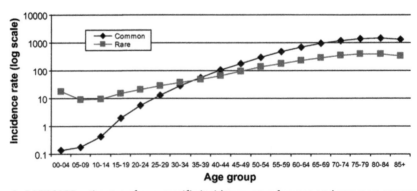

Fig. 4. RARECARE estimates of age-specific incidence rates for rare and common cancers in the European Union. (*From* Gatta G, van der Zwan JM, Casali PG, et al, RARECARE working group. Rare cancers are not so rare: the rare cancer burden in Europe. Eur J Cancer 2011; 47:2493–511; with permission.)

REFERENCES

1. Schaefer R. Rare cancers Europe: joining forces to tackle a common problem. Rare Tumors 2012;4:e24.
2. Miller RC. Problems in rare tumor study: a call for papers. Rare Tumors 2010;2:e16.
3. Gatta G, van der Zwan JM, Casali PG, et al, RARECARE working group. Rare cancers are not so rare: the rare cancer burden in Europe. Eur J Cancer 2011; 47:2493–511.
4. Gatta G, Ciccolallo L, Kunkler I, et al, EUROCARE Working Group. Survival from rare cancer in adults: a population-based study. Lancet Oncol 2006;7:132–40.
5. Greenlee RT, Goodman MT, Lynch CF, et al. The occurrence of rare cancers in U.S. adults, 1995-2004. Public Health Rep 2010;125:28–43.

New Insights into the Pathogenesis, Diagnosis, and Management of Mastocytosis

Stephen J. Fuller, MBBS, PhD, FRACP, FRCPA

KEYWORDS

- Mastocytosis • Myeloid malignancy • Mast cell function • Pathogenesis

KEY POINTS

- Mast cells (MCs) play a role in both innate and adaptive immunity and are an important component of the host response to pathogens and environmental toxins.
- The principal growth factor for MCs is Stem Cell Factor (SCF), which controls differentiation and survival by binding to the KIT receptor tyrosine kinase.
- Somatically acquired mutations in the KIT receptor are central to the pathogenesis of mastocytosis, a myeloid malignancy characterized by the accumulation of malignant MCs.
- Drugs which target KIT have efficacy in the treatment of mastocytosis; however the common activating mutation is resistant to most KIT inhibitors. Identification of other up-regulated signaling pathways will provide additional targets for future therapies.

INTRODUCTION

Mast cells (MCs) are derived from bone marrow progenitor cells,[1] which migrate via the peripheral blood to reside in tissues where they are found closely associated with blood vessels and nerve fibers.[2] In particular, MCs are found in high numbers in the skin and mucosal surfaces where it has been recognized that they play an important role in both innate and adaptive immune responses to pathogens.[3,4] Mastocytosis (MIM 154 800) is a rare myeloid malignancy that is characterized by the abnormal accumulation of malignant MCs in one or several body tissues. Most cases are sporadic and associated with somatically acquired activating mutations in the KIT oncogene.[5–8] However, a small number of familial cases have been described; the occurrence of mastocytosis with concordant clinical features in sets of monozygotic twins indicates that a subset of cases occur as a consequence of an inherited genetic predisposition.[9–13] The disease is divided into 2 main categories: cutaneous mastocytosis (CM), in which the MC infiltrate is confined to one or more lesions on the skin, and systemic mastocytosis (SM), which is characterized by MC infiltration of at least one extracutaneous organ with or

Department of Medicine, Sydney Medical School Nepean, The University of Sydney, Level 5 South Block, Nepean Hospital, PO Box 63, Penrith, New South Wales 2751, Australia
E-mail address: stephen.fuller@sydney.edu.au

Hematol Oncol Clin N Am 26 (2012) 1143–1168
http://dx.doi.org/10.1016/j.hoc.2012.08.008   hemonc.theclinics.com

without evidence of skin involvement.[14] In addition to symptoms and signs attributable to specific organ involvement, most patients report symptoms related to the release of MC mediators that include histamine, various cytokines, and eicosanoid lipid mediators. Although a significant proportion of pediatric cutaneous cases spontaneously regress before adolescence, most MC neoplasms occur in association with a mutation in the catalytic site of KIT, which is refractory to currently available treatments.

BIOLOGIC AND MOLECULAR ASPECTS
MC Function

MCs are widely distributed throughout the body but are particularly found near surfaces exposed to the environment, including the skin, airways, gastrointestinal tract, and genitourinary tract. As a consequence, in conjunction with dendritic cells (DCs) and macrophages, MCs are among the first cells to encounter and help initiate an immune response to pathogens and environmental toxins. MCs can express a range of receptors that detect products generated at sites of infection, such as pathogen-specific antibodies that bind to MC Fc receptors, and they directly recognize pathogens through pattern recognition receptors, including the Toll-like receptors (TLRs) TLR4 and TLR2, which are activated in response to pathogen-associated molecular patterns (PAMPs).[15,16] MCs undergo degranulation in response to exogenous venoms and other antigens that are injected into the skin,[17] which recruits inflammatory cells to the sites of insect bites and may have significance to the immune response against insect-borne pathogens.[18] Finally, several host endogenous peptides and substances generated at sites of inflammation can activate MCs. These substances include neurotensin; substance P; endothelin; and complement components, particularly C5a, which can induce MC degranulation.[19] Following activation, MC populations expand by recruitment and differentiation of circulating MC progenitors. Both innate and acquired immune responses, in particular T_H2-type responses, are associated with increased numbers of MCs at sites of inflammation.[20,21]

MCs share many functions with macrophages, which include host response to damage-associated molecular pattern molecules and PAMPs, antigen presentation, and phagocytosis.[22,23] In a 2-wave process, MCs are able to secrete a large number of preformed and newly synthesized products that can amplify or suppress both the innate and adaptive immune responses. Within seconds of MC activation, preformed mediators, including proteases, histamine, and tumor necrosis factor (TNF), which are stored in cytoplasmic granules, are released at the site of inflammation.[24] This release is followed by the de novo production of eicosanoids, prostaglandins, and leukotrienes, which are released within minutes, and cytokines, including interleukin 4 (IL-4), which are released within hours.[24]

MCs are categorized into 2 groups based on the protease content of their vesicles as either predominantly tryptase (MC_T cells) or, less commonly, tryptase and chymase (MC_{TC} cells).[25] Because these proteases have different substrate specificities,[26,27] factors that regulate the required MC function will determine the predominant MC subtype. MC_T cells are the predominant type found in the respiratory and gastrointestinal mucosa and are increased during inflammation, whereas MC_{TC} cells are found in the connective tissue of the dermis and gastrointestinal tract.[28,29]

Recruitment of immune cells to sites of bacterial infection during the innate immune response is facilitated by MC release of histamine, TNF, vascular endothelial growth factor, and proteases, which contribute to increased local vascular permeability and edema. In addition, chemokines produced by MCs attract other innate immune cells, including neutrophils, eosinophils, and natural killer cells, to inflamed tissues. This process may operate during viral infections and is probably stimulated by double-stranded RNA.[30] In addition, some of the products released by MCs are directly bactericidal, including reactive oxygen species and cathelicidins, which assist in killing group A streptococci.[31]

Following stimulation, MCs participate in modulating the adaptive immune response.[32] At the site of infection, MCs promote the influx of monocyte-derived DCs and, in response to bacterial peptidoglycan and gram-negative bacteria, activate local Langerhans cells.[33] In addition to recruiting antigen-presenting cells (APCs), there is in vivo evidence that MCs themselves function as APCs for major histocompatibility complex class I–restricted CD8+ T cells.[34] Depending on the stimulus, MC function can be altered by the amount and pattern of expression of cell surface receptors, which enhance or suppress particular immune responses. In response to parasitic infections and in allergic disorders, high concentrations of circulating immunoglobulin E (IgE) induce increased surface expression of high-affinity receptor for IgE (FcεRI) by tissue MCs, which enhance IgE-dependent effector functions.[35] However, for allergens, this response is pathologic; FcεRI-mediated MC activation may play a role in the pathogenesis of autoimmune diseases, including bullous pemphigoid, rheumatoid arthritis, and multiple sclerosis.[36–38] There is also evidence that MCs may reduce the duration and response of immune responses either directly through the secretion of IL-10[39] or indirectly via CD4+ CD25+ FoxP3+ regulatory T-cell–dependent peripheral tolerance.[40]

MC Differentiation

Paul Ehrlich first described MCs in 1878; for the subsequent 100 years, it was thought that they were derived from mesenchymal cells and constituted a component of connective tissue. However, in the late 1970s and early 1990s, it was shown that MCs developed from multipotent hematopoietic stem cells,[1,41,42] which are released into the blood as MC precursors and complete their differentiation within connective tissue.[43,44] The principal growth factor for MCs is stem cell factor (SCF) or KIT ligand (Fig. 1), which controls differentiation and survival by binding to the KIT protein tyrosine kinase (CD117).[45] Proliferation of MC progenitors is supported by the presence of IL-6 and IL-11,[46] which both share a common signal-transducing component.[47] In addition to its role as a growth factor, SCF is a potent chemoattractant that induces MC motility and accumulation at sites of infection or inflammation.[48,49] Both MC subtypes, MC$_T$ and MC$_{TC}$, develop from a common precursor cell; MC$_T$ cells maintained in SCF-containing media can be induced to express chymase and upregulate FcεRI after exposure to IL-4.[46,50–52] In addition, in vitro studies have shown SCF in combination with IL-6, IL-1β, transforming growth factor beta 1, or lipopolysaccharide can induce MC$_T$ cells to increase chymase expression.[53,54]

Following SCF binding, KIT is activated by dimerization and autophosphorylation of tyrosine residues. This activation results in the activation of several signaling pathways, including phosphoinositide 3-kinase, phospholipase C, protein kinase C, the Ras–mitogen-activated protein kinase cascade, and the Jak-Stat pathway,[55] which are all critical for MC development.[56–59] The presence in tissues of MCs requires an intact SCF/KIT pathway such that mice with loss-of-function mutations in the Kit gene, which do not express functional Kit receptors, are devoid of MCs.[1] Furthermore, in this murine model, normal MC development and survival can be rescued by retroviral gene transfer of normal wild-type Kit.[60] In addition to playing a central role in migration and differentiation, SCF is involved in the regulation of MC survival by preventing apoptosis. KIT signaling following the treatment of MCs with SCF results in increased levels of the Bcl-2 family proteins, Bcl-2 and Bcl-X$_L$,[61,62] which promote

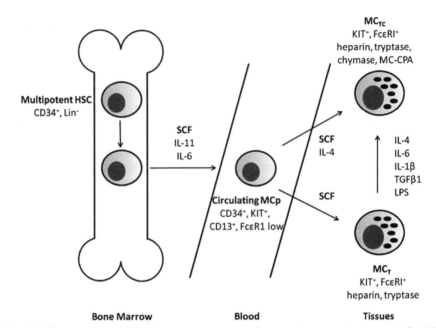

Fig. 1. Differentiation of MCs from a common, multipotent, hematopoietic stem cell. HSC, hematopoietic stem cell; Lin⁻, lineage negative; LPS, lipopolysaccharide; MCp, MC progenitor; MC-CPA, MC carboxypeptidase A; TGFβ1, transforming growth factor beta 1.

MC survival. Furthermore, the levels of the proapoptotic Bcl-2 family members, Bad and Bim, are decreased,[63–66] which in combination with Bcl-2 overexpression prevents MC apoptosis, particularly when associated with growth factor deprivation.[66]

Pathogenesis of Mastocytosis

Considering the crucial role of SCF and KIT signaling for MC survival, several investigators screened for mouse *Kit* and human *KIT* mutations in MC lines and identified several gain-of-function mutations.[67] Moreover, the introduction of an activating murine *Kit* mutation into MCs was found to be sufficient to induce ligand-independent growth, differentiation, and tumorigenicity in vivo.[68]

KIT belongs to the type III transmembrane receptor tyrosine kinase subfamily and contains extracellular, transmembrane, and juxtamembrane domains and an enzymatic pocket domain, which consists of a kinase insert, an adenosine triphosphate–binding site, and an activation loop.[69] Mutations in the human KIT protein at codon 816, which is located within the enzymatic pocket, induce ligand-independent phosphorylation and activation, whereas mutations in the juxtamembrane domain cause disruptions of the regulation of phosphorylation and kinase activity of KIT and are labeled "regulatory type mutations."[70] Based on data using cell line models, investigators screened human mastocytosis cases for KIT mutations and found that aspartic acid to valine at codon 816 (KIT D816V) was the most common activating mutation. This mutated KIT is found in more than 90% of patients with SM, including both indolent and aggressive subgroups.[5–8] In contrast, although activating KIT mutations are found in most pediatric patients with CM, D816V is present in only one-third of patients.[71]

Although mutations in *KIT* clearly play a role in the development of mastocytosis, it has not been shown that the presence of KIT D816V in isolation is sufficient to induce malignant transformation of MCs. The murine equivalent of KIT D816V, the Kit D814V mutation, has transforming activity in vitro and in vivo in tumorigenicity assays; however, these effects have not been observed for the human KIT D816V mutation.[72] Expression of KIT D816V in a murine IL-3–dependent cell line has been shown to induce cluster formation and MC differentiation antigens, which was not observed in wild-type KIT. However, cells were not converted to factor-independent proliferation. Therefore, it has been proposed that D816V in isolation may be sufficient to cause indolent mastocytosis, but additional somatic genetic changes are necessary to induce aggressive mastocytosis.[72] There is evidence that signaling pathways independent of KIT, including phosphorylation of the nonreceptor protein kinases Lyn and Btk,[73] and somatic mutations in the putative tumor suppressor gene TET2[74] provide additional mechanisms for malignant transformation of MCs.

Rare familial mastocytosis cases with germline mutations of KIT have been reported, which include activating mutations in the extracellular and juxtamembrane domains of KIT.[11–13,75] It is important to identify these cases, which (in contrast to D816V cases) may show response to specific tyrosine kinase inhibitors.[12,13,75]

In CM, both activating and inactivating KIT mutations have been detected from MCs in skin samples but rarely from MCs in blood or bone marrow. The reported prevalence in skin samples from pediatric CM cases of codon 816 KIT mutations, which includes KIT D816V, has varied from 0% to 83%[76–79]; initially, it was proposed that the presence of these activating mutations predicted progression to SM.[76] However, this finding has not been replicated in later studies that showed patients with codon 816 mutations, including between 66% and 70% of D816V cases, failed to segregate with progressive or persistent disease.[77,78]

CLASSIFICATION OF MASTOCYTOSIS

Diseases that result from the pathologic accumulation of MCs in various tissues are classified into cutaneous (CM) and systemic forms (SM), which are further subclassified into several variants and subvariants (**Table 1**).[14]

The clinical phenotypes of mastocytosis are heterogeneous; variants are recognized mainly by the distribution of organ involvement and clinical course, which can vary from the presence of benign cutaneous lesions that spontaneously regress to highly aggressive disease with short survival. Mastocytosis is a clonal malignancy; the KIT D816V somatic mutation can be detected in myeloid, non-MC lineage cells. Consequently, mastocytosis is classified as a myeloproliferative neoplasm in the World Health Organization's (WHO) classification of tumors.[14] Following this classification, the diagnosis of mastocytosis requires the presence of typical clinical findings and a histologic demonstration of an abnormal MC infiltrate in tissue biopsies (**Box 1**). In cases of CM, there must be no evidence of systemic disease, such as elevated serum tryptase level or organomegaly. To establish a diagnosis of SM, patients must fulfill at least one major and one minor SM criterion or 3 minor criteria (see **Box 1**).

Following diagnosis, SM is staged as indolent, smoldering, or aggressive based on the presence or absence of B and C findings (**Box 2**).[14] B findings indicate a high MC burden and/or expansion of the genetic defect into other myeloid lineages, whereas C findings result from impaired organ function caused by MC infiltration, which requires confirmation by biopsy in most cases. The criteria for smoldering mastocytosis are fulfilled if 2 or more B findings are present but there is no evidence of impaired organ function. If one or more C findings are present, then patients are classified as either aggressive SM (ASM) or MC leukemia (MCL), and treatment using cytoreductive therapy is considered. Investigations are performed to detect the presence of an additional hematologic non-MC

Table 1
WHO criteria for variants of CM and SM

Variant	Diagnostic Criteria	Subvariants	Prognosis
CM	Typical clinical findings & histologic proof of abnormal MC dermal infiltrate; No systemic involvement (most patients are children)	Urticaria pigmentosa/ maculopapular CM Diffuse CM Solitary mastocytoma of the skin	Good
Indolent SM (ISM)	No impaired organ function; MC burden is low and skin lesions are usually present	Isolated bone marrow mastocytosis - No skin lesions Smoldering SM - High MC burden (2 or more B findings) but no impaired organ function	>16-y expected median survival and not significantly different from age- and sex-matched controls
Systemic mastocytosis with an associated clonal hematologic non-MC lineage disease (SM-AHNMD)	Meets criteria for SM and WHO criteria for an associated, clonal hematological non-MC lineage disorder	SM-AML SM-MDS SM-MPN SM-CEL SM-CMML SM-NHL SM-myeloma	2-y expected median survival, dependent on underlying AHNMD
Aggressive systemic mastocytosis	Meets criteria for SM; existence of signs indicating organ failure secondary to MC infiltration (1 or more C findings): - Bone marrow failure (marked cytopenia) - Palpable hepatomegaly with hepatic failure, ascites, and/or portal hypertension - Palpable splenomegaly with hypersplenism - Osteolysis and pathologic fractures - Malabsorption and weight loss caused by gastrointestinal MC infiltrates	Lymphadenopathic SM with eosinophilia - Progressive lymphadenopathy with blood eosinophilia - Often extensive bone involvement and hepatosplenomegaly - PDGFRA rearrangements excluded	3.5-y expected median survival

MC leukemia	Meets criteria for SM; bone marrow aspirate shows >20% atypical, immature MCs and peripheral blood ≥10% MCs	Aleukemic MCL - <10% white blood cells are MCs	2-mo expected median survival
MCS	Unifocal malignant tumor destroying the soft tissue; no evidence of SM		Very poor; transformation to MCL after a short interval
Extracutaneous mastocytoma	Extremely rare benign tumor; nondestructive growth pattern and low-grade cytology		Good

Abbreviations: AML, acute myeloid leukemia; CEL, chronic eosinophilic leukemia; CMML, chronic myelomonocytic leukemia; MCL, MC leukemia; MCS, MC sarcoma; MDS, myelodysplastic syndrome; MPN, myeloproliferative neoplasm; NHL, non-Hodgkin lymphoma.

Adapted from Horny HP, Metcalfe DD, Bennett JM, et al. Mastocytosis. In: Swerdlow SH, Campo E, Harris NL, et al., editors. WHO classification of tumours of haematopoietic and lymphoid tissues. 4th edition. Lyon (France): International Agency for Research and Cancer (IARC); 2008. p. 54–63; with permission.

Box 1
Diagnostic criteria for CM and SM

CM

There is demonstration of typical skin lesions, which includes urticaria pigmentosa/maculopapular CM, diffuse CM, or solitary mastocytoma, and histologic evidence of an abnormal MC infiltrate in the dermis. There must be insufficient criteria to establish a diagnosis of SM.

SM

The diagnosis of SM can be established if at least one major and one minor or at least 3 minor criteria are fulfilled.

Major criterion

Multifocal dense infiltrates of MCs (>15 MCs in aggregate) are found in tissue sections of bone marrow or other extracutaneous organs.

Minor criteria

Greater than 25% of MCs in bone marrow or extracutaneous organs are spindle-shaped or have abnormal morphology or, in bone marrow smears, more than 25% are immature or atypical.

There is detection of an activating KIT mutation at codon 816 in blood, bone marrow, or another extracutaneous organs.

MCs in bone marrow, blood, or other extracutaneous organs express CD2 and/or CD25.

Serum total tryptase is persistently more than 20 ng/mL (invalid in patients who have associated clonal hematologic non-MC lineage disease).

Adapted from Horny HP, Metcalfe DD, Bennett JM, et al. Mastocytosis. In: Swerdlow SH, Campo E, Harris NL, et al., editors. WHO classification of tumours of haematopoietic and lymphoid tissues. 4th edition. Lyon (France): International Agency for Research and Cancer (IARC); 2008. p. 54-63; with permission.

---

neoplasm (SM-associated clonal hematologic non–mast cell lineage disease [AHNMD]), which will have prognostic implications and specific treatment requirements.

EPIDEMIOLOGY

Mastocytosis occurs in all ethnic groups and may present at any age. CM is more common in children[80]; but a second smaller peak of incidence is seen in adults in the third to fourth decade. About 50% of children develop CM before 6 months of age, and the average duration of disease is estimated at 9.4 years.[81] Improvement or resolution of disease is reported in most of these cases.[82] However, in adults, there is a high risk of CM progressing to SM, which should be suspected in adults with urticaria pigmentosa (UP) skin lesions at presentation.[83] In contrast, SM is more common in adults and usually diagnosed after the second decade. CM has a slight male predominance, whereas SM affects men and women equally.[84]

CLINICAL AND LABORATORY FEATURES AT PRESENTATION

Mastocytosis is comprised of several heterogeneous diseases; consequently, the presenting clinical features are diverse. To a large extent, the clinical manifestations and disease course are related to the age of presentation, which can be classified into pediatric- and adult-onset groups. Mastocytosis in the pediatric group is usually confined to the skin; the most common pattern of disease is UP, which represents

---

Box 2
Staging criteria for SM

B findings

Bone marrow biopsy showing more than 30% MCs and/or serum total tryptase levels more than 200 ng/mL

Bone marrow biopsy showing dysplasia or myeloproliferation in non-MC lineages but without substantial cytopenias or WHO criteria for a myelodysplastic syndrome or myeloproliferative neoplasm

Palpable hepatomegaly, splenomegaly, or lymphadenopathy (on computed tomography or ultrasound >2 cm) without impaired organ function

C findings

Bone marrow dysfunction with one or more cytopenias: absolute neutrophil count less than 1 × 10⁹/l, or hemoglobin less than 100 g/L, or platelets less than 100 × 10⁹/l

Palpable hepatomegaly with impaired liver function, ascites and/or portal hypertension

Palpable splenomegaly with hypersplenism

Skeletal lesions with large osteolytic lesions and/or osteoporosis causing pathologic fracture

Malabsorption with hypoalbuminemia and weight loss caused by gastrointestinal MC infiltration

Adapted from Horny HP, Metcalfe DD, Bennett JM, et al. Mastocytosis. In: Swerdlow SH, Campo E, Harris NL, et al., editors. WHO classification of tumours of haematopoietic and lymphoid tissues. 4th edition. Lyon (France): International Agency for Research and Cancer (IARC); 2008. p. 54-63; with permission.

70% to 90% of cases.[80,85] The clinical course of pediatric CM is variable but tends toward spontaneous resolution before puberty.[80,85] In contrast, mastocytosis in adults usually presents with symptoms and signs of systemic disease that progress over time. Overall, approximately 80% of patients will have signs of skin involvement.[86] The skin is involved in more than 50% of SM cases, which may predict a more indolent course and is usually not a feature of more aggressive SM variants.[87]

The symptoms of SM are usually grouped into 4 categories: (1) constitutional symptoms, which include fatigue, weight loss, sweats, and fever; (2) skin symptoms; (3) MC mediator-related symptoms; and (4) musculoskeletal symptoms, which include bone, muscle, and joint pain. The signs at diagnosis of SM include splenomegaly and, less commonly, lymphadenopathy and hepatomegaly.[88–90] SM cases may also have signs and symptoms of bone marrow infiltration and failure, which include recurrent bacterial infections, bruising and bleeding, and symptoms of anemia.

CM

The WHO classification of CM includes 3 subvariants: UP, diffuse CM, and mastocytoma of the skin. UP is the most common form of CM and usually presents with disseminated brown or red macules and papules that spare the face, palms, and soles of the feet (**Fig. 2**).

Physical stroking of the lesions causes MC degranulation, which is observed as a wheal and flare reaction and constitutes a positive Darier sign. This urticarial reaction, in combination with intraepidermal accumulation of melanin pigment, explains the descriptive term *urticaria pigmentosa* (**Fig. 3**).

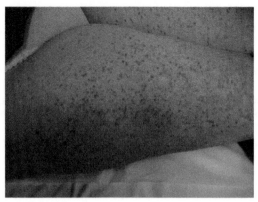

Fig. 2. Urticaria pigmentosa lesions, which consist of multiple, red-brown macules measuring 2 to 3 mm in diameter, located on the legs.

Bullous skin lesions can occur in all forms of pediatric CM but are seen more commonly in children less than 3 years of age and in mastocytoma of the skin and diffuse CM subvariants. In general, pediatric CM is usually asymptomatic or minimally symptomatic.[91] However, all forms of CM can present with systemic symptoms because of the local release of MC mediators, which have both local and systemic effects. Skin symptoms may occur spontaneously or be triggered by mechanical or thermal stimuli and include flushing, pruritus, swelling, and dermatographism.

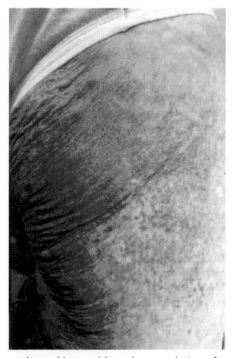

Fig. 3. Erythematous macules and intraepidermal accumulation of melanin pigment on the lateral thigh of a patient with long-standing urticaria pigmentosa.

Systemic symptoms, including diarrhea, wheezing, and syncope, can accompany pediatric UP but seem to be more common in adult-onset UP and, in one series, were reported in 25% of cases.[92] Based on distinct clinical features, several rare subvariants of UP have been described, which include a plaque form, a nodular form, and a telangiectatic variant (telangiectasia macularis eruptiva perstans).[92,93]

Mastocytoma of the skin usually presents in the first 3 months of life with 1 to 3 plaques or nodules that are generally larger than 1 cm in diameter.[92,94] The lesions are brown or orange and are usually located on the extremities but spare the palms and soles of the feet. Bullous lesions, which occur spontaneously or after trauma, can be seen in both mastocytoma of the skin and diffuse CM.[92] Diffuse CM is an extremely rare form of CM, which is characterized by a widespread and heavy skin MC load. Diffuse CM presents in infancy, with erythroderma involving almost the entire body and is often associated with hemorrhage and prominent blister formation.[95] Systemic symptoms are pronounced as a result of the high MC load, although the incidence of systemic involvement by MCs is unknown. In the rare reported cases, acute cutaneous flares of the disease have been associated with significant mortality. However, in those that survive these episodes, spontaneous resolution has usually occurred before 5 years of age.[95,96]

SM

Indolent SM (ISM) is the most frequently diagnosed subvariant of SM[97,98] and composed about half of the cases in the largest series reported by Lim and colleagues.[98] Patients with ISM are younger and experience a longer duration of symptoms before diagnosis compared with other SM subvariants.[98] Patients with ISM are also more likely to have skin involvement with UP lesions and report a higher prevalence of MC mediator-related symptoms.[98] The life expectancy of patients with ISM is not significantly different than age- and sex-matched controls[98]; but those affected can experience a wide variety of symptoms that arise from MC mediator release, which may significantly impact their quality of life. These symptoms can include pruritus, urticaria, angioedema, flushing, bronchoconstriction, abdominal pain, nausea, vomiting, diarrhea, hypotension, and anaphylactoid reactions.[99] Gastric acid secretion is stimulated by histamine, which can cause gastric ulceration and lead to complications, including bleeding and perforation.[100] In addition, it has become increasingly recognized that neuropsychiatric manifestations, particularly the psychological impact of the cosmetic appearance of skin lesions, significantly contribute to disability in mastocytosis.[101]

SM associated with another hematological non-MC disease (SM-AHNMD) and ASM compose 40% and 12%, respectively, of SM cases.[98] In contrast to ISM, ASM and SM-AHNMD are associated with a higher frequency of constitutional symptoms, hepatosplenomegaly, and lymphadenopathy.[98] Patients with SM-AHNMD are generally older and have a shorter survival time compared with ISM,[98,102,103] which is usually related to the underlying AHNMD rather than SM. Almost 90% of cases have an associated myeloid neoplasm, with the remainder associated with lymphoma, myeloma, chronic lymphocytic leukemia, and rarely, primary amyloidosis.[104] Signs and symptoms of hematological abnormalities are seen in both ASM and SM-AHNMD. Approximately one-third of patients with SM-AHNMD and one-quarter of patients with ASM are anemic (hemoglobin <10 g/dL) and thrombocytopenic (platelets <100 × 10^9/L), and 20% to 30% of cases show a prominent eosinophilia (absolute eosinophil count >1500/μL).[98]

MCL is rare and is characterized by circulating MCs and 20% or greater MCs on the bone marrow aspirate smear. Most patients are adults. Cutaneous lesions are typically absent; patients initially present with episodes of mediator-related symptoms and later develop constitutional symptoms, including weight loss and bone pain, and symptoms and signs of organomegaly.

MC sarcoma is extremely rare and characterized by local destructive proliferation of highly atypical MCs, which rapidly progresses to a terminal phase that is indistinguishable from MCL. Reported primary sites of involvement include the larynx, colon, meninges, bone, and skin[105–107]; however the bone marrow is usually not initially affected. At first presentation, it is important to differentiate MC sarcoma from extracutaneous mastocytoma, which is a localized benign MC tumor without systemic involvement. Extracutaneous mastocytomas are characterized by low-grade cytology and a nondestructive growth pattern and have been primarily found in the lungs.[108–110]

Varieties of skeletal changes are associated with SM and differ in frequency depending on the subtype of disease; however, overall, about 50% of patients will have detectable bone involvement.[111] Diffuse osteosclerosis is observed in up to one-third of patients with ASM but is rare in ISM, which is more commonly associated with mixed osteosclerotic and osteolytic lesions.[112] An increased risk of osteopenia and osteoporosis is well described in all forms of SM, with a prevalence between 18% and 31%[111–113]; the prevalence of osteoporotic fractures is significantly higher than controls.[111,113]

DIAGNOSIS
Histology and Immunohistochemistry

CM
Cutaneous MC infiltration can be recognized on hematoxylin and eosin staining (**Fig. 4**A); however, MCs are better visualized using basic dyes, such as Giemsa, toluidine blue, and Astra blue, or by immunocytochemical stains that reveal tryptase and chymase or histochemical techniques with chloroacetate esterase (see **Fig. 4**B). In CM, MCs are spindle shaped or spherical and stain positively for both chymase and tryptase. There are 4 patterns of dermal MC infiltrate that have been described: (1) perivascular in the papillary body and upper dermis; (2) sheetlike within the papillary body and upper reticular dermis; (3) interstitial; and (4) nodular.[114,115] There is a partial correlation between these 4 histologic patterns and the clinical presentations of CM. However, clinical features are related more to the density of the MC infiltrate. For example, the nodular pattern is found in nodular CM but can also be present in larger lesions associated with UP. The pattern of involvement does not predict the course of

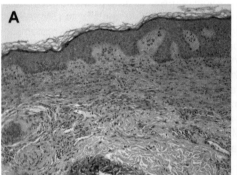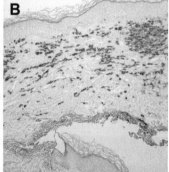

Fig. 4. (A) Superficial dermal perivascular infiltrate comprised predominantly of MCs (hematoxylin- eosin). (B) Leder (naphthol AS-D chloroacetate esterase), original magnification × 10.

the disease or risk of systemic involvement.[116] In CM, the number of MCs in the papillary dermis can be 10-fold higher than for the number found in normal skin[117]; however, the number required to diagnose CM has not been standardized. This point can make it difficult to differentiate between CM with low numbers of MCs and inflammatory conditions associated with an MC infiltrate, such as urticaria or atopic dermatitis. However, the presence of lymphocytes and other inflammatory cells is helpful in distinguishing non-CM inflammatory conditions from CM.[92]

Morphology of MCs in bone marrow smears

SM is usually diagnosed by histologic examination of the bone marrow. Most cases show multifocal, sharply demarcated, compact infiltrates of MCs, which are easily detected in the bone marrow biopsy (**Fig. 5**A, B). The presence of multifocal infiltrates containing 15 or more MCs is sufficient to satisfy the WHO criteria to make a diagnosis of SM. However, in some cases, MCs may be loosely scattered, which can be seen in reactive MC hyperplasia or myelomastocytic leukemia.[118] Consequently, in all cases, immunohistochemical and molecular studies are recommended to distinguish reactive from malignant MC infiltrates. Focal infiltrates are predominantly found in paratrabecular and perivascular locations, intermingled with lymphocytes, eosinophils, histiocytes, and fibroblasts.[119] The bone marrow may be replaced by sheets of MCs; in these cases, marked reticulin or collagen fibrosis is frequently observed.[120,121] Morphologically, the MCs are a mixture of both round and spindle-shaped forms. In SM and isolated mastocytosis of the bone marrow (BM), uninvolved areas of the bone marrow are generally unremarkable; however, some cases show increased cellularity that result from the proliferation of cells of non-MC lineages. Involvement of the marrow surrounding dense MC infiltrates by a diffuse infiltrate is seen in aggressive and leukemic variants. In addition, it is important to examine unaffected areas of the bone marrow for evidence of an associated hematologic disease, such as acute myeloid leukemia, myelodysplasia, a myelodysplastic/myeloproliferative neoplasm, or chronic eosinophilic leukemia. However, in these cases, the associated hematological neoplasm is usually the more dominant feature compared with the MC infiltrate.[97] In addition, a reactive MC hyperplasia may occur in association with myeloid and lymphoid malignancies, in particular, lymphoplasmacytic lymphoma and hairy cell leukemia.[91] Bone marrow involvement is established by examination of the trephine sample; however, the aspirate provides some additional information and is important for the diagnosis of some subvariants of SM-AHNMD.[91] In many patients with SM, the percentage of MCs in the aspirate smear is less than

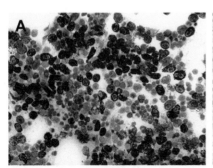
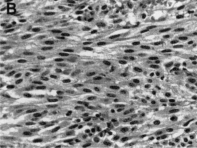

Fig. 5. Bone marrow infiltration by MCs. (A) A bone marrow smear that shows more than 20% MCs (May-Grünwald-Giemsa, original magnification × 40). (B) The bone marrow trephine from the same case (hematoxylin-eosin, original magnification × 40).

5%, even when high levels of infiltration are seen in the trephine sample.[122] However, an MC percentage of 20% or greater of nucleated cells in the aspirate smear is sufficient to establish a diagnosis of MCL (see **Fig. 5**). In most SM cases, MCs in the bone marrow show similar abnormal morphologic changes to MCs in the skin, including a spindle or fusiform shape, eccentric nuclei, and a hypogranulated cytoplasm with focal accumulations of granules.[122]

Immunophenotype of MCs in mastocytosis

Normal MCs coexpress CD9, CD33, CD45, CD68, and high levels of CD117 (KIT) (**Fig. 6**A, B) but lack several myelomonocytic antigens, including CD14, CD15, and CD16, and do not express T- or B-cell–related antigens.[120,123] Antibodies to tryptase will detect all MCs and MC progenitors as well as neoplastic MCs, whereas chymase is expressed in a subpopulation of MCs. Neoplastic MCs have a similar expression profile to normal MCs; however, neoplastic MCs aberrantly coexpress CD2 or CD2 and CD25.[124] Consequently, antibodies to these antigens can be used in immunohistochemical and flow cytometric studies to identify malignant MC populations, which express tryptase/chymase and CD117 and aberrantly coexpress CD2/CD25. However, CD25 expression in SM may be variable and is not detectable in some subvariants, such as well-differentiated SM (WDSM).[75,124]

Serum Tryptase Measurement

The factors that control MC release of tryptase are complex and not fully characterized.[21] More than 95% of patients with SM have elevated serum levels,[98] and a level of 20 ng/mL or greater is included as a minor diagnostic criterion in the WHO classification.[14] In 20% of cases, the serum tryptase is 200 ng/mL or higher (normal range <11.5 ng/mL), with very high levels more frequently observed in patients with ASM and SM-AHNMD compared to patients with ISM.[98,125] Serum tryptase levels have been found to correlate with total MC burden; in patients with CM, who by definition have no evidence of systemic involvement, the levels are normal or only slightly elevated. In contrast, a relationship between serum tryptase levels and symptoms caused by MC mediator release has not been demonstrated. It should also be noted that increased serum tryptase levels are not specific for SM and are also found in association with acute myeloid leukemia, chronic myeloid leukemia, and myelodysplasia.[126]

Molecular and Cytogenetic Tests

Using sensitive molecular techniques, the KIT D816V mutation can be identified in MCs from greater than 90% of adults with SM and about one-third of pediatric CM

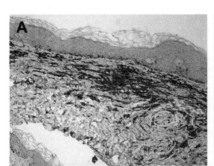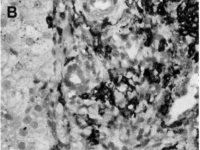

Fig. 6. (*A*) Dermal MC infiltrate (CD117 immunostaining, original magnification × 10). (*B*) Hepatic periportal MC infiltrate (CD117 immunostaining, original magnification × 40).

patients.[8] Other KIT-activating lesions are found in less than 5% of SM patients and include D816Y, D816H, and D816F.[8,127,128] A high frequency of activating KIT mutations is found in all SM subvariants except WDSM, in which less than 30% are positive.[8] Although it had been suggested that the presence of D816V was a prognostic factor in SM, it has been shown that the frequency of the mutation does not differ between aggressive and indolent forms of the disease. However, KIT mutations may be found at a higher frequency in $CD34^+$ hematopoietic progenitor cells isolated from the bone marrow of cases with aggressive forms of SM.[8] Additional genetic mutations should be considered in SM-AHNMD, for example in cases associated with acute myeloid leukemia AML1-ETO (RUNX1-RUNX1T1) can be found and JAK2 V617F can be found in SM associated with myeloproliferative neoplasms.[129,130] The WHO classification distinguishes SM from patients that present with elevated serum tryptase and a BM showing scattered atypical MCs in association with clonal eosinophils carrying a FIP1L1-PDGFRA fusion gene.[131–133] Although initially reported as a variant of SM,[134,135] these cases do not show the presence of compact MC infiltrates in tissues and are classified as a myeloid neoplasm with eosinophilia and rearrangement of PDGFRA.[136,137]

TREATMENT AND PROGNOSIS

The management of all patients with mastocytosis includes specific advice regarding avoidance of factors that trigger MC mediator release; treatment of acute and chronic episodes of MC mediator release; and cytoreductive therapy to treat organ infiltration by MCs, which is indicated by the presence of C findings. The WHO classification is prognostically relevant for SM (see **Table 1**). The life expectancy of ISM patients is not significantly different to age- and sex-matched controls and transformation to acute leukemia occurs rarely.[98] Patients with ASM have a median survival of 2 years; although dependent on the underlying hematological disease, the median survival is 3.5 years for patients with SM-AHNMD.[98] The outlook for MCL is very poor (with a median survival of 2 months) and similarly unfavorable for MCS, which transforms to MCL shortly after diagnosis.[98]

MC Mediator Release

MCs can be activated to release mediators by high and, to a lesser extent, cold temperature. Sudden temperature changes should be avoided, in particular when bathing or swimming, and ambient temperature indoors is best maintained at around 26°C.[138] Rubbing of the skin should be avoided; a skin moisturizer, such as water-soluble sodium cromoglycate cream, should be applied topically to prevent dryness.[139]

In symptomatic patients, a combination of histamine receptor 1 and 2 (HR1 and HR2) antagonists is used, which in most patients controls cutaneous manifestations, such as pruritus, flushing, and gastric hypersecretion, and is effective for prophylaxis of hypotensive episodes.[140–142] Corticosteroids may be prescribed to control malabsorption, abdominal pain, nausea and vomiting, and for the prevention or treatment of anaphylaxis.[143] However, corticosteroids should only be used for short periods as a second- or third-line therapy because long-term use may contribute to the development of osteopenia or osteoporosis. Because of the risk of osteopathy associated with mastocytosis, routine measurements of bone mineral density should be performed and oral or intravenous bisphosphonate therapy is recommended for cases of severe osteopenia or overt osteoporosis.[143]

The prevalence of atopy in patients with mastocytosis does not differ from the general population; however, reactions are more severe in those patients who suffer from both allergy and mastocytosis. The cumulative incidence of anaphylaxis in adults has been reported to be as high as 49% and, of these, 38% will result in unconsciousness.[144] Consequently, an emergency medication plan that includes epinephrine as a self-injector (EpiPen, Dey Pharma, L.P., Napa, CA) is recommended; treatment of refractory hypotension and shock requires standard resuscitation measures, including intravenous fluids and other pharmacologic agents.[145] Fatal anaphylaxis may follow hymenoptera stings; foods; and medications, such as nonsteroidal antiinflammatory drugs, codeine, and narcotics.[146–149] Venom immunotherapy has been used to treat patients with mastocytosis; however, therapy has been associated with a higher frequency of side effects, including fatal anaphylaxis, and lower efficacy compared with the general insect-venom allergic population.[150] Nevertheless, patients with mastocytosis with a known allergic trigger and specific IgE demonstrable should be considered for specific immunotherapy.[143]

MC mediator release may be triggered by drugs used in general anesthesia, which is considered a high-risk procedure in patients with mastocytosis.[151,152] Several perioperative protocols have been proposed for the management of patients with mastocytosis, which include avoidance of β-adrenergic blockers, α-adrenergic blockers, and cholinergic receptor antagonists, and the monitoring of serum tryptase levels and coagulation profiles during surgery and anesthesia.[153–157]

Symptomatic Cutaneous Disease

Unless patients are concerned about the cosmetic appearance of lesions, asymptomatic cutaneous disease does not require any therapy apart from prophylaxis using H1 and H2 histamine receptor antagonists. Topical therapy using water-soluble cromolyn sodium cream in addition to aqueous-based cromolyn sodium skin lotion is used to decrease pruritus and flaring of skin lesions but should not be used on denuded lesions, which may require topical antibacterials.[138,139] Topical steroids are also used to prevent blistering and denuded areas require dressing with sterile gauze and application of zinc sulfate.[138] In pediatric CM, systemic therapy is rarely required; but for severe symptoms, antihistamines, oral cromolyn sodium, and leukotriene receptor antagonists may be required.[138] In cases of bullous diffuse CM that are refractory to these treatments, oral psoralen with UV-A radiation has been reported to be effective.[158,159] Consideration may be given to the treatment of solitary mastocytomas on skin flexures, the soles, palm, or scalp with surgical excision.[138]

Cytoreductive Therapy

Advanced stages of mastocytosis are recognized by the presence of B or C findings as defined by the WHO classification (see **Box 2**).[14] B findings indicate a high burden of MCs and 2 or more of these, with no C findings, is diagnostic of smoldering SM. However, the presence of smoldering myeloma is not an indication for treatment with cytoreductive therapy. The presence of one or more C findings, indicating impaired organ function caused by MC infiltration, is diagnostic of aggressive SM, in which case cytoreductive therapy should be considered. Once a decision is made to commence treatment, the first objective is to find targets for drug therapy, such as wild-type KIT or KIT D816V, and to exclude an AHNMD as the cause for C findings. For patients carrying the KIT D816V mutation, interferon-α (IFN-α) in combination with glucocorticoids is used as initial therapy; if no response is seen or patients are intolerant of IFN-α, then treatment is changed to cladribine.[160–164] In highly aggressive or relapsed cases, combination chemotherapy followed by a hematopoietic stem cell transplant should be considered.[165] Several chemotherapeutic agents have activity in the treatment of ASM or MCL, including cytarabine, fludarabine, and hydroxyurea.[160,165,166] Those patients who are negative for D816V but have non–codon 816 mutations or wild-type KIT may show a response to specific tyrosine kinase inhibitors, such as imatinib, or other tyrosine kinase inhibitors.[167-169]

Although the D816V mutant is resistant to KIT kinase inhibition by imatinib, masitinib, bafetinib, and others,[170,171] several tyrosine kinase inhibitors, including midostaurin, dasatinib, and nilotinib, have in vitro blocking activity.[169,172,173] Midostaurin and dasatinib inhibit MC growth in patients with advanced SM[174,175]; however, the effects are mild and transient, which may occur as a result of upregulation of KIT-independent oncogenic pathways. At present, the results of clinical trials studying the efficacy of these agents are awaited.

In patients with SM-AHNMD, both underlying disease components should be treated as if they existed in isolation. If no C findings can be attributed to the SM component, then no SM-directed therapy is required; however, treatment of the AHNMD should commence if indicated. The AHNMD is treated with standard therapy for that component, and complete remissions have been reported in patients with SM and acute myeloid leukemia.[176,177]

FUTURE DEVELOPMENTS

Much progress has been made in understanding the role of activating mutations in the KIT receptor and the pathogenesis of mastocytosis. This progress has led to the development of drug therapies with therapeutic efficacies that target both wild-type KIT and mutated KIT. However, the common activating KIT mutation D816V is resistant to most tyrosine kinase inhibitors, and KIT-independent pathways contribute to disease progression. It is hoped that a better understanding of the mechanisms whereby constitutively activated KIT promotes MC proliferation and survival will lead to the identification of additional signaling pathways that can be molecularly targeted to treat mastocytosis. It is predicted that these new targeted treatments will be used together in combinations and in synergy with conventional cytoreductive agents to provide an individualized treatment of each patient.

REFERENCES

1. Kitamura Y, Go S, Hatanaka K. Decrease of mast cells in W/Wv mice and their increase by bone marrow transplantation. Blood 1978;52(2):447–52.
2. Metcalfe DD. Mast cells and mastocytosis. Blood 2008;112(4):946–56.
3. Feger F, Varadaradjalou S, Gao Z, et al. The role of mast cells in host defense and their subversion by bacterial pathogens. Trends Immunol 2002;23(3): 151–8.
4. Hofmann AM, Abraham SN. New roles for mast cells in modulating allergic reactions and immunity against pathogens. Curr Opin Immunol 2009;21(6): 679–86.
5. Nagata H, Worobec AS, Oh CK, et al. Identification of a point mutation in the catalytic domain of the proto-oncogene c-kit in peripheral blood mononuclear cells of patients who have mastocytosis with an associated hematologic disorder. Proc Natl Acad Sci U S A 1995;92(23):10560–4.
6. Longley BJ, Tyrrell L, Lu SZ, et al. Somatic c-KIT activating mutation in urticaria pigmentosa and aggressive mastocytosis: establishment of clonality in a human mast cell neoplasm. Nat Genet 1996;12(3):312–4.
7. Fritsche-Polanz R, Jordan JH, Feix A, et al. Mutation analysis of C-KIT in patients with myelodysplastic syndromes without mastocytosis and cases of systemic mastocytosis. Br J Haematol 2001;113(2):357–64.

8. Garcia-Montero AC, Jara-Acevedo M, Teodosio C, et al. KIT mutation in mast cells and other bone marrow hematopoietic cell lineages in systemic mast cell disorders: a prospective study of the Spanish Network on Mastocytosis (REMA) in a series of 113 patients. Blood 2006;108(7):2366–72.

9. Hartmann K, Henz BM. Mastocytosis: recent advances in defining the disease. Br J Dermatol 2001;144(4):682–95.

10. Boyano T, Carrascosa T, Val J, et al. Urticaria pigmentosa in monozygotic twins. Arch Dermatol 1990;126(10):1375–6.

11. Tang X, Boxer M, Drummond A, et al. A germline mutation in KIT in familial diffuse cutaneous mastocytosis. J Med Genet 2004;41(6):e88.

12. Zhang LY, Smith ML, Schultheis B, et al. A novel K509I mutation of KIT identified in familial mastocytosis-in vitro and in vivo responsiveness to imatinib therapy. Leuk Res 2006;30(4):373–8.

13. Hartmann K, Wardelmann E, Ma Y, et al. Novel germline mutation of KIT associated with familial gastrointestinal stromal tumors and mastocytosis. Gastroenterology 2005;129(3):1042–6.

14. Swerdlow SH. International Agency for Research on Cancer., World Health Organization. WHO classification of tumours of haematopoietic and lymphoid tissues. 4th edition. Lyon (France): International Agency for Research on Cancer; 2008.

15. Trinchieri G, Sher A. Cooperation of Toll-like receptor signals in innate immune defence. Nat Rev Immunol 2007;7(3):179–90.

16. Supajatura V, Ushio H, Nakao A, et al. Differential responses of mast cell Toll-like receptors 2 and 4 in allergy and innate immunity. J Clin Invest 2002;109(10):1351–9.

17. Hirai Y, Kuwada M, Yasuhara T, et al. A new mast cell degranulating peptide homologous to mastoparan in the venom of Japanese hornet (Vespa xanthoptera). Chem Pharm Bull (Tokyo) 1979;27(8):1945–6.

18. Demeure CE, Brahimi K, Hacini F, et al. Anopheles mosquito bites activate cutaneous mast cells leading to a local inflammatory response and lymph node hyperplasia. J Immunol 2005;174(7):3932–40.

19. Abraham SN, St John AL. Mast cell-orchestrated immunity to pathogens. Nat Rev Immunol 2010;10(6):440–52.

20. Ryan JJ, Kashyap M, Bailey D, et al. Mast cell homeostasis: a fundamental aspect of allergic disease. Crit Rev Immunol 2007;27(1):15–32.

21. Galli SJ, Kalesnikoff J, Grimbaldeston MA, et al. Mast cells as "tunable" effector and immunoregulatory cells: recent advances. Annu Rev Immunol 2005;23:749–86.

22. Malaviya R, Ikeda T, Ross E, et al. Mast cell modulation of neutrophil influx and bacterial clearance at sites of infection through TNF-alpha. Nature 1996;381(6577):77–80.

23. Malaviya R, Ross EA, MacGregor JI, et al. Mast cell phagocytosis of FimH-expressing enterobacteria. J Immunol 1994;152(4):1907–14.

24. Kalesnikoff J, Galli SJ. New developments in mast cell biology. Nat Immunol 2008;9(11):1215–23.

25. Welle M. Development, significance, and heterogeneity of mast cells with particular regard to the mast cell-specific proteases chymase and tryptase. J Leukoc Biol 1997;61(3):233–45.

26. Pejler G, Abrink M, Ringvall M, et al. Mast cell proteases. Adv Immunol 2007;95:167–255.

27. Caughey GH. Mast cell tryptases and chymases in inflammation and host defense. Immunol Rev 2007;217:141–54.

28. Irani AM, Schwartz LB. Human mast cell heterogeneity. Allergy Proc 1994;15(6): 303–8.
29. Schwartz LB. Mediators of human mast cells and human mast cell subsets. Ann Allergy 1987;58(4):226–35.
30. Burke SM, Issekutz TB, Mohan K, et al. Human mast cell activation with virus-associated stimuli leads to the selective chemotaxis of natural killer cells by a CXCL8-dependent mechanism. Blood 2008;111(12):5467–76.
31. Di Nardo A, Vitiello A, Gallo RL. Cutting edge: mast cell antimicrobial activity is mediated by expression of cathelicidin antimicrobial peptide. J Immunol 2003; 170(5):2274–8.
32. McLachlan JB, Hart JP, Pizzo SV, et al. Mast cell-derived tumor necrosis factor induces hypertrophy of draining lymph nodes during infection. Nat Immunol 2003;4(12):1199–205.
33. Jawdat DM, Rowden G, Marshall JS. Mast cells have a pivotal role in TNF-independent lymph node hypertrophy and the mobilization of Langerhans cells in response to bacterial peptidoglycan. J Immunol 2006;177(3):1755–62.
34. Stelekati E, Bahri R, D'Orlando O, et al. Mast cell-mediated antigen presentation regulates CD8+ T cell effector functions. Immunity 2009;31(4):665–76.
35. Kawakami T, Galli SJ. Regulation of mast-cell and basophil function and survival by IgE. Nat Rev Immunol 2002;2(10):773–86.
36. Secor VH, Secor WE, Gutekunst CA, et al. Mast cells are essential for early onset and severe disease in a murine model of multiple sclerosis. J Exp Med 2000; 191(5):813–22.
37. Lee DM, Friend DS, Gurish MF, et al. Mast cells: a cellular link between autoantibodies and inflammatory arthritis. Science 2002;297(5587):1689–92.
38. Chen R, Ning G, Zhao ML, et al. Mast cells play a key role in neutrophil recruitment in experimental bullous pemphigoid. J Clin Invest 2001;108(8):1151–8.
39. Grimbaldeston MA, Nakae S, Kalesnikoff J, et al. Mast cell-derived interleukin 10 limits skin pathology in contact dermatitis and chronic irradiation with ultraviolet B. Nat Immunol 2007;8(10):1095–104.
40. Lu LF, Lind EF, Gondek DC, et al. Mast cells are essential intermediaries in regulatory T-cell tolerance. Nature 2006;442(7106):997–1002.
41. Nabel G, Galli SJ, Dvorak AM, et al. Inducer T lymphocytes synthesize a factor that stimulates proliferation of cloned mast cells. Nature 1981;291(5813):332–4.
42. Kirshenbaum AS, Kessler SW, Goff JP, et al. Demonstration of the origin of human mast cells from CD34+ bone marrow progenitor cells. J Immunol 1991;146(5):1410–5.
43. Rodewald HR, Dessing M, Dvorak AM, et al. Identification of a committed precursor for the mast cell lineage. Science 1996;271(5250):818–22.
44. Chen CC, Grimbaldeston MA, Tsai M, et al. Identification of mast cell progenitors in adult mice. Proc Natl Acad Sci U S A 2005;102(32):11408–13.
45. Okayama Y, Kawakami T. Development, migration, and survival of mast cells. Immunol Res 2006;34(2):97–115.
46. Nakahata T, Toru H. Cytokines regulate development of human mast cells from hematopoietic progenitors. Int J Hematol 2002;75(4):350–6.
47. Yin T, Taga T, Tsang ML, et al. Involvement of IL-6 signal transducer gp130 in IL-11-mediated signal transduction. J Immunol 1993;151(5):2555–61.
48. Meininger CJ, Yano H, Rottapel R, et al. The c-kit receptor ligand functions as a mast cell chemoattractant. Blood 1992;79(4):958–63.
49. Matsuura N, Zetter BR. Stimulation of mast cell chemotaxis by interleukin 3. J Exp Med 1989;170(4):1421–6.

50. Toru H, Eguchi M, Matsumoto R, et al. Interleukin-4 promotes the development of tryptase and chymase double-positive human mast cells accompanied by cell maturation. Blood 1998;91(1):187–95.

51. Toru H, Ra C, Nonoyama S, et al. Induction of the high-affinity IgE receptor (Fc epsilon RI) on human mast cells by IL-4. Int Immunol 1996;8(9):1367–73.

52. Xia HZ, Du Z, Craig S, et al. Effect of recombinant human IL-4 on tryptase, chymase, and Fc epsilon receptor type I expression in recombinant human stem cell factor-dependent fetal liver-derived human mast cells. J Immunol 1997; 159(6):2911–21.

53. Kirshenbaum AS, Swindle E, Kulka M, et al. Effect of lipopolysaccharide (LPS) and peptidoglycan (PGN) on human mast cell numbers, cytokine production, and protease composition. BMC Immunol 2008;9:45.

54. Gebhardt T, Lorentz A, Detmer F, et al. Growth, phenotype, and function of human intestinal mast cells are tightly regulated by transforming growth factor beta1. Gut 2005;54(7):928–34.

55. Roskoski R Jr. Signaling by Kit protein-tyrosine kinase–the stem cell factor receptor. Biochem Biophys Res Commun 2005;337(1):1–13.

56. Koyasu S. The role of PI3K in immune cells. Nat Immunol 2003;4(4):313–9.

57. Ali K, Bilancio A, Thomas M, et al. Essential role for the p110delta phosphoinositide 3-kinase in the allergic response. Nature 2004;431(7011):1007–11.

58. Li Z, Jiang H, Xie W, et al. Roles of PLC-beta2 and -beta3 and PI3Kgamma in chemoattractant-mediated signal transduction. Science 2000;287(5455):1046–9.

59. Shelburne CP, McCoy ME, Piekorz R, et al. Stat5 expression is critical for mast cell development and survival. Blood 2003;102(4):1290–7.

60. Alexander WS, Lyman SD, Wagner EF. Expression of functional c-kit receptors rescues the genetic defect of W mutant mast cells. EMBO J 1991;10(12):3683–91.

61. Mekori YA, Gilfillan AM, Akin C, et al. Human mast cell apoptosis is regulated through Bcl-2 and Bcl-XL. J Clin Immunol 2001;21(3):171–4.

62. Baghestanian M, Jordan JH, Kiener HP, et al. Activation of human mast cells through stem cell factor receptor (KIT) is associated with expression of bcl-2. Int Arch Allergy Immunol 2002;129(3):228–36.

63. Datta SR, Dudek H, Tao X, et al. Akt phosphorylation of BAD couples survival signals to the cell-intrinsic death machinery. Cell 1997;91(2):231–41.

64. Blume-Jensen P, Janknecht R, Hunter T. The kit receptor promotes cell survival via activation of PI 3-kinase and subsequent Akt-mediated phosphorylation of Bad on Ser136. Curr Biol 1998;8(13):779–82.

65. del Peso L, Gonzalez-Garcia M, Page C, et al. Interleukin-3-induced phosphorylation of BAD through the protein kinase Akt. Science 1997;278(5338):687–9.

66. Alfredsson J, Puthalakath H, Martin H, et al. Proapoptotic Bcl-2 family member Bim is involved in the control of mast cell survival and is induced together with Bcl-XL upon IgE-receptor activation. Cell Death Differ 2005;12(2):136–44.

67. Furitsu T, Tsujimura T, Tono T, et al. Identification of mutations in the coding sequence of the proto-oncogene c-kit in a human mast cell leukemia cell line causing ligand-independent activation of c-kit product. J Clin Invest 1993; 92(4):1736–44.

68. Piao X, Bernstein A. A point mutation in the catalytic domain of c-kit induces growth factor independence, tumorigenicity, and differentiation of mast cells. Blood 1996;87(8):3117–23.

69. Longley BJ, Reguera MJ, Ma Y. Classes of c-KIT activating mutations: proposed mechanisms of action and implications for disease classification and therapy. Leuk Res 2001;25(7):571–6.

70. Feger F, Ribadeau Dumas A, Leriche L, et al. Kit and c-kit mutations in mastocytosis: a short overview with special reference to novel molecular and diagnostic concepts. Int Arch Allergy Immunol 2002;127(2):110–4.

71. Bodemer C, Hermine O, Palmerini F, et al. Pediatric mastocytosis is a clonal disease associated with D816V and other activating c-KIT mutations. J Invest Dermatol 2010;130(3):804–15.

72. Mayerhofer M, Gleixner KV, Hoelbl A, et al. Unique effects of KIT D816V in BaF3 cells: induction of cluster formation, histamine synthesis, and early mast cell differentiation antigens. J Immunol 2008;180(8):5466–76.

73. Gleixner KV, Mayerhofer M, Cerny-Reiterer S, et al. KIT-D816V-independent oncogenic signaling in neoplastic cells in systemic mastocytosis: role of Lyn and Btk activation and disruption by dasatinib and bosutinib. Blood 2011; 118(7):1885–98.

74. Tefferi A, Levine RL, Lim KH, et al. Frequent TET2 mutations in systemic mastocytosis: clinical, KITD816V and FIP1L1-PDGFRA correlates. Leukemia 2009; 23(5):900–4.

75. Akin C, Fumo G, Yavuz AS, et al. A novel form of mastocytosis associated with a transmembrane c-kit mutation and response to imatinib. Blood 2004;103(8): 3222–5.

76. Longley BJ Jr, Metcalfe DD, Tharp M, et al. Activating and dominant inactivating c-KIT catalytic domain mutations in distinct clinical forms of human mastocytosis. Proc Natl Acad Sci U S A 1999;96(4):1609–14.

77. Sotlar K, Escribano L, Landt O, et al. One-step detection of c-kit point mutations using peptide nucleic acid-mediated polymerase chain reaction clamping and hybridization probes. Am J Pathol 2003;162(3):737–46.

78. Yanagihori H, Oyama N, Nakamura K, et al. c-kit Mutations in patients with childhood-onset mastocytosis and genotype-phenotype correlation. J Mol Diagn 2005;7(2):252–7.

79. Buttner C, Henz BM, Welker P, et al. Identification of activating c-kit mutations in adult-, but not in childhood-onset indolent mastocytosis: a possible explanation for divergent clinical behavior. J Invest Dermatol 1998;111(6):1227–31.

80. Kettelhut BV, Metcalfe DD. Pediatric mastocytosis. J Invest Dermatol 1991; 96(Suppl 3):15S–8S [discussion: 8S, 60S–5S].

81. Azana JM, Torrelo A, Mediero IG, et al. Urticaria pigmentosa: a review of 67 pediatric cases. Pediatr Dermatol 1994;11(2):102–6.

82. Middelkamp Hup MA, Heide R, Tank B, et al. Comparison of mastocytosis with onset in children and adults. J Eur Acad Dermatol Venereol 2002;16(2):115–20.

83. Czarnetzki BM, Kolde G, Schoemann A, et al. Bone marrow findings in adult patients with urticaria pigmentosa. J Am Acad Dermatol 1988;18(1 Pt 1):45–51.

84. Parwaresch MR, Horny HP, Lennert K. Tissue mast cells in health and disease. Pathol Res Pract 1985;179(4–5):439–61.

85. Hannaford R, Rogers M. Presentation of cutaneous mastocytosis in 173 children. Australas J Dermatol 2001;42(1):15–21.

86. Pardanani A, Akin C, Valent P. Pathogenesis, clinical features, and treatment advances in mastocytosis. Best Pract Res Clin Haematol 2006;19(3):595–615.

87. Horny HP, Parwaresch MR, Lennert K. Bone marrow findings in systemic mastocytosis. Hum Pathol 1985;16(8):808–14.

88. Horny HP, Kaiserling E, Campbell M, et al. Liver findings in generalized mastocytosis. A clinicopathologic study. Cancer 1989;63(3):532–8.

89. Horny HP, Ruck MT, Kaiserling E. Spleen findings in generalized mastocytosis. A clinicopathologic study. Cancer 1992;70(2):459–68.

90. Horny HP, Kaiserling E, Parwaresch MR, et al. Lymph node findings in generalized mastocytosis. Histopathology 1992;21(5):439–46.
91. Valent P, Horny HP, Escribano L, et al. Diagnostic criteria and classification of mastocytosis: a consensus proposal. Leuk Res 2001;25(7):603–25.
92. Wolff K, Komar M, Petzelbauer P. Clinical and histopathological aspects of cutaneous mastocytosis. Leuk Res 2001;25(7):519–28.
93. Topar G, Staudacher C, Geisen F, et al. Urticaria pigmentosa: a clinical, hematopathologic, and serologic study of 30 adults. Am J Clin Pathol 1998;109(3):279–85.
94. Scheck O, Horny HP, Ruck P, et al. Solitary mastocytoma of the eyelid. A case report with special reference to the immunocytology of human tissue mast cells, and a review of the literature. Virchows Arch A Pathol Anat Histopathol 1987; 412(1):31–6.
95. Orkin M, Good RA, Clawson CC, et al. Bullous mastocytosis. Arch Dermatol 1970;101(5):547–64.
96. Golitz LE, Weston WL, Lane AT. Bullous mastocytosis: diffuse cutaneous mastocytosis with extensive blisters mimicking scalded skin syndrome or erythema multiforme. Pediatr Dermatol 1984;1(4):288–94.
97. Horny HP, Sotlar K, Sperr WR, et al. Systemic mastocytosis with associated clonal haematological non-mast cell lineage diseases: a histopathological challenge. J Clin Pathol 2004;57(6):604–8.
98. Lim KH, Tefferi A, Lasho TL, et al. Systemic mastocytosis in 342 consecutive adults: survival studies and prognostic factors. Blood 2009;113(23):5727–36.
99. Castells M, Austen KF. Mastocytosis: mediator-related signs and symptoms. Int Arch Allergy Immunol 2002;127(2):147–52.
100. Cherner JA, Jensen RT, Dubois A, et al. Gastrointestinal dysfunction in systemic mastocytosis. A prospective study. Gastroenterology 1988;95(3):657–67.
101. Hermine O, Lortholary O, Leventhal PS, et al. Case-control cohort study of patients' perceptions of disability in mastocytosis. PLoS One 2008;3(5):e2266.
102. Horny HP, Ruck M, Wehrmann M, et al. Blood findings in generalized mastocytosis: evidence of frequent simultaneous occurrence of myeloproliferative disorders. Br J Haematol 1990;76(2):186–93.
103. Travis WD, Li CY, Yam LT, et al. Significance of systemic mast cell disease with associated hematologic disorders. Cancer 1988;62(5):965–72.
104. Pardanani A, Lim KH, Lasho TL, et al. Prognostically relevant breakdown of 123 patients with systemic mastocytosis associated with other myeloid malignancies. Blood 2009;114(18):3769–72.
105. Brcic L, Vuletic LB, Stepan J, et al. Mast-cell sarcoma of the tibia. J Clin Pathol 2007;60(4):424–5.
106. Horny HP, Parwaresch MR, Kaiserling E, et al. Mast cell sarcoma of the larynx. J Clin Pathol 1986;39(6):596–602.
107. Kojima M, Nakamura S, Itoh H, et al. Mast cell sarcoma with tissue eosinophilia arising in the ascending colon. Mod Pathol 1999;12(7):739–43.
108. Charrette EE, Mariano AV, Laforet EG. Solitary mast cell "tumor" of lung. Its place in the spectrum of mast cell disease. Arch Intern Med 1966;118(4):358–62.
109. Sherwin RP, Kern WH, Jones JC. Solitary mast cell granuloma (histiocytoma) of the lung; a histopathologic, tissue culture and time-lapse cinematographic study. Cancer 1965;18:634–41.
110. Kudo H, Morinaga S, Shimosato Y, et al. Solitary mast cell tumor of the lung. Cancer 1988;61(10):2089–94.
111. Barete S, Assous N, de Gennes C, et al. Systemic mastocytosis and bone involvement in a cohort of 75 patients. Ann Rheum Dis 2010;69(10):1838–41.

112. Escribano L, Alvarez-Twose I, Sanchez-Munoz L, et al. Prognosis in adult indolent systemic mastocytosis: a long-term study of the Spanish Network on Mastocytosis in a series of 145 patients. J Allergy Clin Immunol 2009;124(3): 514–21.

113. van der Veer E, van der Goot W, de Monchy JG, et al. High prevalence of fractures and osteoporosis in patients with indolent systemic mastocytosis. Allergy 2012;67(3):431–8.

114. Tharp MD, Glass MJ, Seelig LL Jr. Ultrastructural morphometric analysis of human mast cells in normal skin and pathological cutaneous lesions. J Cutan Pathol 1988;15(2):78–83.

115. Weidner N, Austen KF. Ultrastructural and immunohistochemical characterization of normal mast cells at multiple body sites. J Invest Dermatol 1991; 96(Suppl 3):26S–30S [discussion: S–1S, 60S–5S].

116. Travis WD, Li CY, Bergstralh EJ, et al. Systemic mast cell disease. Analysis of 58 cases and literature review. Medicine (Baltimore) 1988;67(6):345–68.

117. Garriga MM, Friedman MM, Metcalfe DD. A survey of the number and distribution of mast cells in the skin of patients with mast cell disorders. J Allergy Clin Immunol 1988;82(3 Pt 1):425–32.

118. Sperr WR, Drach J, Hauswirth AW, et al. Myelomastocytic leukemia: evidence for the origin of mast cells from the leukemic clone and eradication by allogeneic stem cell transplantation. Clin Cancer Res 2005;11(19 Pt 1):6787–92.

119. Krokowski M, Sotlar K, Krauth MT, et al. Delineation of patterns of bone marrow mast cell infiltration in systemic mastocytosis: value of CD25, correlation with subvariants of the disease, and separation from mast cell hyperplasia. Am J Clin Pathol 2005;124(4):560–8.

120. Horny HP, Valent P. Diagnosis of mastocytosis: general histopathological aspects, morphological criteria, and immunohistochemical findings. Leuk Res 2001;25(7):543–51.

121. Horny HP, Valent P. Histopathological and immunohistochemical aspects of mastocytosis. Int Arch Allergy Immunol 2002;127(2):115–7.

122. Sperr WR, Escribano L, Jordan JH, et al. Morphologic properties of neoplastic mast cells: delineation of stages of maturation and implication for cytological grading of mastocytosis. Leuk Res 2001;25(7):529–36.

123. Li WV, Kapadia SB, Sonmez-Alpan E, et al. Immunohistochemical characterization of mast cell disease in paraffin sections using tryptase, CD68, myeloperoxidase, lysozyme, and CD20 antibodies. Mod Pathol 1996;9(10): 982–8.

124. Patnaik MM, Rindos M, Kouides PA, et al. Systemic mastocytosis: a concise clinical and laboratory review. Arch Pathol Lab Med 2007;131(5):784–91.

125. Sperr WR, Jordan JH, Fiegl M, et al. Serum tryptase levels in patients with mastocytosis: correlation with mast cell burden and implication for defining the category of disease. Int Arch Allergy Immunol 2002;128(2):136–41.

126. Sperr WR, El-Samahi A, Kundi M, et al. Elevated tryptase levels selectively cluster in myeloid neoplasms: a novel diagnostic approach and screen marker in clinical haematology. Eur J Clin Invest 2009;39(10):914–23.

127. Sotlar K, Marafioti T, Griesser H, et al. Detection of c-kit mutation Asp 816 to Val in microdissected bone marrow infiltrates in a case of systemic mastocytosis associated with chronic myelomonocytic leukaemia. Mol Pathol 2000;53(4): 188–93.

128. Valent P, Akin C, Sperr WR, et al. Mastocytosis: pathology, genetics, and current options for therapy. Leuk Lymphoma 2005;46(1):35–48.

129. Pullarkat V, Bedell V, Kim Y, et al. Neoplastic mast cells in systemic mastocytosis associated with t(8;21) acute myeloid leukemia are derived from the leukemic clone. Leuk Res 2007;31(2):261–5.
130. Thachil J, Hawkins S, Woodcock B. JAK2-positive myeloproliferative neoplasm co-existing with systemic mastocytosis. Br J Haematol 2011;152(6):675.
131. Bain BJ. Relationship between idiopathic hypereosinophilic syndrome, eosinophilic leukemia, and systemic mastocytosis. Am J Hematol 2004;77(1):82–5.
132. Klion AD, Noel P, Akin C, et al. Elevated serum tryptase levels identify a subset of patients with a myeloproliferative variant of idiopathic hypereosinophilic syndrome associated with tissue fibrosis, poor prognosis, and imatinib responsiveness. Blood 2003;101(12):4660–6.
133. Pardanani A. Systemic mastocytosis in adults: 2012 update on diagnosis, risk stratification, and management. Am J Hematol 2012;87(4):401–11.
134. Pardanani A, Ketterling RP, Brockman SR, et al. CHIC2 deletion, a surrogate for FIP1L1-PDGFRA fusion, occurs in systemic mastocytosis associated with eosinophilia and predicts response to imatinib mesylate therapy. Blood 2003;102(9): 3093–6.
135. Florian S, Esterbauer H, Binder T, et al. Systemic mastocytosis (SM) associated with chronic eosinophilic leukemia (SM-CEL): detection of FIP1L1/PDGFRalpha, classification by WHO criteria, and response to therapy with imatinib. Leuk Res 2006;30(9):1201–5.
136. Valent P, Akin C, Metcalfe DD. FIP1L1/PDGFRA is a molecular marker of chronic eosinophilic leukaemia but not for systemic mastocytosis. Eur J Clin Invest 2007; 37(2):153–4.
137. Maric I, Robyn J, Metcalfe DD, et al. KIT D816V-associated systemic mastocytosis with eosinophilia and FIP1L1/PDGFRA-associated chronic eosinophilic leukemia are distinct entities. J Allergy Clin Immunol 2007;120(3):680–7.
138. Castells M, Metcalfe DD, Escribano L. Diagnosis and treatment of cutaneous mastocytosis in children: practical recommendations. Am J Clin Dermatol 2011;12(4):259–70.
139. Welch EA, Alper JC, Bogaars H, et al. Treatment of bullous mastocytosis with disodium cromoglycate. J Am Acad Dermatol 1983;9(3):349–53.
140. Marone G, Spadaro G, Granata F, et al. Treatment of mastocytosis: pharmacologic basis and current concepts. Leuk Res 2001;25(7):583–94.
141. Kettelhut BV, Berkebile C, Bradley D, et al. A double-blind, placebo-controlled, crossover trial of ketotifen versus hydroxyzine in the treatment of pediatric mastocytosis. J Allergy Clin Immunol 1989;83(5):866–70.
142. Frieri M, Alling DW, Metcalfe DD. Comparison of the therapeutic efficacy of cromolyn sodium with that of combined chlorpheniramine and cimetidine in systemic mastocytosis. Results of a double-blind clinical trial. Am J Med 1985;78(1):9–14.
143. Valent P, Akin C, Escribano L, et al. Standards and standardization in mastocytosis: consensus statements on diagnostics, treatment recommendations and response criteria. Eur J Clin Invest 2007;37(6):435–53.
144. Brockow K, Jofer C, Behrendt H, et al. Anaphylaxis in patients with mastocytosis: a study on history, clinical features and risk factors in 120 patients. Allergy 2008;63(2):226–32.
145. Worobec AS, Metcalfe DD. Mastocytosis: current treatment concepts. Int Arch Allergy Immunol 2002;127(2):153–5.
146. Butterfield JH, Kao PC, Klee GC, et al. Aspirin idiosyncrasy in systemic mast cell disease: a new look at mediator release during aspirin desensitization. Mayo Clin Proc 1995;70(5):481–7.

147. Oude Elberink JN, de Monchy JG, Kors JW, et al. Fatal anaphylaxis after a yellow jacket sting, despite venom immunotherapy, in two patients with mastocytosis. J Allergy Clin Immunol 1997;99(1 Pt 1):153–4.

148. Pumphrey RS. Lessons for management of anaphylaxis from a study of fatal reactions. Clin Exp Allergy 2000;30(8):1144–50.

149. Desborough JP, Taylor I, Hattersley A, et al. Massive histamine release in a patient with systemic mastocytosis. Br J Anaesth 1990;65(6):833–6.

150. Niedoszytko M, de Monchy J, van Doormaal JJ, et al. Mastocytosis and insect venom allergy: diagnosis, safety and efficacy of venom immunotherapy. Allergy 2009;64(9):1237–45.

151. Marone G, Stellato C. Activation of human mast cells and basophils by general anaesthetic drugs. Monogr Allergy 1992;30:54–73.

152. Stellato C, Marone G. Mast cells and basophils in adverse reactions to drugs used during general anesthesia. Chem Immunol 1995;62:108–31.

153. Scott HW Jr, Parris WC, Sandidge PC, et al. Hazards in operative management of patients with systemic mastocytosis. Ann Surg 1983;197(5):507–14.

154. James PD, Krafchik BR, Johnston AE. Cutaneous mastocytosis in children: anaesthetic considerations. Can J Anaesth 1987;34(5):522–4.

155. Greenblatt EP, Chen L. Urticaria pigmentosa: an anesthetic challenge. J Clin Anesth 1990;2(2):108–15.

156. Lerno G, Slaats G, Coenen E, et al. Anaesthetic management of systemic mastocytosis. Br J Anaesth 1990;65(2):254–7.

157. Borgeat A, Ruetsch YA. Anesthesia in a patient with malignant systemic mastocytosis using a total intravenous anesthetic technique. Anesth Analg 1998;86(2):442–4.

158. Mackey S, Pride HB, Tyler WB. Diffuse cutaneous mastocytosis. Treatment with oral psoralen plus UV-A. Arch Dermatol 1996;132(12):1429–30.

159. Smith ML, Orton PW, Chu H, et al. Photochemotherapy of dominant, diffuse, cutaneous mastocytosis. Pediatr Dermatol 1990;7(4):251–5.

160. Lim KH, Pardanani A, Butterfield JH, et al. Cytoreductive therapy in 108 adults with systemic mastocytosis: outcome analysis and response prediction during treatment with interferon-alpha, hydroxyurea, imatinib mesylate or 2-chlorodeoxyadenosine. Am J Hematol 2009;84(12):790–4.

161. Kluin-Nelemans HC, Jansen JH, Breukelman H, et al. Response to interferon alfa-2b in a patient with systemic mastocytosis. N Engl J Med 1992;326(9):619–23.

162. Casassus P, Caillat-Vigneron N, Martin A, et al. Treatment of adult systemic mastocytosis with interferon-alpha: results of a multicentre phase II trial on 20 patients. Br J Haematol 2002;119(4):1090–7.

163. Kluin-Nelemans HC, Oldhoff JM, Van Doormaal JJ, et al. Cladribine therapy for systemic mastocytosis. Blood 2003;102(13):4270–6.

164. Tefferi A, Li CY, Butterfield JH, et al. Treatment of systemic mast-cell disease with cladribine. N Engl J Med 2001;344(4):307–9.

165. Hennessy B, Giles F, Cortes J, et al. Management of patients with systemic mastocytosis: review of M. D. Anderson Cancer Center experience. Am J Hematol 2004;77(3):209–14.

166. Samorapoompichit P, Steiner M, Lucas T, et al. Induction of apoptosis in the human mast cell leukemia cell line HMC-1 by various antineoplastic drugs. Leuk Lymphoma 2003;44(3):509–15.

167. Pardanani A, Elliott M, Reeder T, et al. Imatinib for systemic mast-cell disease. Lancet 2003;362(9383):535–6.

168. Droogendijk HJ, Kluin-Nelemans HJ, van Doormaal JJ, et al. Imatinib mesylate in the treatment of systemic mastocytosis: a phase II trial. Cancer 2006;107(2): 345–51.

169. Shah NP, Lee FY, Luo R, et al. Dasatinib (BMS-354825) inhibits KITD816V, an imatinib-resistant activating mutation that triggers neoplastic growth in most patients with systemic mastocytosis. Blood 2006;108(1):286–91.

170. Dubreuil P, Letard S, Ciufolini M, et al. Masitinib (AB1010), a potent and selective tyrosine kinase inhibitor targeting KIT. PLoS One 2009;4(9):e7258.

171. Paul C, Sans B, Suarez F, et al. Masitinib for the treatment of systemic and cutaneous mastocytosis with handicap: a phase 2a study. Am J Hematol 2010; 85(12):921–5.

172. Growney JD, Clark JJ, Adelsperger J, et al. Activation mutations of human c-KIT resistant to imatinib mesylate are sensitive to the tyrosine kinase inhibitor PKC412. Blood 2005;106(2):721–4.

173. Gleixner KV, Mayerhofer M, Aichberger KJ, et al. PKC412 inhibits in vitro growth of neoplastic human mast cells expressing the D816V-mutated variant of KIT: comparison with AMN107, imatinib, and cladribine (2CdA) and evaluation of cooperative drug effects. Blood 2006;107(2):752–9.

174. Gotlib J, Berube C, Growney JD, et al. Activity of the tyrosine kinase inhibitor PKC412 in a patient with mast cell leukemia with the D816V KIT mutation. Blood 2005;106(8):2865–70.

175. Verstovsek S, Tefferi A, Cortes J, et al. Phase II study of dasatinib in Philadelphia chromosome-negative acute and chronic myeloid diseases, including systemic mastocytosis. Clin Cancer Res 2008;14(12):3906–15.

176. Sperr WR, Horny HP, Lechner K, et al. Clinical and biologic diversity of leukemias occurring in patients with mastocytosis. Leuk Lymphoma 2000;37(5–6): 473–86.

177. Sperr WR, Walchshofer S, Horny HP, et al. Systemic mastocytosis associated with acute myeloid leukaemia: report of two cases and detection of the c-kit mutation Asp-816 to Val. Br J Haematol 1998;103(3):740–9.

Epidemiology and Management of Uveal Melanoma

Yoshihiro Yonekawa, MD, Ivana K. Kim, MD*

KEYWORDS

- Uveal melanoma • Choroidal melanoma • Proton beam irradiation • Brachytherapy
- Enucleation

KEY POINTS

- Uveal melanoma is the most common primary intraocular malignancy in adults.
- Most affected patients are Caucasian.
- Most cases can be treated with eye-conserving local irradiation, but enucleation is sometimes necessary.
- The pathogenesis of uveal melanoma involves the mitogen-activated protein kinase pathway.
- Risk of metastatic disease can be predicted by molecular diagnostic testing.
- There is currently no effective treatment of metastatic uveal melanoma.

INTRODUCTION

Uveal melanoma is the most common primary intraocular malignancy in adults. The tumors arise from the uveal tract, which is comprised of the iris, ciliary body, and choroid. Although both cutaneous and uveal melanomas share the melanocyte as their common origin, their clinical behavior and underlying molecular mechanisms are significantly different. Substantial advances in the diagnosis and local treatment of uveal melanoma have been made in the past few decades, shifting from enucleation to eye-conserving treatments as the primary treatment modalities, without compromising survival.[1]

EPIDEMIOLOGY
Incidence

Uveal melanoma is relatively rare. A study based on the National Cancer Data Base of the United States reviewed 84,836 cases of cutaneous and noncutaneous melanomas

Disclosure statement: No conflicting relationship exists for any author.
Department of Ophthalmology, Harvard Medical School, Retina Service, Massachusetts Eye and Ear Infirmary, 243 Charles Street, Boston, MA 02114, USA
* Corresponding author.
E-mail address: ivana_kim@meei.harvard.edu

diagnosed between 1985 and 1994.[2] Ocular melanomas comprised 5.2%, of which 85% were uveal melanomas. In an analysis of the Surveillance, Epidemiology, and End Results (SEER) program of the National Cancer Institute, which covers approximately 28% of the US population, Singh and colleagues[3] reported 4070 cases of uveal melanoma from 1973 to 2008. This rate represented 3.1% of all recorded cases of melanoma. The mean age-adjusted incidence was calculated to be 5.1 per million per year (95% confidence interval [CI], 4.8–5.3). The incidence remained unchanged from 1973 to 2008. Similar rates, or slightly higher, have been reported from Canada,[4] Denmark,[5] Finland,[6] Israel,[7] Norway,[8] and the Netherlands,[9] which have predominantly white populations.

Age

The average age at initial diagnosis of uveal melanoma is approximately 60 years.[2,3] Unlike other malignancies, uveal melanoma may plateau or decrease in incidence in older patients.[8,10] Pediatric cases are rare. In several large series of patients with uveal melanoma, only 0.5% to 1.3% were 20 years of age or younger.[11–13] Compared with older patients, younger patients are more likely to have associated ocular melanocytosis, present with iris melanomas, and lower risk of metastatic disease.[11] Congenital cases have been reported, but seldom occur.[14]

Gender

It is uncertain whether there is a difference in the incidence of uveal melanoma between men and women. Data from the SEER program indicate that the age-adjusted incidence is slightly higher in men: 5.8 per million (95% CI, 5.5–6.2) for men, and 4.4 per million (95% CI, 4.2–4.7) for women.[3] However, a review of 8033 eyes from Wills Eye Institute did not note a difference.[11] The authors also have not observed a gender predisposition at the Massachusetts Eye and Ear Infirmary.[15]

The Collaborative Ocular Melanoma Study (COMS) was a set of multicenter randomized clinical trials in the United States and Canada (**Table 1**). In the medium-sized melanoma trial, comparing enucleation to brachytherapy, there was no gender imbalance: 1478 men (51%) and 1398 women (49%) were eligible for the study.[16] However, in the large-sized melanoma trial, comparing enucleation with or without preenucleation radiation therapy, there was a slight predominance of men: 731 (56%) men and 567 (44%) women were eligible for the study, but there was no difference in those who were not eligible.[17] An interesting finding from Sweden notes that while there was a decrease in the incidence of uveal melanoma in men between 1960 and 1998, the incidence remained stable in women.[18] In a study of 6673 cases from

Table 1
Collaborative Ocular Melanoma Study classification of choroidal melanoma sizes[a]

Size Category	Apical Height (mm)	Longest Basal Diameter (mm)
Small	1.0 to <2.5	5.0 to 16.0
Medium	2.5 to 10.0	≤16.0
Large	≥2.0	>16.0
	>10.0	any

Abbreviation: mm, millimeters.
[a] Criteria since November 1990. Please see references for peripapillary tumor criteria.
Data from Refs.[16,17,100]

European registries from 1983 to 1994, there were more men with uveal melanoma than women (incidence rate ratio 1.22, 95% CI, 1.16–1.28).[10]

Race and Ethnicity

Uveal melanoma predominantly affects the white population. In the recent SEER study, 97.8% of affected patients were white, with a white:black incidence ratio of 196:1.[3] In a smaller analysis of the SEER database from 1992 to 2000, Hu and colleagues[19] reported that of 1352 uveal melanomas, the annual age-adjusted incidence per million was 0.31 in blacks, 0.38 in Asian and Pacific Islanders, 1.67 in Hispanics, and 6.02 in non-Hispanic whites. The relative risks compared with black individuals were 1.2 for Asian and Pacific Islanders, 5.4 for Hispanics, and 19.2 for non-Hispanic whites. At Wills Eye Institute, of 2586 patients with posterior uveal melanoma from 1974 to 1987, only 10 (0.39%) were black.[20] A study from the Armed Forces Institute of Pathology reported 39 black individuals out of 3876 (1.0%) with ciliary body and choroidal melanomas before 1975.[21] The investigators noted that compared with a control group of white subjects, black subjects were more likely to have secondary glaucoma and inflammation before enucleation.

Uveal melanoma is rare in Asian populations but may occur at an earlier age.[22–24] A review of 65 cases of uveal melanoma from Shanghai between 1956 and 1979 noted that 20% occurred in patients between 19 and 30 years of age.[23] Most cases occurred in the fifth decade, but only 5 occurred in the sixth decade, which is the highest risk age group in white populations. A high number of epithelioid tumors were noted, which often portends a poorer prognosis.

Among the white population, ancestry from northern latitudes appears to be a risk factor for developing uveal melanoma.[25] Our group investigated 197 white individuals with uveal melanoma with matched population controls and found that compared with subjects with parents of both Southern European or Mediterranean ancestry (Greece, Italy, Portugal, Spain, Yugoslavia, or Middle East), the adjusted relative risks were 2 (95% CI, 0.96–4.2) for those of central European decent (other European countries and Russia), 2.4 (95% CI, 1.02–5.5) for those of mixed ancestry, 2.4 (95% CI, 1.1–5.1) for those of British decent, and 6.5 (95% CI, 1.9–22.4) for those of northern European decent (Finland and Scandinavian and Baltic countries, including Lithuania, Latvia, and Estonia). Similar results were found in the European Cancer Registry-based study on survival and care of cancer patients (EUROCARE) study that examined 67 cancer registries from 22 European countries.[10] Five thousand five hundred sixty-six cases of uveal melanoma were reported from 1983 to 1994, and standardized incidence rates increased from southern to northern registries, with a minimum of less than 2 per million in Spain and southern Italy, up to greater than 8 per million in Norway and Denmark.

In addition to ethnicity, intrinsic host factors that appear to predispose white individuals to uveal melanoma include light eye color, light skin color, and the inability to tan. A meta-analysis of 10 case-control studies of white populations found that the blue or gray eye color (odds ratio [OR] 1.75 [95% CI, 1.31–2.34]), fair skin color (OR 1.80 [95% CI, 1.31–2.47]), and a propensity to sunburn (OR 1.64 [95% CI, 1.29–2.09]) were statistically significant risk factors.[26]

Choroidal Nevi

Cutaneous nevi are a well-known risk factor for developing cutaneous melanoma.[27] Uveal melanomas are thought to arise from choroidal nevi as well, but the evidence is not as robust. Approximately 3% of individuals older than 30 years of age have nevi in the posterior half of the choroid, and it has been estimated that 1 out of every

4800 choroidal nevi may transform into a melanoma per year.[28] Similarly, the Blue Mountains Eye Study estimated the rate of malignant transformation to be 1 melanoma per 4300 nevi per year.[29] A systematic literature review noted the prevalence of choroidal nevi to be 4.6% to 7.9% in the white US population and estimated the annual malignant transformation to be 1 in 8845.[30] In clinical practice, benign-appearing choroidal nevi are monitored on regular eye examinations. Fundus photography and ultrasonography are valuable adjuncts to the clinical examination in determining if there has been significant growth.

Ocular/Oculodermal Melanocytosis

Ocular melanocytosis is a diffuse congenital melanosis of the episclera and uvea that is more common in black, Hispanic, and Asian populations. Half of the patients also have ipsilateral dermal melanocytosis (nevus of Ota), and the combination is termed oculodermal melanocytosis. Ocular/oculodermal melanocytosis affects approximately 0.04% of the general white population, whereas about 1.4% of patients with uveal melanoma have ocular melanosis, indicating that ocular melanosis is approximately 35 times more common in patients with uveal melanoma.[31] One in 400 patients with ocular melanosis is thought to develop uveal melanoma in their lifetimes.[31] The increased number of melanocytes in the uveal tract appears to predispose these patients to uveal melanoma, as evidenced by their propensity to develop the tumors in sectoral areas affected by the melanocytosis.[32]

Other Risk Factors

Development of uveal melanoma is usually considered a sporadic event. However, approximately 90 cases of familial uveal melanoma have been reported in the literature,[33,34] and recently, germline BAP1 (BRCA1 [breast cancer 1, early onset]-associated protein 1) mutations have been shown to predispose to uveal melanoma, cutaneous melanocytic tumors, and other malignancies.[35–37] Pregnancy,[38,39] ovarian cancer,[40] and history of malignancy in women[41] have been implicated as well but without substantial evidence. Some reports indicate that sun exposure may increase the risk of uveal melanoma, but study results are conflicting.[25,42,43] Dietary factors[44] and smoking[45] have not been found to be contributory risk factors.

PATHOGENESIS

Advances in understanding the molecular mechanisms of uveal melanoma have been made in recent years. Cutaneous and uveal melanomas differ in their pathogenesis, despite sharing the melanocyte as their common origin. For example, BRAF (v-raf murine sarcoma viral oncogene homolog B1) mutations are found in up to 62% of cutaneous melanomas but rarely implicated in uveal melanoma.[46–48] The mitogen-activated protein kinase (MAPK) pathway, of which BRAF is a key component, has been shown to be activated in 86% of primary uveal melanoma specimens.[49] Therefore, cutaneous and uveal melanomas appear to activate the MAPK pathway, but through different mechanisms.

The upstream modulator of the MAPK pathway in uveal melanoma was unknown until recently. Van Raamsdonk and colleagues[50] reported that guanine nucleotide binding protein q polypeptide (GNAQ) or GNA11 mutations occurred in 83% of the 186 uveal melanomas that they analyzed. Both GNAQ and GNA11 encode the alpha subunit of G proteins, which are a family of heterotrimeric proteins bound to cell membrane receptors. These proteins modulate the signaling pathway that lead to activation of downstream components including Raf, MEK, and ERK. GNAQ/11 mutations are found in blue nevi and are not associated with survival in uveal melanoma and therefore, represent early or perhaps initiating mutations that require further genetic aberrations for malignant transformation.[50]

Specific genetic alterations have been associated with increased risk of metastasis of uveal melanoma. Monosomy 3 occurs in approximately half of uveal melanomas and has been strongly correlated with poor histopathologic factors and metastasis-related death.[51–53] Recently, Harbour and colleagues[54] reported that 26 (84%) of 31 metastasizing uveal melanomas contained BAP1 mutations. BAP1 is located on chromosome 3, and biallelic inactivation of this gene likely accounts for the noted association between monosomy 3 and risk of metastasis.

CLINICAL PRESENTATION AND DIAGNOSIS

Uveal melanomas are either detected on routine eye examinations, or when patients present with visual symptoms. Common symptoms include blurry vision, photopsias (flashing lights), and visual-field defects. Loss of vision is usually caused by tumor involvement of the macula or by exudative retinal detachments.

A dilated fundus examination by an ophthalmologist with experience in ocular oncology is the most important factor in accurately diagnosing uveal melanoma. Classically, melanomas appear as pigmented, dome or collar-button shaped masses (**Fig. 1**). The collar-button configuration occurs when the tumor breaks through Bruch membrane, which is the basement membrane of the retinal pigment epithelium (RPE) and choriocapillaris. Larger tumors may be associated with dilated episcleral vessels, visible externally.

The color, shape, and number of lesions are important considerations in diagnosis. Jet-black pigmentation is not characteristic of uveal melanoma, and other diagnoses should be considered, such as RPE hyperplasia, RPE hypertrophy, and melanocytoma. Amelanotic uveal melanomas do occur, but choroidal hemangioma, choroidal osteoma,

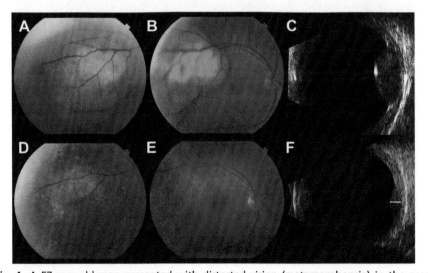

Fig. 1. A 57-year-old man presented with distorted vision (metamorphopsia) in the nasal visual field of the right eye for 2 weeks. (*A, B*) Fundus photograph of a lightly pigmented dome-shaped choroidal melanoma. (*C*) B-scan ultrasonography shows a choroidal lesion measuring 6.5 mm in height. (*D–F*) Two years after proton beam irradiation. The tumor has regressed to 2.1 mm, and vision remains 20/20.

and choroidal metastasis should be included in the differential diagnosis of amelanotic lesions (**Fig. 2**). Multifocal and bilateral lesions are also more consistent with choroidal metastasis. Hemorrhage, inflammation, and pain are rare but may be seen in large tumors. An atypical presentation is the "diffuse" melanoma, which by definition, is less than 5 mm thick and encompasses more than a quarter of the uvea. Other choroidal tumors that can appear similar to uveal melanoma are listed in **Box 1**.

Small lesions are difficult to diagnose definitively. Indeterminate lesions are monitored for growth. Signs suggestive of malignancy include tumor thickness greater than 2.0 mm, posterior tumor margin abutting the optic disc, visual symptoms, orange pigment (representing lipofuscin deposits at the level of the RPE), and subretinal fluid.[55,56]

Ultrasonography is the most important ancillary imaging modality in diagnosing and monitoring uveal melanoma. B-scan ultrasonography is useful for characterizing the tumor and for obtaining tumor dimensions. Typical findings in larger melanomas include choroidal excavation and orbital shadowing. High-resolution ultrasound (ultrasound biomicroscopy) allows excellent visualization of iris and ciliary body tumors, which are difficult to fully appreciate on the clinical examination. A-scan ultrasonography classically reveals low to medium internal echogenicity in uveal melanomas, allowing differentiation from tumors with typically high internal reflectivity, such as choroidal hemangiomas.

Fluorescein angiography can also aid in the diagnosis, especially if other lesions that mimic uveal melanomas may be under consideration. Larger melanomas may exhibit an intrinsic tumor circulation called a "double circulation." Although most cases of uveal melanoma can be accurately diagnosed noninvasively, fine-needle aspiration for cytological studies may be warranted for diagnostic dilemmas, especially if it alters

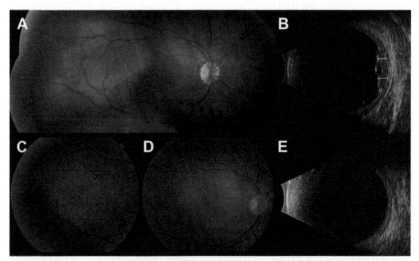

Fig. 2. A 47-year-old woman with a history of HER-2 positive invasive ductal carcinoma of the right breast, treated with lumpectomy, axillary dissection, and chemoradiation, presented with blurriness of the nasal visual field of the right eye and was diagnosed with choroidal metastasis. (*A*) Fundus photograph of an amelanotic lesion in the right eye involving the temporal macula. (*B*) B-scan ultrasonography shows an elevated choroidal lesion measuring 2.5 mm in height, associated with an inferior retinal detachment. (*C–E*) Eleven months after proton beam irradiation. The tumor has almost completely regressed, the retinal detachment has resolved, and vision remains 20/20.

Box 1
Choroidal tumors that may mimic choroidal melanoma

- Metastatic carcinoma
- Choroidal hemangioma
- Combined hamartoma of the retina and RPE
- Choroidal osteoma
- Intraocular or metastatic lymphoma
- Hemangiopericytoma
- Leiomyoma
- Neurilemmoma
- Adenoma of the pigmented ciliary epithelium
- Reactive lymphoid hyperplasia

Abbreviation: RPE, retinal pigment epithelium.

---

subsequent management.[57] Posterior tumors are accessed via transvitreal approaches and anterior tumors via direct transscleral approaches. Tumor seeding of the biopsy tract does not occur if properly performed by experienced ocular oncologists and retina surgeons.

TREATMENT

The main treatment options for uveal melanoma are radiation therapy or enucleation. Local resection has been performed for selected tumors. Currently, most patients undergo radiation treatment, and enucleation is reserved for large tumors in which radiation would have high ocular morbidity with little chance of globe or vision retention. The COMS confirmed equivalent survival rates in patients treated with enucleation versus I-125 brachytherapy. The trial enrolled 1317 patients with medium-sized tumors, and the 5-year survival rate for enucleation was 81% (95% CI, 77%–84%), and 82% (95% CI, 79%–84%) in the brachytherapy arm.[58] This rate was not a statistically significant difference. Further analysis indicated that 12.5% (95% CI, 10.0–15.6%) of eyes initially treated with brachytherapy required enucleation in the first 5 years.[59] Visual acuity loss to 20/200 or worse occurred in 43% (95% CI, 38%–48%) of eyes in the first 3 years.[60] The 12-year follow-up data confirmed that enucleation does not confer a survival advantage.[61]

Brachytherapy

Radiation therapy has become the most commonly used treatment modality for choroidal melanoma since the COMS trials. Brachytherapy is the most frequently treatment because of its wide availability. Cobalt-60 was initially used in the 1970s and 1980s, but the high-energy gamma emission did not allow adequate shielding of surrounding tissue and operating room staff.[62] The lower-energy iodine-125 plaque was subsequently developed and has largely replaced Cobalt-60 as the isotype of choice in the United States. Other isotopes include palladium-103 and ruthenium-106, but clinical experience is limited.

Ophthalmologists determine the exact location, size, and shape of the melanoma, and physicists subsequently design patient-specific plaques based on such parameters. The plaques are fixated onto the globe in the operating room under intravenous sedation and retrobulbar block. The conjunctiva is first dissected 360°, and the rectus muscles are isolated with sutures for traction. Transillumination is then performed to visualize the tumor borders, which are marked. The plaques are oversized so that they are slightly larger than the actual tumor. A plastic template is first sutured to optimize positioning. The template is then removed, and the radioactive plaque is sutured onto the sclera. Rectus muscles may need to be temporarily disinserted for proper plaque placement. The eye is covered by a lead shield throughout the treatment period, and contact with others are limited to prevent radiation dissemination. The plaque is subsequently removed in the operating room after several days of treatment.

Proton Beam Irradiation

The second major radiation treatment modality for uveal melanoma is charged particle irradiation using protons[63] and helium.[64] Unlike conventional external beam radiation therapy, charged particles allow tightly localized radiation. Helium ion irradiation has been largely replaced by proton beam irradiation because of its cost. Protons and helium ions are charged particles with a property called the Bragg peak, which allows a uniform radiation dose at desired depths, with a sudden drop off of radiation, thus theoretically limiting irradiation of surrounding tissues. Large tumors and posterior tumors that cannot be accessed by conventional plaque therapy are often referred to proton centers.[65] The gamma knife is an alternative stereotactic option to proton beam irradiation, but there is limited data, and the dose distributions are less favorable compared with proton therapy.[66,67]

Proton treatment requires tumor localization surgery in which tantalum rings are sutured on the sclera to outline the tumor. The relative position of the rings as seen on radiograph are used in a treatment planning program, which creates a 3-dimensional model of the eye and the tumor to help determine the best gaze direction and specify beam parameters. Standard treatment of uveal melanoma uses 70 cobalt gray equivalents delivered in 5 fractions over 5 to 7 days. Individualized facemasks and bite blocks are mounted onto the treatment frame for immobilization, and the patient is asked to gaze at a fixation light. Fluoroscopy is used to confirm positioning, and eye movement is monitored by a closed-circuit television system.

Most tumors show regression by 6 months and continue to regress thereafter.[68] The risk factors for poor visual outcome include proximity to the macula and optic nerve, tumor height and diameter, baseline visual acuity, retinal detachment, and history of diabetes.[15] For example, for patients with tumors less than 5 mm in height and located more than 2 disc diameters away from the optic nerve and fovea, approximately 75% of patients retain vision of 20/200 or better at 10 years, whereas the rate is only 3% for those with tall tumors close to both the optic disc and fovea.[69]

Local recurrence is observed in 2% to 5% of eyes treated with charged particle irradiation.[15,70–73] At the Massachusetts Eye and Ear Infirmary, of 2069 tumors treated with proton beam irradiation, 2.2% showed growth between 5 months and 11 years after treatment.[15] This recurrence rate is favorable compared with rates reported with brachytherapy.[59,74] Main risk factors for tumor recurrence are larger tumor diameter[15,70] and tumors that involve the ciliary body.[15,70,72] Local recurrences are typically treated with repeat proton irradiation or with enucleation. However, recurrences are associated with an increased risk of death from metastatic disease.[70,71,73]

Complications of Radiation Treatment

Radiation retinopathy is a slowly progressive disease caused by radiation-induced endothelial damage and capillary occlusion, which results in retinal hemorrhage, macular edema, vascular sheathing, microaneurysms, retinal exudation, telangiectasias, retinal pigment epithelial atrophy, and cotton wool spots.[75] Radiation optic neuropathy is characterized by optic disc hemorrhage, disc pallor, and/or disc edema and was present in 27.4% of subjects in the COMS trial at 5 years.[75] In a review of 1300 patients treated with brachytherapy, 42% (95% CI, 38%–45%) developed radiation retinopathy at 5 years.[76] Major risk factors for developing retinopathy were high radiation dose and proximity of the tumor to the fovea and/or optic disc.[75,76] In patients treated with proton beam irradiation, the incidence of radiation retinopathy and optic neuropathy peaks at 2 to 3 years after treatment, and at 10 years, approximately 50% patients have retinopathy and 25% have optic neuropathy.[77] Diabetes mellitus has been shown to be a significant risk factor for developing radiation retinopathy.[75,76,78]

The main treatment of radiation retinopathy is panretinal photocoagulation for proliferative disease (in which there is retinal neovascularization).[79] Emerging therapeutic modalities for macular edema in this setting include intravitreal or periocular steroids,[80,81] intravitreal anti-vascular endothelial growth factor (VEGF) agents,[82] and photodynamic therapy.[83] There is no proven treatment of radiation optic neuropathy; mixed results have been reported for corticosteroids, hyperbaric oxygen, and anticoagulation.[84,85] Intravitreal anti-VEGF treatment has been proposed as a possible treatment option, but the evidence is lacking.[84] The authors' study investigating the natural history of radiation optic neuropathy in eyes with parapapillary melanomas treated with proton beam irradiation showed that of 93 patients, 42% retained visual acuity at counting fingers or better at 5 years, and 31% had spontaneous visual improvement of 3 or more lines, indicating that the natural history of radiation optic neuropathy after proton irradiation may be better than generally assumed.[86]

Metastatic Disease

Overall, approximately half of patients with posterior uveal melanoma will die from the disease. Uveal melanoma metastasizes hematogenously because there are no lymphatics in the uveal tract. Unlike cutaneous melanoma, the liver is the most common site for metastasis, accounting for 90% of cases.[87,88] The factors associated with metastasis include tumor size and location (see **Table 1**), histologic grade, and genetic composition.[89] Ciliary body-involving tumors are more likely to metastasize,[15] whereas iris melanomas are significantly more indolent,[90] and epithelioid tumors are more aggressive than spindle tumors. Two TNM staging systems exist (one for all uveal melanomas and one for ciliary body/choroidal melanomas), based on size and location (ciliary body vs choroidal), and presence of extrascleral extention.[91] However, TNM staging has limited clinical application.

Risk of metastasis can be most accurately predicted by molecular profiling of fine-needle aspiration biopsy samples of the ocular tumor before irradiation. Cytogenetic analysis for monosomy 3 status and expression profiling are the 2 most commonly used methods for risk profiling. A 15 gene expression profiling assay has been shown to have better accuracy in predicting risk of metastasis than monosomy 3 status (**Fig. 3**).[92] Expression profiling defines 2 classes of uveal melanoma: class 1: tumors which have extremely low rates of metastasis and class 2: tumors in which approximately 50% of patients have metastatic disease at 3 years after diagnosis.[93]

Although the authors can provide molecular prognostication with respect to metastatic risk, they have not made significant advances in treatment of metastatic disease. In the COMS trials, the 5- and 10-year cumulative metastasis rates were 25% and 34%, respectively.[87] Eighty percent died within 1 year of diagnosis of metastasis and 92% within 2 years. The median time until death was less than 6 months. The

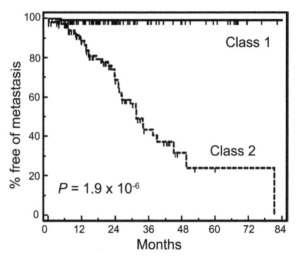

Fig. 3. Kaplan-Meier analysis of metastasis-free survival of 172 patients with uveal melanoma. The subjects are divided into class 1 and class 2 based on a 15 gene expression assay. Class 2 uveal melanomas are significantly more likely to metastasize. (*Reprinted from* Onken MD, Worley LA, Tuscan MD, et al. An accurate, clinically feasible multi-gene expression assay for predicting metastasis in uveal melanoma. J Mol Diagn 2010;12(4): 461–8; with permission from Elsevier.)

baseline size of the uveal melanoma did not change outcomes, and unfortunately, treatment of the metastatic disease did not increase survival after adjusting for age.

Systemic chemotherapies thus far have no benefit in metastatic uveal melanoma. The Eastern Cooperative Oncology Group trials for metastatic cutaneous melanoma also included patients with metastatic ocular melanoma and examined various combinations of lomustine, hydroxyurea, dacarbazine, Bacillus Calmette-Guerin vaccine, zinostatin, dibromodulcitol, dihydroxy anthracenedione, and aziridinyl benzoquinone. Of the 662 patients with cutaneous or unknown primary tumors, 74 showed response to treatment. However, of 51 patients with metastatic ocular melanoma, none responded to any chemotherapy.[94]

Given the lack of treatment of metastatic disease, it is controversial whether to aggressively pursue early detection of metastasis. Several uncontrolled studies investigated focal hepatic resection and hepatic artery infusion chemotherapy with some improved survival, suggesting that earlier detection may be beneficial.[95–98] The authors compared the survival outcomes of 90 presymptomatic patients who were diagnosed with metastatic disease (early diagnosis) to 259 patients who were diagnosed after becoming symptomatic (late diagnosis).[99] There were no baseline differences in the risk factors for metastasis, including age and tumor size. Melanoma-associated death occurred more frequently in the symptomatic group in the first year after diagnosis (88% compared with 69%), but by the second year, there was no difference. The median time from diagnosis of the primary melanoma to death was 40.6 months in the asymptomatic group, and 45.1 months in the symptomatic group. It appears that with the currently available treatments, early diagnosis confers a survival benefit only in the first year, representing a lead-time bias. However, molecular prognostic testing and advances in understanding of the genetics of uveal melanoma are likely to aid in the development of new therapies. High-risk patients can now be identified for clinical trials that may lead to effective therapies for metastatic disease and adjuvant therapy to prevent metastatic disease.

SUMMARY

Uveal melanoma is the most common primary intraocular malignancy in adults. Most affected patients are Caucasian. Historically, enucleation was the definitive treatment, but currently eye-conserving irradiation is the most common treatment. There is currently no effective treatment of metastatic disease, but potential therapeutic targets have been identified and clinical trials are anticipated.

REFERENCES

1. Trends in size and treatment of recently diagnosed choroidal melanoma, 1987-1997: findings from patients examined at collaborative ocular melanoma study (COMS) centers: COMS report no. 20. Arch Ophthalmol 2003;121:1156–62.
2. Chang AE, Karnell LH, Menck HR. The National Cancer Data Base report on cutaneous and noncutaneous melanoma: a summary of 84,836 cases from the past decade. The American College of Surgeons Commission on Cancer and the American Cancer Society. Cancer 1998;83:1664–78.
3. Singh AD, Turell ME, Topham AK. Uveal melanoma: trends in incidence, treatment, and survival. Ophthalmology 2011;118:1881–5.
4. Birdsell JM, Gunther BK, Boyd TA, et al. Ocular melanoma: a population-based study. Can J Ophthalmol 1980;15:9–12.
5. Osterlind A. Trends in incidence of ocular malignant melanoma in Denmark 1943-1982. Int J Cancer 1987;40:161–4.
6. Teikari JM, Raivio I. Incidence of choroidal malignant melanoma in Finland in the years 1973-1980. Acta Ophthalmol (Copenh) 1985;63:661–5.
7. Iscovich J, Ackerman C, Andreev H, et al. An epidemiological study of posterior uveal melanoma in Israel, 1961-1989. Int J Cancer 1995;61:291–5.
8. Mork T. Malignant neoplasms of the eye in Norway. Incidence, treatment and prognosis. Acta Ophthalmol (Copenh) 1961;39:824–31.
9. Koomen ER, de Vries E, van Kempen LC, et al. Epidemiology of extracutaneous melanoma in the Netherlands. Cancer Epidemiol Biomarkers Prev 2010;19:1453–9.
10. Virgili G, Gatta G, Ciccolallo L, et al. Incidence of uveal melanoma in Europe. Ophthalmology 2007;114:2309–15.
11. Shields CL, Kaliki S, Furuta M, et al. Clinical Spectrum and Prognosis of Uveal Melanoma Based on Age at Presentation in 8,033 Cases. Retina 2012;32(7):1363–72.
12. Singh AD, Shields CL, Shields JA, et al. Uveal melanoma in young patients. Arch Ophthalmol 2000;118:918–23.
13. Vavvas D, Kim I, Lane AM, et al. Posterior uveal melanoma in young patients treated with proton beam therapy. Retina 2010;30:1267–71.
14. Greer CH. Congenital melanoma of the anterior uvea. Arch Ophthalmol 1966;76:77–8.
15. Gragoudas E, Li W, Goitein M, et al. Evidence-based estimates of outcome in patients irradiated for intraocular melanoma. Arch Ophthalmol 2002;120:1665–71.
16. Diener-West M, Earle JD, Fine SL, et al. The COMS randomized trial of iodine 125 brachytherapy for choroidal melanoma, II: characteristics of patients enrolled and not enrolled. COMS Report No. 17. Arch Ophthalmol 2001;119:951–65.
17. The Collaborative Ocular Melanoma Study (COMS) randomized trial of pre-enucleation radiation of large choroidal melanoma I: characteristics of patients

enrolled and not enrolled. COMS report no. 9. Am J Ophthalmol 1998;125: 767–78.

18. Bergman L, Seregard S, Nilsson B, et al. Incidence of uveal melanoma in Sweden from 1960 to 1998. Invest Ophthalmol Vis Sci 2002;43:2579–83.

19. Hu DN, Yu GP, McCormick SA, et al. Population-based incidence of uveal melanoma in various races and ethnic groups. Am J Ophthalmol 2005;140:612–7.

20. Phillpotts BA, Sanders RJ, Shields JA, et al. Uveal melanomas in black patients: a case series and comparative review. J Natl Med Assoc 1995;87:709–14.

21. Margo CE, McLean IW. Malignant melanoma of the choroid and ciliary body in black patients. Arch Ophthalmol 1984;102:77–9.

22. Biswas J, Krishnakumar S, Shanmugam MP. Uveal melanoma in Asian Indians: a clinicopathological study. Arch Ophthalmol 2002;120:522–3.

23. Kuo PK, Puliafito CA, Wang KM, et al. Uveal melanoma in China. Int Ophthalmol Clin 1982;22:57–71.

24. Sakamoto T, Sakamoto M, Yoshikawa H, et al. Histologic findings and prognosis of uveal malignant melanoma in japanese patients. Am J Ophthalmol 1996;121: 276–83.

25. Seddon JM, Gragoudas ES, Glynn RJ, et al. Host factors, UV radiation, and risk of uveal melanoma. A case-control study. Arch Ophthalmol 1990;108:1274–80.

26. Weis E, Shah CP, Lajous M, et al. The association between host susceptibility factors and uveal melanoma: a meta-analysis. Arch Ophthalmol 2006;124:54–60.

27. Grob JJ, Gouvernet J, Aymar D, et al. Count of benign melanocytic nevi as a major indicator of risk for nonfamilial nodular and superficial spreading melanoma. Cancer 1990;66:387–95.

28. Ganley JP, Comstock GW. Benign nevi and malignant melanomas of the choroid. Am J Ophthalmol 1973;76:19–25.

29. Sumich P, Mitchell P, Wang JJ. Choroidal nevi in a white population: the Blue Mountains Eye Study. Arch Ophthalmol 1998;116:645–50.

30. Singh AD, Kalyani P, Topham A. Estimating the risk of malignant transformation of a choroidal nevus. Ophthalmology 2005;112:1784–9.

31. Singh AD, De Potter P, Fijal BA, et al. Lifetime prevalence of uveal melanoma in white patients with oculo(dermal) melanocytosis. Ophthalmology 1998;105: 195–8.

32. Gonder JR, Shields JA, Albert DM, et al. Uveal malignant melanoma associated with ocular and oculodermal melanocytosis. Ophthalmology 1982;89:953–60.

33. Smith JH, Padnick-Silver L, Newlin A, et al. Genetic study of familial uveal melanoma: association of uveal and cutaneous melanoma with cutaneous and ocular nevi. Ophthalmology 2007;114:774–9.

34. Young LH, Egan KM, Walsh SM, et al. Familial uveal melanoma. Am J Ophthalmol 1994;117:516–20.

35. Wiesner T, Obenauf AC, Murali R, et al. Germline mutations in BAP1 predispose to melanocytic tumors. Nat Genet 2011;43:1018–21.

36. Abdel-Rahman MH, Pilarski R, Cebulla CM, et al. Germline BAP1 mutation predisposes to uveal melanoma, lung adenocarcinoma, meningioma, and other cancers. J Med Genet 2011;48:856–9.

37. Njauw CN, Kim I, Piris A, et al. Germline BAP1 inactivation is preferentially associated with metastatic ocular melanoma and cutaneous-ocular melanoma families. PLoS One 2012;7:e35295.

38. Seddon JM, MacLaughlin DT, Albert DM, et al. Uveal melanomas presenting during pregnancy and the investigation of oestrogen receptors in melanomas. Br J Ophthalmol 1982;66:695–704.

39. Shields CL, Shields JA, Eagle RC Jr, et al. Uveal melanoma and pregnancy. A report of 16 cases. Ophthalmology 1991;98:1667–73.
40. Travis LB, Curtis RE, Boice JD Jr, et al. Second malignant neoplasms among long-term survivors of ovarian cancer. Cancer Res 1996;56:1564–70.
41. Turner BJ, Siatkowski RM, Augsburger JJ, et al. Other cancers in uveal melanoma patients and their families. Am J Ophthalmol 1989;107:601–8.
42. Li W, Judge H, Gragoudas ES, et al. Patterns of tumor initiation in choroidal melanoma. Cancer Res 2000;60:3757–60.
43. Schwartz LH, Ferrand R, Boelle PY, et al. Lack of correlation between the location of choroidal melanoma and ultraviolet-radiation dose distribution. Radiat Res 1997;147:451–6.
44. Tallberg T, Uusitalo R, Sarna S, et al. Improvement of the recurrence-free interval using biological adjuvant therapy in uveal melanoma. Anticancer Res 2000;20: 1969–75.
45. Egan KM, Gragoudas ES, Seddon JM, et al. Smoking and the risk of early metastases from uveal melanoma. Ophthalmology 1992;99:537–41.
46. Davies H, Bignell GR, Cox C, et al. Mutations of the BRAF gene in human cancer. Nature 2002;417:949–54.
47. Edmunds SC, Cree IA, Di Nicolantonio F, et al. Absence of BRAF gene mutations in uveal melanomas in contrast to cutaneous melanomas. Br J Cancer 2003;88: 1403–5.
48. Rimoldi D, Salvi S, Lienard D, et al. Lack of BRAF mutations in uveal melanoma. Cancer Res 2003;63:5712–5.
49. Weber A, Hengge UR, Urbanik D, et al. Absence of mutations of the BRAF gene and constitutive activation of extracellular-regulated kinase in malignant melanomas of the uvea. Lab Invest 2003;83:1771–6.
50. Van Raamsdonk CD, Griewank KG, Crosby MB, et al. Mutations in GNA11 in uveal melanoma. N Engl J Med 2010;363:2191–9.
51. Prescher G, Bornfeld N, Hirche H, et al. Prognostic implications of monosomy 3 in uveal melanoma. Lancet 1996;347:1222–5.
52. Scholes AG, Damato BE, Nunn J, et al. Monosomy 3 in uveal melanoma: correlation with clinical and histologic predictors of survival. Invest Ophthalmol Vis Sci 2003;44:1008–11.
53. Shields CL, Ganguly A, Bianciotto CG, et al. Prognosis of uveal melanoma in 500 cases using genetic testing of fine-needle aspiration biopsy specimens. Ophthalmology 2011;118:396–401.
54. Harbour JW, Onken MD, Roberson ED, et al. Frequent mutation of BAP1 in metastasizing uveal melanomas. Science 2010;330:1410–3.
55. Shields CL, Cater J, Shields JA, et al. Combination of clinical factors predictive of growth of small choroidal melanocytic tumors. Arch Ophthalmol 2000;118: 360–4.
56. Shields CL, Shields JA, Kiratli H, et al. Risk factors for growth and metastasis of small choroidal melanocytic lesions. Ophthalmology 1995;102:1351–61.
57. Augsburger JJ, Shields JA, Folberg R, et al. Fine needle aspiration biopsy in the diagnosis of intraocular cancer. Cytologic-histologic correlations. Ophthalmology 1985;92:39–49.
58. Diener-West M, Earle JD, Fine SL, et al. The COMS randomized trial of iodine 125 brachytherapy for choroidal melanoma, III: initial mortality findings. COMS Report No. 18. Arch Ophthalmol 2001;119:969–82.
59. Jampol LM, Moy CS, Murray TG, et al. The COMS randomized trial of iodine 125 brachytherapy for choroidal melanoma: IV. Local treatment failure and

enucleation in the first 5 years after brachytherapy. COMS report no. 19. Ophthalmology 2002;109:2197–206.

60. Melia BM, Abramson DH, Albert DM, et al. Collaborative ocular melanoma study (COMS) randomized trial of I-125 brachytherapy for medium choroidal melanoma. I. Visual acuity after 3 years COMS report no. 16. Ophthalmology 2001; 108:348–66.

61. The COMS randomized trial of iodine 125 brachytherapy for choroidal melanoma: V. Twelve-year mortality rates and prognostic factors: COMS report No. 28. Arch Ophthalmol 2006;124:1684–93.

62. Shields CL, Shields JA, Gunduz K, et al. Radiation therapy for uveal malignant melanoma. Ophthalmic Surg Lasers 1998;29:397–409.

63. Gragoudas ES, Seddon J, Goitein M, et al. Current results of proton beam irradiation of uveal melanomas. Ophthalmology 1985;92:284–91.

64. Char DH, Saunders W, Castro JR, et al. Helium ion therapy for choroidal melanoma. Ophthalmology 1983;90:1219–25.

65. Lane AM, Kim IK, Gragoudas ES. Proton irradiation for peripapillary and parapapillary melanomas. Arch Ophthalmol 2011;129:1127–30.

66. Modorati G, Miserocchi E, Galli L, et al. Gamma knife radiosurgery for uveal melanoma: 12 years of experience. Br J Ophthalmol 2009;93:40–4.

67. Mueller AJ, Talies S, Schaller UC, et al. Stereotactic radiosurgery of large uveal melanomas with the gamma-knife. Ophthalmology 2000;107:1381–7 [discussion: 7–8].

68. Wilkes SR, Gragoudas ES. Regression patterns of uveal melanomas after proton beam irradiation. Ophthalmology 1982;89:840–4.

69. Gragoudas E, Lane A, Collier J. Charged particle irradiation of uveal melanoma. In: Albert DM, Miller JW, Azar D, et al, editors. Albert & Jakobiec's principles & practice of ophthalmology. 3rd edition. New York: Saunders; 2008. p. 4887–98.

70. Dendale R, Lumbroso-Le Rouic L, Noel G, et al. Proton beam radiotherapy for uveal melanoma: results of Curie Institut-Orsay proton therapy center (ICPO). Int J Radiat Oncol Biol Phys 2006;65:780–7.

71. Egger E, Schalenbourg A, Zografos L, et al. Maximizing local tumor control and survival after proton beam radiotherapy of uveal melanoma. Int J Radiat Oncol Biol Phys 2001;51:138–47.

72. Gragoudas ES, Egan KM, Seddon JM, et al. Intraocular recurrence of uveal melanoma after proton beam irradiation. Ophthalmology 1992;99:760–6.

73. Kodjikian L, Roy P, Rouberol F, et al. Survival after proton-beam irradiation of uveal melanomas. Am J Ophthalmol 2004;137:1002–10.

74. Char DH, Quivey JM, Castro JR, et al. Helium ions versus iodine 125 brachytherapy in the management of uveal melanoma. A prospective, randomized, dynamically balanced trial. Ophthalmology 1993;100:1547–54.

75. Boldt HC, Melia BM, Liu JC, et al. I-125 brachytherapy for choroidal melanoma photographic and angiographic abnormalities: the Collaborative Ocular Melanoma Study: COMS Report No. 30. Ophthalmology 2009;116:106–15.e1.

76. Gunduz K, Shields CL, Shields JA, et al. Radiation retinopathy following plaque radiotherapy for posterior uveal melanoma. Arch Ophthalmol 1999;117:609–14.

77. Gragoudas ES, Marie Lane A. Uveal melanoma: proton beam irradiation. Ophthalmol Clin North Am 2005;18:111–8, ix.

78. Gragoudas ES, Li W, Lane AM, et al. Risk factors for radiation maculopathy and papillopathy after intraocular irradiation. Ophthalmology 1999;106:1571–7 [discussion: 7–8].

79. Kinyoun JL, Lawrence BS, Barlow WE. Proliferative radiation retinopathy. Arch Ophthalmol 1996;114:1097–100.
80. Horgan N, Shields CL, Mashayekhi A, et al. Periocular triamcinolone for prevention of macular edema after plaque radiotherapy of uveal melanoma: a randomized controlled trial. Ophthalmology 2009;116:1383–90.
81. Shields CL, Demirci H, Dai V, et al. Intravitreal triamcinolone acetonide for radiation maculopathy after plaque radiotherapy for choroidal melanoma. Retina 2005;25:868–74.
82. Mason JO 3rd, Albert MA Jr, Persaud TO, et al. Intravitreal bevacizumab treatment for radiation macular edema after plaque radiotherapy for choroidal melanoma. Retina 2007;27:903–7.
83. Bakri SJ, Beer PM. Photodynamic therapy for maculopathy due to radiation retinopathy. Eye (Lond) 2005;19:795–9.
84. Finger PT, Chin KJ. Antivascular endothelial growth factor bevacizumab for radiation optic neuropathy: secondary to plaque radiotherapy. Int J Radiat Oncol Biol Phys 2012;82:789–98.
85. Lessell S. Friendly fire: neurogenic visual loss from radiation therapy. J Neuroophthalmol 2004;24:243–50.
86. Kim IK, Lane AM, Egan KM, et al. Natural history of radiation papillopathy after proton beam irradiation of parapapillary melanoma. Ophthalmology 2010;117: 1617–22.
87. Diener-West M, Reynolds SM, Agugliaro DJ, et al. Development of metastatic disease after enrollment in the COMS trials for treatment of choroidal melanoma: Collaborative Ocular Melanoma Study Group Report No. 26. Arch Ophthalmol 2005;123:1639–43.
88. Gragoudas ES, Egan KM, Seddon JM, et al. Survival of patients with metastases from uveal melanoma. Ophthalmology 1991;98:383–9 [discussion: 90].
89. Coupland SE, Campbell I, Damato B. Routes of extraocular extension of uveal melanoma: risk factors and influence on survival probability. Ophthalmology 2008;115:1778–85.
90. Shields CL, Shields JA, Materin M, et al. Iris melanoma: risk factors for metastasis in 169 consecutive patients. Ophthalmology 2001;108:172–8.
91. AJCC cancer staging handbook from the AJCC cancer staging manual. 7th edition. New York: Springer; 2010. p. 611–22.
92. Onken MD, Worley LA, Char DH, et al. Collaborative ocular oncology group report number 1: prospective validation of a multi-gene prognostic assay in uveal melanoma. Ophthalmology 2012;119(8):1596–603.
93. Onken MD, Worley LA, Tuscan MD, et al. An accurate, clinically feasible multi-gene expression assay for predicting metastasis in uveal melanoma. J Mol Diagn 2010;12:461–8.
94. Albert DM, Ryan LM, Borden EC. Metastatic ocular and cutaneous melanoma: a comparison of patient characteristics and prognosis. Arch Ophthalmol 1996;114:107–8.
95. Aoyama T, Mastrangelo MJ, Berd D, et al. Protracted survival after resection of metastatic uveal melanoma. Cancer 2000;89:1561–8.
96. Kodjikian L, Grange JD, Rivoire M. Prolonged survival after resection of liver metastases from uveal melanoma and intra-arterial chemotherapy. Graefes Arch Clin Exp Ophthalmol 2005;243:622–4.
97. Peters S, Voelter V, Zografos L, et al. Intra-arterial hepatic fotemustine for the treatment of liver metastases from uveal melanoma: experience in 101 patients. Ann Oncol 2006;17:578–83.

98. Voelter V, Schalenbourg A, Pampallona S, et al. Adjuvant intra-arterial hepatic fotemustine for high-risk uveal melanoma patients. Melanoma Res 2008;18: 220–4.

99. Kim IK, Lane AM, Gragoudas ES. Survival in patients with presymptomatic diagnosis of metastatic uveal melanoma. Arch Ophthalmol 2010;128:871–5.

100. Mortality in patients with small choroidal melanoma. COMS report no. 4. The Collaborative Ocular Melanoma Study Group. Arch Ophthalmol 1997;115: 886–93.

Esthesioneuroblastoma
A Contemporary Review of Diagnosis and Management

Matthew Bak, MD[a], Richard O. Wein, MD[b],*

KEYWORDS

- Esthesioneuroblastoma • Olfactory neuroblastoma • Craniofacial resection

KEY POINTS

- For selected presentations, endoscopy-assisted craniofacial resections and "endoscopic-only" resections have demonstrated success with long-term results comparable to those of conventional open craniofacial resection techniques.
- Most series advocate combined modality therapy (surgery and radiation therapy with or without chemotherapy) in the management of esthesioneuroblastoma (ENB).
- Neoadjuvant chemotherapy has been advocated for locally invasive and advanced staged ENBs and has demonstrated the capacity to significantly decrease gross tumor volume before definitive surgery and/or radiation.
- Elective management of the neck in patients with ENB remains a controversial topic. Early surgical salvage of patients with regional recurrence is possible in a portion of patients.
- ENB requires long-term follow-up (>10 years) given the extended time to local and regional recurrence.

INTRODUCTION

Esthesioneuroblastoma (ENB), also known as olfactory neuroblastoma, is an uncommon malignancy of the head and neck, representing only 3% to 6% of nasal cavity and sinonasal neoplasms.[1] First described by Berger, Luc, and Richard in 1924,[2] ENB is a tumor of neural crest origin that is considered to arise from the olfactory neuroepithelium of the olfactory cleft in the superior nasal cavity at the anterior skull base.[3] Local spread of tumor can extend throughout the paranasal sinuses and skull base with invasion of the orbit, cavernous sinus, and brain.

Several treatment approaches for ENB have been described in the literature, but rigorous, prospective treatment studies are absent given the tumor's rarity and pattern of recurrence that requires an extended posttreatment observation period. The

Conflict of Interest: Richard O. Wein, MD, FACS, Speaker's Bureau for Bristol Myers Squibb. Matthew Bak, MD - Nil.
[a] Eastern Virginia Medical School, 600 Gresham Drive Suite 1100, Norfolk, VA 23507, USA;
[b] Tufts Medical Center, 800 Washington Street, Box 850, Boston, MA 02111, USA
* Corresponding author.
E-mail address: rwein@tuftsmedicalcenter.org

behavior of the tumor varies from an indolent slow-growing neoplasm to that of a highly aggressive and locally invasive malignancy with a capacity for regional and distant metastases. Unfortunately, ENB is typically diagnosed after extensive local spread. However, the advances in surgical and radiation techniques and the use of novel chemotherapeutic approaches have lead to the development of an evolving array of encouraging treatment options reported on this diagnosis.

Traditionally, surgery using a craniofacial resection (with a transfacial approach and craniotomy) and adjuvant radiation therapy have been the mainstay of treatment of patients with resectable disease. Endoscopic resection has gained popularity for selected lesions and can spare some patients the morbidity of facial incisions and even craniotomy while remaining an oncologically sound operation. Neoadjuvant, concurrent, and adjuvant chemotherapy (single agent and combination) has been used in combination with surgery and radiation therapy to exploit ENBs' biologically similarity to other tumors of neural crest cell origin that are also chemosensitive.

This article will review the typical presentation, diagnostic assessment, and various treatment options that have been advocated for ENB, while illustrating the limitations of staging and the impact of long-term recurrence on advocated treatment strategies.

EPIDEMIOLOGY

ENBs represent only 0.3% of all upper aerodigestive tract malignancies and 3% to 6% of all sinonasal malignancies. A bimodal age distribution has classically been described for ENB, but recent Surveillance Epidemiology and End Results (SEER) data and meta-analyses support a unimodal age distribution with a reported mean age of presentation ranging from 45 to 56 years of age.[1,4–7]

Of note, approximately 7% to 20% of patients present at between 10 and 24 years of age.[1,5,6] The impact of age on prognosis is unclear, with one study showing no impact,[8] whereas univariate analyses in other studies suggest an impact on survival in patients diagnosed older than 65.[9] One study suggests that pediatric patients with ENB present with more aggressive local disease that typically requires combined modality care.[10] There is no defined cause and no sex or race predilection. There is no specific laterality that is more common in presentation.[5]

PATIENT EVALUATION
Clinical Presentation

Patients with ENB present with symptoms related to the local extension of their tumor. Initial symptoms are typically unilateral nasal obstruction (53%–100%), epistaxis (10%–52%), headache (10%–20%), and hyposomia/anosmia (6%–35%).[8,11–16] With extension of disease outside the nasal cavity and paranasal sinuses, symptoms of orbital and cranial involvement can manifest. Up to 20% of patients will present with orbital symptoms, including visual loss, diplopia, epiphora with nasolacrimal obstruction, and proptosis.[14] Headaches, nausea, and vomiting can be indicative of dural or intracranial involvement.[8] Rarely, patients will present with frontal lobe symptoms, seizures, or symptoms of syndrome of inappropriate antidiuretic hormone secretion.[12]

Advanced stage presentation is common because of the subtlety of the initial presenting symptoms, which may be initially mistaken as inflammatory or infectious sinonasal disease. The average reported delay between the appearance of first symptoms and diagnosis is 6 months[17]; however, the median time to diagnosis by radiographic imaging after onset of first symptoms was as long as 23.1 months in one study.[8]

A listing of differential diagnoses (clinical and histopathologic) for ENB is given in **Box 1.**

Box 1
Differential diagnosis for sinonasal pathologic conditions with a similar presentation (clinical and histopathologic) as ENB

Sinonasal undifferentiated carcinoma (SNUC)

Sinonasal squamous cell carcinoma

Neuroendocrine carcinoma (NEC)

Merkel cell carcinoma

Ewing's sarcoma

Metastatic pulmonary small cell NEC

Small cell lymphoma

Atypical extracranial meningioma

Rhabdomyosarcoma

Pituitary adenoma

Melanoma

Diagnosis

Clinical examination

Rigid nasal endoscopy often reveals a reddish gray pedunculated mass with a smooth surface that readily bleeds with manipulation (**Fig. 1**). Given the enhanced vascularity of ENBs, biopsy is typically performed in the operating room to control potential hemorrhage. Additionally, the tumor's close proximity to the orbit and anterior cranial fossa warrant obtaining imaging before endoscopic biopsy.

Most series report that less than 15% of individuals present with regional nodal metastasis at the time of initial evaluation.[5,11,17] Zafereo and colleagues[16] noted that 22% their patients were stage N+ at diagnosis. Office-based fine needle aspiration may assist in appropriate staging and establishing the need for treatment of the neck in these patients.

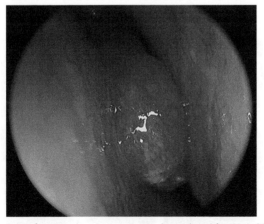

Fig. 1. Endoscopic view of ENB appearing as a vascular polypoid mass with irregular surface in the left nasal cavity between septum (*left*) and inferior turbinate (*right*).

Imaging

Initially, imaging is obtained to distinguish between inflammatory and neoplastic causes given a patient's symptoms and clinical examination findings. This is usually accomplished with a fine-cut computed tomography (CT) scan of the paranasal sinuses. If a neoplastic process is suspected, CT can be used to identify bony erosion of the cribriform plate and lamina papyracea, but magnetic resonance (MR) imaging is also needed for a thorough evaluation. On CT, ENB can display isodensity or slight hyperdensity with scattered necroses and marginal cysts.[18]

MR imaging is superior to CT scanning at delineating the extent of the tumor and distinguishing it from inspissated sinonasal secretions, which can have a significant impact on the surgical approach or treatment planning for radiation. Fine-cut cross-sectional imaging for coronal and sagittal reconstructions aid in identifying intracranial, orbital, and pterygopalatine fossa involvement. MR imaging is also superior at showing dural enhancement, perineural spread, and submucosal extension.[19] ENB is best evaluated with fat-suppressed, contrast-enhanced T1-weighted images and will be hypointense on T1-weighted images and have a heterogeneous hyperintensity on T2-weighted images with variable enhancement.[18]

Figs. 2–5 feature various levels of Kadish staging of ENB imaged with CT and MR imaging.

Intracalverial invasion is generally considered poor prognostic finding.[8] Using pretreatment CT and MR imaging, Yu and colleagues[18] classified direct intracranial extension in Kadish stage C ENB into 3 different categories based on extent of invasion. These patterns of invasion were cranio-orbital-nasal-communicating ENB, cranio-nasal-communicating ENB (most common), and orbital-nasal-communicating ENB. Response to therapy was not correlated to pattern of invasion in this series.

Clinical staging should be completed with a metastatic assessment for cases with advanced local disease or regional metastasis on presentation. In one meta-analysis, 1.5% of patients presented with distant metastases at initial diagnosis.[5] Wu and colleagues[20] showed ENB was positron-emission tomography (PET) positive in 7 of 9 patients (77.7%) with a maximal standard uptake value (SUV_{max}) of 6.37 ± 4.22 in primary tumors. Tracer uptake did not correlate with tumor size. PET/CT detected regional metastases in 2 (cervical and parapharyngeal) patients and distant metastases in 4 (lung, liver, and bone). PET/CT altered the clinical staging in 3 of the 9 patients. The use of pretreatment PET/CT has also been advocated by other authors.[21]

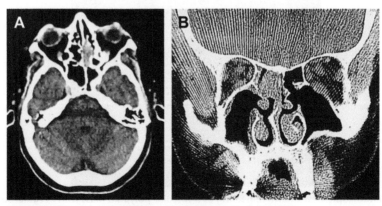

Fig. 2. CT axial (*A*) and coronal (*B*) cuts illustrating a Kadish A ENB.

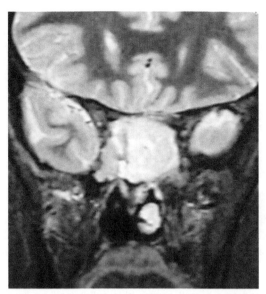

Fig. 3. MR imaging coronal cut illustrating the findings of a Kadish B ENB.

Pathologic Conditions

Olfactory epithelium contains 3 types of cells: basal, olfactory neurosensory, and sustentacular.[22] ENB is thought to arise from the mitotically active basal cells that give rise to neuronal and sustentacular cells.[22,23] Molecular studies have suggested ENB may be a member of the Ewing sarcoma/primitive neuroectodermal tumor group of tumors.[22,23]

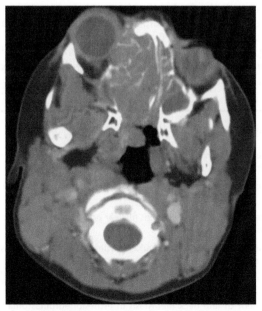

Fig. 4. CT axial cut of a Kadish C ENB presenting in a pediatric patient with regional metastatic lymphadenopathy with orbital extension of tumor.

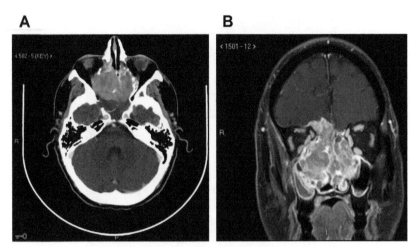

Fig. 5. CT axial (*A*) and MR imaging coronal (*B*) images of a Kadish C ENB with frontal lobe involvement.

ENB is categorized as a "small, round, blue cell tumor" on light microscopy. The cells can have indistinct cytoplasmic borders, hyperchromatic nuclei, infrequent mitoses, and rare nucleoli.[23] Additionally, ENB demonstrates a highly vascularized stroma that is infiltrated with nests of cells. Two types of rosettes are seen. Homer-Wright (HW) rosettes, also known as pseudorosettes, are present in approximately 30%–50% of cases. They are characterized by neurofibrillary and edematous stroma in the center of a cuffing arrangement of cells.[1,22] Flexner-Wintersteiner rosettes, also known as true rosettes, are seen in up to 5% of cases and distinguished by a tight annular arrangement with glandlike spaces.[22]

The extent of differentiation is classified by the Hyams grading system[24] based on histologic features including architecture, mitotic activity, nuclear pleomorphism, rosettes and necrosis (**Box 2**, **Figs. 6** and **7**).

The literature typically refers to ENB as low grade, consistent with Hyams grade 1 or 2, or high grade (grades 3 or 4). The diagnosis of a high-grade ENB has been shown to have a significant impact on survival.[9,25,26] In a retrospective review by Dias and

---

Box 2
Hyams' histopathologic grading

Grade 1 – Well differentiated with lobular preservation, prominent fibrillary matrix, no nuclear pleomorphism, Homer-Wright (HW) rosettes

Grade 2 – Low mitotic index, moderate nuclear polymorphism, fibrillary matrix present, HW rosettes

Grade 3 – Moderate mitotic index, prominent nuclear polymorphism, low fibrillary matrix, HW rosettes, rare necrosis

Grade 4 – High mitotic index, anaplasia, marked nuclear pleomorphism, absence of fibrillary matrix and HW rosettes, frequent necrosis

Data from Jiang GY, Li FC, Chen WK, et al. Therapy and prognosis of intracranial invasive olfactory neuroblastoma. Otolaryngol Head Neck Surg 2011;145(6):951–5; and Gore MR, Zanation AM. Salvage treatment of late neck metastasis in esthesioneuroblastoma. Arch Otolaryngol Head Neck Surg 2009;135(10):1030–4.

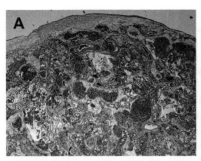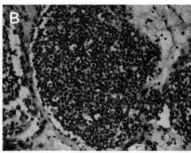

Fig. 6. Pathologic examination of a low-grade ENB. (*A*) Biopsy specimen with nasal mucosa noted on superior aspect, demonstrating lobular growth pattern with small hyperchromatic nuclei (hematoxylin and eosin, original magnification ×2). (*B*) Lobules featuring fibrillary matrix and lacking nuclear pleomorphism with focal cytoplasmic clearing (hematoxylin and eosin, original magnification ×20).

colleagues,[27] the 5-year disease-specific survival (DSS) for patients with low-grade tumors was 64%, whereas for patients with high-grade tumors it was 43%.

The importance of a patient's tumor histopathologic findings, as they relate to prognosis, vary among reports. Levine and colleagues[11] found no valuable pathologic or molecular indicators to predict aggressive clinical behavior in their series of patients. Morita and colleagues[28] examined the pathologic findings of 49 patients with ENB and noted the pathologic grade correlated with prognosis. Patients with low-grade lesions were able to undergo surgery alone if negative margins were obtained with resection. The authors advocated that patients with high-grade lesions be treated with surgery and postoperative radiation with a consideration for the inclusion of chemotherapy.

Care must be taken when interpreting older studies in which the histopathologic differentiation of similar yet distinctly unique sinonasal tumors, such as SNUC or neuroendocrine carcinoma (NEC), may have been combined under the diagnosis of ENB. Some authors have even suggested the seemingly dichotomous behavior of the tumor may be an indication of this problem. ENBs are typically considered low-grade tumors that respond well to treatment. However, when an ENB is considered a high-grade or anaplastic variant and actively progresses despite standard combined modality therapy, the potential for initial misdiagnosis should be considered.[9]

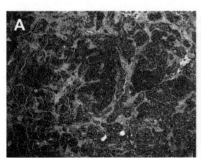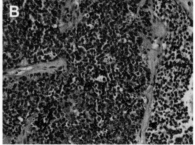

Fig. 7. Pathologic examination of a high-grade ENB. (*A*) Poorly defined lobules with hyperchromatic nuclei with absence of fibrillary matrix and Homer-Wright rosettes (hematoxylin and eosin, original magnification ×4). (*B*) Frequent mitosis, anaplasia, marked nuclear pleomorphism, absence of fibrillary matrix and Homer-Wright rosettes, frequent necrosis (hematoxylin and eosin, original magnification ×20).

Cohen and colleagues,[29] at MD Anderson Cancer Center (MDACC), reviewed the pathologic findings of 12 previously diagnosed cases of ENB and were able to confirm diagnosis in only 2. Misdiagnoses included 2 cases of melanoma, 3 cases of NEC, 3 cases of pituitary adenoma, and 2 cases of SNUC. The change in diagnosis would have lead to a significant alteration in the patient's original treatment plan in 8 of the 10 patients.

Immunohistochemistry demonstrates that greater than 90% of ENB cells are neuron-specific enolase positive. Approximately 80% of cases are positive for S-100, staining cell nests, and synaptophysin.[30] Cytokeratin AE1/AE3 and epithelial membrane antigen are typically negative with ENB.[18] SNUC demonstrates greater pleomorphism than ENB, may contain enlarged nucleoli, and is EMA positive and S-100 negative.[1]

Kim and colleagues[31] examined 17 ENB specimens for staining with bcl-2, p53, MIC-2, and N-myc. Of note, 70% of specimens were positive for bcl-2. All specimens were negative for N-myc. MIC-2 and p53 staining was noted in only one specimen. The results suggested a potential survival advantage and improved response to chemotherapy with bcl-2 positivity in patients with ENB, yet this finding was not statistically significant.

In patients with regional lymphadenopathy, fine needle aspiration can be considered a diagnostic aid. Mahooti and Wakely[1] reviewed 6 fine needle aspiration samples for cytopathologic features of ENB and noted specimens were typically nonspecific. However, if fibrillar neuropil was identified in the context of a patient with an established diagnosis of ENB, the confirmation of metastatic spread could be confirmed with cytometry. The histologic findings noted on aspirates can be mistaken for rhabdomyosarcoma, Ewing sarcoma, lymphoma, extracranial meningioma, poorly differentiated NEC, or pituitary adenoma.

Clinical Staging

There are 2 major clinical staging systems for ENB. The Kadish staging system,[32] originally reported in 1976 with the pretreatment assessment of 17 patients with ENB, has traditionally been the one most commonly reported. Proposed by Morita,[28] and later used by Jethanamest and colleagues,[5] a modification to the initial 3-tier Kadish staging system was created that included an additional stage for patients who had distant metastases at the time of diagnosis (stage D). Tumors are staged based on their anatomic involvement (**Box 3**).

The Kadish system has been shown to correlate with survival.[5,27,33–35] A criticism of the Kadish system is that it fails to completely stratify patients. Very few patients actually present at stage A and a wide spectrum of presentations can be grouped within stage C. Reports that were published before the addition of stage D with the modified

---

Box 3
Modified Kadish tumor staging

Stage A: Limited to the nasal cavity

Stage B: Involves the paranasal sinuses

Stage C: Extends outside the sinonasal cavity, including involvement of the base of skull, orbit and intracranial cavity

Stage D: Distant metastases at diagnosis

Data from Refs.[7,10,11]

system allowed patients with intracranial extension and distant metastases to be initially staged identically. An additional weakness cited in the Kadish system was that it did not allow for stratification of patients with pathologic adenopathy.[14]

It should be noted that radiologic staging and tumor grading are not directly related. In one report, only 14% of Kadish A tumors were low grade based on Hyams' grading.[9]

Dulguerov[17,36] proposed a TNM style of staging system for ENB that allowed for the inclusion of nodal status (**Box 4**). Some authors have commented that the Dulguerov classification more closely correlates with survival and recurrence.[14]

TREATMENT

The rarity of presentation and lack of controlled trials have resulted in a wide variation in the management of ENB. As a general rule, sinonasal malignancies are best managed with a multidisciplinary approach. There is a sufficient body of evidence to suggest that for advanced-stage ENB, such as Kadish C lesions, a combined modality approach improves disease free survival (DFS) and overall survival (OS) compared with surgery or radiation alone.

For Kadish A lesions, the consensus for treatment approach diverges significantly and monomodality care has been explored. Surgical management has evolved beyond open approaches to now include endoscopic management options. Radiation has expanded to include approaches that now use proton therapy. Controversy continues to exist relative to the role of chemotherapy, the most appropriate agents to use, and the timing of administration. The following section provides a review of the published literature as it applies to these various issues.

Surgical Management

Most of the literature examining the treatment of ENB consists of retrospective institutional reviews. Surgery, primarily using a craniofacial resection (CFR) approach, has been the traditional treatment modality in the initial care of these patients.[37] Exposure is obtained through a coronal scalp incision and bifrontal craniotomy (**Fig. 8**) from above and through a lateral rhinotomy facial incision with potential extension under the ipsilateral eyelid (Weber-Ferguson approach) from below. This approach can allow for excellent exposure and en bloc resection of the tumor (**Fig. 9**). Reconstruction typically involves placement of a pericranial flap to create a vascularized flap separation

---

Box 4
Dulguerov TNM staging

T1: limited to the sinonasal cavity excluding the sphenoid sinus

T2: involves the cribriform plate or sphenoid sinus

T3: involves the orbit or anterior cranial fossa without dural involvement

T4: tumors with intracranial involvement

N1: any lymph node metastasis

M1: any distant metastasis

Data from Jiang GY, Li FC, Chen WK, et al. Therapy and prognosis of intracranial invasive olfactory neuroblastoma. Otolaryngol Head Neck Surg 2011;145(6):951–5; and Zanation AM, Ferlito A, Rinaldo A, et al. When, how and why to treat in patients with esthesioneuroblastoma: a review. Eur Arch Otorhinolaryngol 2010;267(11):1667–71.

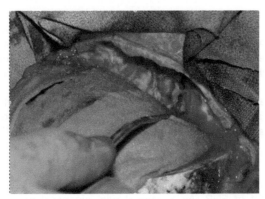

Fig. 8. Exposure to the site of the cribriform plate from a craniotomy approach before resection.

of the nasal cavity from the intracranial contents (**Fig. 10**). Criticisms of this approach include cosmesis-related concerns from the mid-facial incision and frontal lobe trauma from intraoperative retraction.

Shah and colleagues[38] reported on 23-year experience with the use of CFR at Memorial Sloan-Kettering Cancer Center in 115 consecutive patients for malignant tumors of the anterior skull base. The 5- and 10-year DSS rates for ENB (14/115) were 100%. The need for orbital exenteration was associated with a reduction in survival in the group overall. Absolute contraindications to CFR were considered involvement of the cavernous sinus and carotid artery.

Alternative open approaches include the transglabellar-subcranial approach and the transfrontal sinus approach. Pioneered by Raveh and associates in 1998, the sub-frontal approach provides wide exposure to the cribriform plate for en bloc resection but avoids facial incisions and lessens the need for frontal lobe retraction. This is accomplished by removing the nasal root and supraorbital rims with a bifrontal crani-otomy.[12] With this approach the clival-sphenoidal region can be viewed, allowing for potential optic nerve decompression and exposure to the medial aspect of each

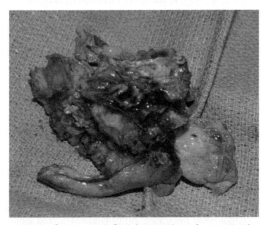

Fig. 9. Operative specimen from craniofacial resection demonstrating frontal lobe/dura resection with cribriform plate bisecting the midpoint of ENB and lateral paranasal sinus anatomy inferiorly (including lamina papyracea, septum, and middle turbinates).

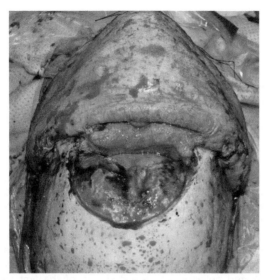

Fig. 10. Exposure from craniotomy approach (after removal of tumor) showing frontal lobe and superior orbital access after placement of a pericranial flap to reconstruct the resection site and separate the nasal and intracranial cavity.

cavernous sinus. In the report of their 13-year experience with the technique in 104 patients, 8 specifically for ENB, Raveh and colleagues[39] reported a low complication rate for cerebrospinal fluid (CSF) leak (2.9%), flap necrosis (1.9%), pneumocranium (1.9%), and epidural infection (1.9%).

Ward and colleagues[12] reported on the use of the subcranial approach in 15 patients with ENB (Kadish B, 13; C, 2). None of the patients experienced a decrease in the Karnovsky performance status after surgery. Median time to recurrence in the study was 82.1 months. Patients who underwent surgery alone had 5- and 15-year DFS rates of 26.7% and 0%, respectively. Individuals who underwent surgery and adjuvant radiation therapy had 5- and 15-year DFS rates of 83.3%. As a result, the authors concluded that low-grade disease and negative margins were not sufficient to warrant foregoing postoperative radiation therapy.

Kane and colleagues[9] performed a Kaplan-Meier analysis reviewing 205 published reports, which included 956 ENB patients, on the treatment outcomes. In contrast to the findings of other studies, no difference in survival was noted for patients who underwent surgery alone versus surgery and adjuvant radiation therapy at 5 (78% vs 75%) and 10 years (67% vs 61%) ($P = .3$). Univariate analysis demonstrated a negative impact on survival in patients who were Kadish stage C, Hyams grade 3 or 4 lesions, or older than 65 years. The authors concluded that unimodal and combined modality treatment options demonstrated equivalent survival. This finding was also noted with Kadish C and Hyams grade 2 to 4 tumors; however, consideration for the use of chemotherapy was advocated for patients with high-grade ENB. Of note, the median follow-up within the review was only 3 years.

Resto and colleagues[7] reported on 16 patients at Johns Hopkins Hospital during a 17-year period who underwent CFR as part of their treatment of ENB. Complete surgical resection was achieved in 62% patients. Adjuvant radiation was used in the setting of positive margins. In cases of complete resection with negative margins, 80% of patients demonstrated no evidence of disease at a mean follow-up of 5.6 years.

The transfrontal sinus approach, as described in 14 patients by Ducic,[40] is considered a minimally invasive modification of the subfrontal approach that eliminates the need for craniotomy and orbitonasal osteotomy. Patients with a well-pneumatized frontal sinus and limited superior and lateral extent of tumor are capable of complete resection of ENB and require a smaller scope of reconstruction. It also differs from the subfrontal approach in that it is not necessary to reestablish the nasal root position, address lacrimal drainage, and perform canthal repositioning.

Endoscopic Management

CFR has traditionally entailed a craniotomy (superior approach) with a transfacial incision (inferior approach) using a lateral rhinotomy. With the evolution of endoscopic sinus surgery, substitution of the lateral rhinotomy with an endoscopic approach for the inferior resection cuts has been a significant improvement in the traditional technique for appropriate cases. One of the earliest reports detaining this approach for ENB was in 1997.[34]

Endoscopic techniques have progressed to the use of purely endoscopic approaches for early-stage lesions with limited anterior skull base involvement. As experience has grown with tumor resection and dural repair, endoscopic skull base surgeons have become more aggressive with the purely endoscopic approach. In 1999, Stammberger and colleagues[41] reported one of the first series of patients, including 8 with ENB, to undergo endoscopic resection with no evidence of disease at a mean observation time of 37.2 months.

In a retrospective review from MDACC, Hanna and colleagues[42] reported on the endoscopic resection of sinonasal cancers from 1992 to 2007. Within the group, 93 patients underwent endoscope-only resection and 27 underwent an endoscope-assisted CFR. ENB was the primary diagnosis in 17% of the patients. Two-thirds of the patients who had an endoscope-only approach had stage T1 or T2 disease, whereas 95% in the endoscope-assisted group had advanced-stage tumors (T3 or T4). No survival difference was noted between the 2 groups. It was considered that acceptable outcomes were achieved with an endoscope-only approach for selected low-grade/early-stage malignancies with appropriate adjuvant therapy. Their indications for adjuvant radiation therapy were high-grade tumors, advanced T stage, bone invasion, perineural spread, intracranial extension, dural or brain involvement, or positive margins. For patients undergoing radiation, 90% were treated with intensity-modulated radiation therapy (IMRT) to optimize tumor dose and minimize toxicity to local structures.

Castelnuovo and colleagues[4] examined the use of endoscopic techniques in the treatment of ENB in a series of 10 patients of various staging (Kadish A, 3; B, 5; C, 2). En bloc excision was possible only for smaller lesions and piecemeal resection was required for larger tumors. Microscopic negative margins were obtained in all patients. Duraplasty was performed as needed dependent on the extent of resection. Most of the patients (9/10) underwent adjuvant radiation therapy. No recurrences were noted at a mean follow-up of 38.1 months. The authors advocated conversion to an open approach if a negative margin resection is not possible during an endoscopic approach and emphasized the importance of selection criteria.

Gallia and colleagues[21] reported on the use of a purely endoscopic approach in 8 patients with ENB at Johns Hopkins Hospital. Their technique uses 2 surgeons, an otolaryngologist and neurosurgeon, with a 3- and 4-handed technique. During the procedure, a lumbar drain is placed and a neuronavigation system is used. Resection involves initial debulking of tumor to gain access to the tumor margins, followed by maxillary antrostomies, ethmoidectomies, sphenoidotomies, and frontal sinusotomies. Next, septal transfixation incisions are made and the ventral skull base is exposed from the planum sphenoidale to the frontal sinus. With tumor resection, circumferential contiguous intraoperative margins are taken with the goal of obtaining negative margins. Reconstruction is performed with a nasal septal flap or dural/dermal inlay grafting. All patients in this series underwent postoperative radiation therapy and have demonstrated no evidence of disease with a mean follow-up of 27 months.

A meta-analysis reviewing the treatment options of 361 patients (from 1992 to 2008) demonstrated an equivalent survival rate for patients undergoing endoscopic surgery compared with those who had open CFR. Additionally, it was also noted that patients who underwent any surgery, as part of their care, experienced a significant benefit in disease-free outcome and survival compared with patients treated with nonsurgical modalities. The authors concluded that endoscope-only and endoscope-assisted surgery was a valid treatment method with comparable survival to open surgical techniques.[43] Criticisms of the study include that the analysis did not control for Kadish staging, limited follow-up (<5 years), and the bias inherent in retrospective reviews of institutional experiences.[3]

Contraindications to using an exclusively endoscopic approach include involvement of the facial soft tissues.[16] Relative contraindications include highly vascular tumors, the need for orbital exenteration, significant intracranial/intraparenchyma involvement, and lateral extension into the infratemporal fossa.[4,16,21] Complete surgical resection remains the expectation of the surgical procedure chosen and if not possible with endoscopic techniques should be considered a contraindication to using this approach.[3]

Complications from endoscopic resections are related to extent of tumor resection and the creation of a connection between the sinonasal cavity and intracranial contents. If an endoscopic dural resection is performed, failure to adequately reconstruct this defect can result in a CSF leak and potential meningitis. Folbe and colleagues[44] reported a CSF leak rate of 17% in their series of 23 patients. Other potential complications include frontal sinusitis, dacrocystitis, epistaxis, and chronic crusting from large areas of mucosal injury.

Randomized controlled clinical trials comparing the efficacy of CFR, endoscope-assisted, and purely endoscopic techniques are unlikely to ever occur. The ultimate goal of endoscopic resection remains the same as with open craniofacial resection: complete resection with a limited associated morbidity.[3] Independent of technique, negative margins should be pursued and abandoned only if critical neurovascular structures are involved, such as the optic nerves or the internal carotid artery. In an editorial on the topic endoscopic resection for ENB, Snyderman[45] advocated that until major skull base centers have treated adequate numbers with endoscopic technique with extended follow-up, open surgical procedures should remain the standard for care.

Combined Modality Therapy - Surgery and Radiation Therapy With or Without Chemotherapy

A common theme in the treatment of ENB is the importance of combined modality therapy. The way in which therapy is delivered may differ between institutions; however, the use of surgery in combination with radiation, with or without chemotherapy, remains the standard of care.[8,15,25,26,35,46–48]

Controversy does exist over the need for adjuvant radiation therapy for patients with Kadish stage A lesions that are resected with negative margins. Of interest, in the original report describing the staging that carries his name, Kadish advocated for adjuvant radiation therapy for stage A ENB secondary to concerns over local recurrence.[32] The use of adjuvant radiation to reduce the risk of local recurrence, independent of the margin status of resection, is a widely accepted concept.[33,46]

In a meta-analysis examining 26 studies (from 1990 to 2000) with 390 patients, Dulguerov and colleagues[8] attempted to assess for new developments in the treatment of ENB. The authors established that tumor stage (Kadish or Dulguerov), histopathologic grade (Hyams' classification), and treatment modality (surgery with or without adjuvant therapy) were important determinants of DFS. Five-year OS within the group was 45%. Based on the review of this group of patients, they concluded that surgery with adjuvant radiation therapy was the optimum treatment strategy for ENB.

In contrast, Platek and colleagues,[6] performing a SEER database review (from 1973 to 2006) of 511 patients with ENB came to a different conclusion. The 5-year OS for surgery with adjuvant radiation therapy, surgery alone, and radiation therapy alone were 73%, 68%, and 35% respectively (P<.01). At 10-years post-treatment, the authors concluded there was no significant improvement experienced in survival with the addition of radiation to surgery. A prior report by Jethananest also showed no benefit of adjuvant radiation therapy in OS.[5]

Despite this question of survival benefit with the routine use of adjuvant radiation, the practice standard of several institutions that have reported their retrospective experiences is to include adjuvant radiation or chemoradiation in their treatment algorithms.

Levine and colleagues[11] described the surgical management of 35 patients with ENB during a 21-year period. At diagnosis, 62.9% of patients had Kadish stage C disease and 6% presented with regional lymphadenopathy. Patients were treated with standard CFR and adjuvant radiation with or without chemotherapy (vincristine and etoposide). The local recurrence rate was 14.3% and occurred at an average of 6 years after diagnosis; 25.7% developed cervical metastases and the rate of distant metastatic spread was 11.4%. DFS was 80.4% at 8 years.

Dias and colleagues[27] reported on 36 patients with ENB in a 17-year review. Most patients were treated with surgery and adjuvant radiation or radiation alone. The rate of neck metastasis (early and late) was 14%. The authors noted that Kadish staging correlated with DFS and the development of regional or distant metastasis significantly affected prognosis. CFR with adjuvant radiation therapy was associated with the best 5-year DFS (86%).

Diaz and colleagues,[33] reporting the 22-year experience at the MDACC, reviewed the treatment of 30 patients with ENB. In the group, 77% were treated with surgery and adjuvant radiation therapy. The 5- and 10-year OS rates were 89% and 81%, respectively. Relapse-free survival and OS in early-stage (Kadish A/B) lesions was 100%. All of the recurrences in the series occurred in Kadish C patients with a mean time to recurrence of 4.67 years. Salvage was considered successful in prolonging survival in this group. The authors advocated complete surgical resection with postoperative radiation therapy regardless of initial Kadish stage.

Smee and colleagues,[49] reviewing a group of 24 patients with ENB, attempted to use neoadjuvant chemotherapy to direct subsequent treatment. All newly diagnosed patients with surgically resectable disease underwent 2 to 4 cycles of cisplatin/etoposide (cisplatin 100 mg/m^2 day 1, etoposide 100 mg/m^2 days 1, 2, and 3 every 3 weeks) and were then reimaged and rebiopsied. If both parameters were negative, patients would proceed to radiotherapy as definitive local treatment. If either were positive, patients underwent surgery with adjuvant radiation therapy. Only 2 of the initial 6 patients were locally controlled with this approach and avoided surgery. As a result, the authors did not advocate this form of neoadjuvant chemoselection and believed surgery and adjuvant radiation was required to achieve the best local control.

Jiang and colleagues[8] reviewed the treatment of 25 patients with invasive intracranial ENB. The worse survival rates were seen in the subgroups of patients who did not undergo surgery. Without any treatment, no patient lived longer than 1 year. Patients treated with standard CFR (opposed to endoscopic resection) with postoperative radiation therapy (with or without chemotherapy) had the best prognosis, with OS rates of 100%, 88%, and 66% at 1, 3, and 5 years. In a review by Argiris and colleagues[26] of 16 patients, 50% of whom had brain involvement at diagnosis, similar findings and recommendations were made for combined modality treatment with complete surgical resection.

Gruber and colleagues[35] examined the use of radical radiation therapy (with dosing up to 73 Gy) in the primary treatment of ENB in 28 patients. The authors concluded that primary radiation could not replace surgery and recommended complete surgical resection, followed by high-dose radiation therapy (median dose, 60 Gy) and simultaneous chemotherapy. When surgery was included in care, patients experienced a significantly better local progression-free survival and DFS than did patients treated with radiation alone.

In one of the largest retrospective reviews, Ozsahin and colleagues[48] examined the outcomes of 77 patients with nonmetastatic ENB from the Rare Cancer Network. On univariate analysis, favorable prognostic factors included Kadish stage A/B, T1 to T3 tumors, N0 status, "curative surgery," negative or microscopic positive resection margins (R0/R1), and radiation dosing to 54 Gy or greater. Favorable prognostic factors on multivariate analysis included T1 to T3 tumors, N0 status, R0/R1 resection, and total radiation dose to 54 Gy or greater. Median follow-up was 72 months. For the entire group, the 5-year local-regional control was 62% and OS was 64%. The authors advocated combined modality treatment and suggest that novel chemotherapeutic strategies and alternative radiation dosing should be investigated in an attempt to improve local control.

Radiation Therapy

Monomodality "radiation-alone" protocols have generally been reserved for patients considered inappropriate for surgery or with selected small lesions below the cribriform plate (Kadish A). Meta-analysis and SEER data reviews have shown decreased survival in patients with ENB receiving monomodality radiation therapy compared with combined modality care.[6,17]

Radiation therapy used in combination with chemotherapy before surgical resection has been shown to be an effective adjunct in a combined modality care plan.[11] Preoperative radiation has advocated as a tool to aid in orbital preservation and decrease gross tumor volume with invasive tumors.[50,51] Adjuvant radiation can improve local control after surgery, decreasing local recurrence rates in one study from 71% to 17%, as well as decrease the risk of regional recurrence.[52] The timing of radiation, before or after surgery, does not seem to impact the benefit it offers to local disease control.[14]

Nichols and colleagues[13] reported on the use of proton beam radiation after CFR in 10 patients with ENB with predominantly Kadish stage C disease. With a median follow-up of 52.8 months, 5-year DFS and OS rates were 90% and 85.7%, respectively. Proton beam radiation was considered safe and effective with ENB and potentially less toxic than photon radiation because of the capacity to lower radiotoxicity to critical adjacent structures (brain, optic nerve, orbit).

In a more aggressive combination of proton therapy with neoadjuvant chemotherapy, Fitzek and colleagues reported on the multimodality treatment of malignant neuroendocrine tumors of the sinonasal tract using high-dose proton-photon radiotherapy. In this series of 19 patients, which included patients with ENB 9 and NEC 10, most tumors were Kadish stage C (15/19). Treatment included 2 cycles of cisplatin/etoposide followed by high-dose proton-photon radiotherapy to 69.2 cGy equivalents using 1.6–1.8 cobalt-Gray equivalents per fraction twice daily in a concomitant boost schedule. Responders (68%) received 2 additional adjuvant courses of chemotherapy. Nonresponders underwent surgery. The actuarial 5-year survival was 74%. The authors noted that secondary to the precision of the radiation delivered with stereotactic guidance, no radiation-induced visual loss was observed.[53]

Role of Chemotherapy

A definitive role for the use of chemotherapy in the treatment of ENB has not been explicitly defined, but there is an abundance of evidence to support its use in a multi-modality approach. Whether chemotherapy is best used as a neoadjuvant regimen or as an adjuvant treatment in combination with radiation remains a topic of debate. Chemotherapy has been generally accepted for patients with ENB with high-grade, recurrent, or unresectable disease.[12]

Some of the most cited evidence for the use of chemotherapy in the treatment of ENB comes from the experience of University of Virginia Health System. Patients with Kadish stage A or B disease received preoperative radiation therapy, whereas patients with Kadish stage C disease (22/50) were treated with preoperative sequential chemoradiation. Surgery in both settings was standard CFR. The preoperative sequential chemotherapy involved 1 cycle of cyclophosphamide (650 mg/m^2) and vincristine (1.5 mg/m^2) with the addition of doxorubicin in a select group of patients. In patients who experienced a good response, a second cycle given. In the series overall, a 5- and 15-year DFS rate of 86.5% and 82.6%, respectively, was noted with a mean follow-up of 93 months. Recurrence occurred in 17 (34%) with a mean interval to recurrence of 6 years. In patients with a locoregional recurrence (12/17), 41% were capable of undergoing successful salvage surgery.[54]

The authors based their treatment regimen on a philosophy that ENB has biologic characteristics similar to those of other chemosensitive tumors of neural crest origin such as high-grade NEC and primitive neuroectodermal tumor.[50,54] A similar consideration led to the use of 2 neoadjuvant cycles of cisplatin (33 mg/m^2 daily) and etoposide (100 mg/m^2 daily) before definitive proton therapy (45 Gy during 5 weeks) for 9 patients with ENB and NEC by Bhattacharyya and colleagues[55] After treatment, 8 of 9 patients achieved a complete response and avoided surgical resection. In contrast, Smee and colleagues[49] described the unsuccessful use of neoadjuvant cisplatin/etoposide as a predictive tool for selecting nonsurgical candidates with ENB.

The combination of cisplatin and etoposide represents a popular regimen that has been successfully used in the neoadjuvant and adjuvant setting. A review from the Mayo Clinic, involving 12 patients with Kadish stage C high-grade ENB, examined the use of adjuvant cisplatin and etoposide after complete surgical resection. Six patients received adjuvant chemotherapy with radiation and 6 received only postoperative radiation. The addition of adjuvant chemotherapy improved median time to relapse from 10.5 to 35 months yet did not significantly affect OS.[56] Neoadjuvant cisplatin/etoposide, CFR, and adjuvant chemoradiation with IMRT have also been described with successful use in a Kadish C patient with frontal lobe invasion.[57] Use of neoadjuvant chemoradiation (with cisplatin/etoposide) demonstrated a complete pathologic response in 2 Kadish stage C patients who underwent subsequent CFR.[58]

Kim and colleagues[59] described the use of 4 cycles of neoadjuvant etoposide (75 mg/m^2), ifosfamide (1000 mg/m^2), and cisplatin (20 mg/m^2) (VIP) in 11 previously untreated patients with ENB. The induction regimen demonstrated a partial response in 64% of patients and complete responses in 18%. Radiation therapy was used in partial responders and surgery with radiation was offered for nonresponders. Other reports have failed to demonstrate a significant response to neoadjuvant use of the VIP regimen.[60]

Presentation of ENB in younger patients is frequently associated with advanced-stage presentations and has provoked interest in chemotherapy-associated regimens in an attempt to potentially limit the extent of surgical intervention. Mishima and colleagues[61] reviewed the care of 12 treated patients with adolescent-onset ENB. Most patients enrolled had advanced-stage disease (Kadish staging A, 1; B, 1; C, 6; D, 4). Patients were treated with 2 cycles of chemotherapy (cyclophosphamide, doxorubicin, vincristine with continuous-infusion cisplatin, and etoposide), radiation therapy, and peripheral blood stem cell transplantation (PBSCT). A partial response was seen in 75% after induction chemotherapy and 50% experienced a complete response after radiation with or without PBSCT. All patients undergoing PBSCT experienced a CR.

Bisogno and colleagues[10] reported on the experience of 9 patients (age 0.9–18 years, median 9.9) who were identified by the Italian Association of Pediatric Hematology and Oncology registry. Local invasion was extensive at diagnosis in all patients. Complete surgical resection was considered challenging but the addition of chemotherapy (vincristine, doxorubicin, ifosfamide, actinomycin D or vincristine, doxorubicin, and cyclophosphamide alternated with the cisplatin-etoposide combination) and radiotherapy (48.5–60 Gy) enabled tumor control in 8 patients. With a median follow-up of 13.4 years (range 9.2–22.9), 7 patients were still alive.

Novel approaches have been described using various chemotherapeutic combinations with unique presentations and settings. Gupta and colleagues[62] reported a patient, incapable of obtaining CFR, in whom limited endoscopic excision was performed after 6 cycles of cisplatin, etoposide, and bleomycin and radiation therapy (56 Gy). The patient was free of recurrence at 5 years posttreatment.

Kiyota and colleagues[63] reported on 12 patients with advanced or metastatic ENB treated with irinotecan and docetaxol and radiation therapy (1 photon, 6 protons). The 7 patients with advanced locoregional disease treated with CRT had a 2-year survival of 100%. The authors noted that younger patients had a better response to therapy.

Management of the Neck

Cervical lymph node metastases are infrequent at presentation for patients diagnosed with ENB with reported rates between 5% and 10%.[11,17,52,64] The natural history of ENB requires long-term follow-up as many patients (18–33%) may subsequently develop regional lymph node metastases. Demiroz and colleagues[52] reported regional recurrence in 27% of their series with a median time to regional failure of 74 months. The lymphatic vessels of the lateral cribriform plate and anterior nasal cavity pass superficially to join the external nasal skin. Nodal metastases are found most commonly in level II, but metastases have also been seen in levels IB, III, and IV and in retropharyngeal nodes. Bilateral or contralateral spread is also common and should be considered during treatment planning.[52,54]

Patients who present with N+ disease have a clinically and statistically worse prognosis. Dulguerov and colleagues[17] noted that N+ patients (5%) at initial presentation were less likely to be treated successfully compared with patients with N0 disease (29% vs 64%). These findings were reinforced by Jethanamest showing only a 40% DSS at 5 years for patients with N+ disease, which was significantly less than that for patients with N0 disease.[5]

Monroe and colleagues[64] examined the rationale for elective neck radiation in ENB as regional failure correlates with prognosis for distant failure and DFS. In their study, 22 patients with ENB were treated, 2 had positive neck disease at presentation, and 11 of the remaining 20 underwent elective neck radiation. No patients developed regional disease after elective treatment; however, 4 of the remaining 9 who did not receive elective neck treatment developed regional disease. The authors suggest these findings justify elective regional nodal XRT in Kadish B and C patients.

Demiroz and colleagues[52] report regional failure in 27% of cases in their series with a median time to failure of 74 months. They use their data to support the consideration of elective treatment in the N0 neck. Of their 7 neck failures, only 3 could be salvaged. Salvage rates for isolated neck metastases range between 27% and 80%. Currently, there are no good data to show that elective neck treatment improves survival, and some authors argue that isolated, late neck recurrences are easily salvaged. Given the relatively high reported rates of late regional failures and limited morbidity-associated IMRT, elective neck radiation may warrant consideration in patients with high-grade Kadish C disease.

Management of Recurrence

Local recurrence of ENB can occur more than a decade after definitive treatment.[46,52,54] The rate of local recurrence depends on the primary treatment. Lund and colleagues[46] report a 17% local recurrence rate for all patients. A study from the University of Michigan showed 10 of 14 (71%) patients treated with surgery alone developed a local recurrence within 5 years, whereas 2 of 12 (17%) treated with surgery followed by radiation had local recurrences at 72 and 115 months.[52] Of the 12 patients with local recurrence 7 were capable of salvage treatment that included surgery. Success of salvage treatment of local disease depends on the extent of disease and location of recurrence. Careful follow-up examination with rigid nasal endoscopy is of great importance because early recurrences may be successfully treated by endoscopic resection.[46]

For intracranial recurrence, a report of an intracavitary chemotherapy wafer placed in the field of a recurrent ENB undergoing re-resection showed acceptable results. Gliadel is a biodegradable polymer of carmustine (BCNU) allowing for the controlled release and local delivery of the chemotherapeutic agent with minimal systemic side effects.[65]

Lymph node metastases are uncommon at presentation, but up to 27% of patients with ENB will develop neck disease. A meta-analysis reviewing 33 articles revealed 137 of 678 (20.2%) patients developed neck metastases and 79 (61.7%) of those were recurrences that presented 6 months or later after initial diagnosis. Salvage rate for these recurrences, defined by 1 year of DFS, was 31.2%. Combined therapy with surgery and radiation increased salvage rates compared with either treatment alone (OR 8.6 vs 3).[66] Additional reports confirm these findings in the setting of recurrence showing an advantage in DFS for combined modality therapy versus monomodality treatment.[67,68]

Distant metastasis occurs to brain, bone, lungs, viscera, trachea, and heart. Distant disease may develop in up to 10%. One study reported the development of distant metastases at a mean of 13.4 months after primary treatment.[54] Despite the poor prognosis of distant metastatic disease, when possible, salvage therapy can offer symptom palliation and extend overall survival.[54] Gabory and colleagues[15] reported that 3 of 28 patients developed distant metastases at 6-, 168-, and 243-month follow-up.

McElroy and colleagues[69] reviewed a series of 10 patients with recurrent ENB. Cisplatin-based chemotherapy was noted to be active in advanced high-grade ENB and was considered a reasonable choice for systemic therapy. Mean duration of regression was noted to be 9.3 months.

Complications

Treatment of ENB is not without significant procedure- and therapy-related morbidities. Complications, short and long term, vary with the therapeutic intervention used and are more likely when extensive local invasion is seen at initial presentation.

Levine and colleagues[11] reported a central nervous system complication rate of 25.7% (1 patient with elevated intracranial pressure, 2 with pneumocephalus, 5 with CSF leaks) in patients who underwent CFR. Orbital complications were encountered in 22.9% and included epiphora, radiation-associated cataracts, radiation keratopathy, and transient diplopia with cranial nerve IV dysfunction. Shah and colleagues[38] reported an operative mortality of 3.5% with 115 consecutive patients undergoing limited or extended CFR. The major complication rate was 35% (frontal bone osteomyelitis, local sepsis, delayed return of neurologic function, meningitis) and 4 patients died as a result of perioperative complications.

Kryzanski and colleagues[70] reported on 58 patients undergoing surgery for a midline anterior skull base lesions (including 4 ENB, 29 meningioma) that required a craniotomy or craniofacial approach. Most of the patients underwent a narrow 2-piece biorbitofrontal craniotomy. Dura was typically repaired before the nasal cavity was entered in an attempt to prevent infection. Their complication rates were 2% for CSF leak, 2% for meningitis, 3% for bone flap necrosis, and 3% for symptomatic pneumocephalus. No deaths occurred and no reoperations for CSF leak were necessary. There were no new permanent neurologic deficits experienced by patients beyond anosmia. The authors concluded that transcranial approaches for anterior skull base lesions can be associated with low complication rates.

Bisogno and colleagues reported on 9 pediatric patients (age 0.9–18 years, median 9.9) with ENB treated with neoadjuvant chemotherapy, surgery, and adjuvant chemoradiation therapy. Treatment-related complications included 4 patients with subsequent endocrinologic dysfunction (hypogonadism, hypothyroidism), and 4 patients experienced craniofacial growth impairments (hypoplasia).[10]

LONG-TERM RECOMMENDATIONS

Multiple authors have advocated extended follow-up because of the average time to recurrence. Follow-up for ENB patients that extends longer than 15 years after the completion of treatment is recommended.[11,14,15,17,28,33]

Routine clinical examination augmented with nasal endoscopy should be expected during reevaluation. Abnormal findings on clinical examination, including new-onset lymphadenopathy, should provoke a low threshold for biopsy. Follow-up imaging with contrast-enhanced MR imaging at 4-month intervals for the first 1 to 3 years, then every 6 months for 3 years, and followed by every 9 to 12 months thereafter has been advocated (**Fig. 11**A, B).[12,54]

A　　　**B**

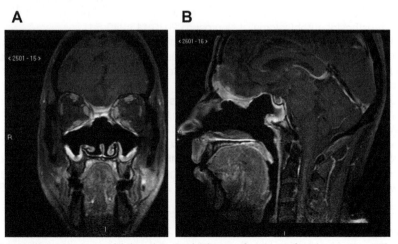

Fig. 11. MR imaging coronal (A) and sagittal (B) cuts after craniofacial resection with pericranial flap reconstruction for a Kadish C ENB.

SUMMARY

For selected presentation, endoscope-assisted craniofacial resections and "endo-scope-only" resections have demonstrated success with long-term results compa-rable to those of conventional open craniofacial resection techniques. Most series advocate combined modality therapy (surgery and radiation therapy with or without chemotherapy) in the management of ENB. Neoadjuvant chemotherapy has been advocated for locally invasive and advanced-staged ENBs and has demonstrated the capacity to significantly decrease gross tumor volume before definitive surgery and/or radiation. Elective management of the neck in patients with ENB remains a controversial topic. Early surgical salvage of patients with regional recurrence is possible in a portion of patients. ENB requires long-term follow-up (>10 years) given the extended time to local and regional recurrence.

REFERENCES

1. Mahooti S, Wakely PE. Cytopathologic features of olfactory neuroblastoma. Cancer 2006;108:86–92.
2. Berger L, Luc H, Richard R. L'esthesioneuro epitheliome olfactif. Bull Assoc Fr Etud Cancer 1924;13:410–20.
3. Soler ZM, Smith TL. Endoscopic versus open craniofacial resection of esthesio-neuroblastoma: what is the evidence? Laryngoscope 2012;122:244–5.
4. Castelnuovo PG, Delu G, Sberze F, et al. Esthesioneuroblastoma: endonasal endoscopic treatment. Skull Base 2006;16(1):25–9.
5. Jethananest D, Morris LG, Sikora AG, et al. Esthesioneuroblastoma: a population-based analysis of survival and prognostic factors. Arch Otolaryngol Head Neck Surg 2007;133:276–80.
6. Platek ME, Merzianu M, Mashtare TL, et al. Improved survival following surgery and radiation therapy for olfactory neuroblastoma: analysis of the SEER data-base. Radiat Oncol 2011;6:41.
7. Resto VA, Eisele DW, Forastiere A, et al. Esthesioneuroblastoma: the Johns Hopkins experience. Head Neck 2000;22:550–8.
8. Jiang GY, Li FC, Chen WK, et al. Therapy and prognosis of intracranial invasive olfactory neuroblastoma. Otolaryngol Head Neck Surg 2011;145(6):951–5.
9. Kane AJ, Sughrue ME, Rutkowski MJ, et al. Posttreatment prognosis of patients with esthesioneuroblastoma. J Neurosurg 2010;113:340–51.
10. Bisogno G, Soloni P, Conte M, et al. Esthesioneuroblastoma in pediatric and adolescent age. A report from the TREP project in cooperation with the Italian Neuroblastoma and Soft tissue sarcoma Committees. BMC Cancer 2012;12(1): 117 [Epub ahead of print].
11. Levine PA, Gallagher R, Cantrell RW. Esthesioneuroblastoma: reflections of a 21-year experience. Laryngoscope 1999;109:1539–43.
12. Ward PD, Heth JA, Thompson BG, et al. Esthesioneuroblastoma: results and outcomes of a single institution's experience. Skull Base 2009;19:133–40.
13. Nichols AC, Chan AW, Curry WT, et al. Esthesioneuroblastoma: the Massachu-setts Eye and Ear Infirmary and Massachusetts General Hospital experience with craniofacial resection, proton beam radiation, and chemotherapy. Skull Base 2008;18:327–37.
14. Bachar G, Goldstein DP, Shah M, et al. Esthesioneuroblastoma: the Princess Margaret Hospital experience. Head Neck 2008;30(12):1607–14.
15. Gabory L, Abdulkhaleq HM, Darrouzet V, et al. Long-term results of 28 esthesio-neuroblastomas managed over 35 years. Head Neck 2011;33:82–6.

16. Zafereo ME, Fakhi S, Prayson R, et al. Esthesioneuroblastoma: 25-year experience at a single institution. Otolaryngol Head Neck Surg 2008;138:452–8.
17. Dulguerov P, Allal AS, Calcaterra TC. Esthesioneuroblastoma: a meta-analysis and review. Lancet Oncol 2001;11:683–90.
18. Yu T, Xu YK, Li L, et al. Esthesioneuroblastoma methods of intracranial extension: CT and MR imaging findings. Neuroradiology 2009;51:841–50.
19. Madani G, Beale TJ, Lund VJ. Imaging of sinonasal tumors. Semin Ultrasound CT MR 2009;30:25–38.
20. Wu HB, Wang QS, Zhing JM, et al. Preliminary study of the evaluation of olfactory neuroblastoma using PET/CT. Clin Nucl Med 2011;36(10):894–8.
21. Gallia GL, Reh DD, Salmasi V, et al. Endonasal endoscopic resection of esthesioneuroblastoma: the Johns Hopkins Hospital experience and review of the literature. Neurosurg Rev 2011;34:465–75.
22. Thompson LD. Olfactory neuroblastoma. Head Neck Pathol 2009;3:252–9.
23. Richardson MS. Pathology of skull base tumors. Otolaryngol Clin North Am 2001; 34(6):1025–41.
24. Hyams VJ. Tumors of the upper respiratory tract and ear. In: Hyams V, Batsakis JG, Michaels L, editors. *Atlas of Tumor Pathology.* Washington (DC): Armed Forces Institute of Pathology; 1988. p. 240–8.
25. McLean JN, Nunley SR, Klass C, et al. Combined modality therapy of esthesioneuroblastoma. Otolaryngol Head Neck Surg 2007;136:998–1002.
26. Argiris A, Dutra J, Tseke P, et al. Esthesioneuroblastoma: the Northwestern experience. Laryngoscope 2003;113(1):155–60.
27. Dias FL, Sa GM, Lima RA, et al. Patterns of failure and outcome in esthesioneuroblastoma. Arch Otolaryngol Head Neck Surg 2003;129:1186–92.
28. Morita A, Ebersold MJ, Olsen KD, et al. Esthesioneuroblastoma: prognosis and management. Neurosurgery 1993;32(5):706–15.
29. Cohen ZR, Marmor R, Fuller GN, et al. Misdiagnosis of olfactory neuroblastoma. Neurosurg Focus 2002;12(5):1–6.
30. Patel SG, Singh B, Stambuk HE, et al. Craniofacial surgery for esthesioneuroblastoma: Report of an international collaborative study. J Neurol Surg B 2012;73: 208–20.
31. Kim JW, Kong IG, Lee CH, et al. Expression of Bcl-2 in olfactory neuroblastoma and its association with chemotherapy and survival. Otolaryngol Head Neck Surg 2008;139:708–12.
32. Kadish S, Goodman M, Wang CC. Olfactory neuroblastoma. A clinical analysis of 17 cases. Cancer 1976;37(3):1571–6.
33. Diaz EM Jr, Johnigan RH 3rd, Pero C, et al. Olfactory neuroblastoma: the 22-year experience at one comprehensive cancer center. Head Neck 2005;27(2):138–49.
34. Yuen AP, Fung CF, Hung KN. Endoscopic cranionasal resection of anterior skull base tumor. Am J Otolaryngol 1997;18:431–3.
35. Gruber G, Laedrach K, Baumert B, et al. Esthesioneuroblastoma: irradiation alone and surgery alone are not enough. Int J Radiat Oncol Biol Phys 2002; 54(2):486–91.
36. Dulguerov P, Calcaterra T. Esthesioneuroblastoma: the UCLA experience 1970–1990. Laryngoscope 1992;102:843–9.
37. Tufano RP, Mokadam NA, Montone KT, et al. Malignant tumors of the nose and paranasal sinuses: hospital of the University of Pennsylvania experience 1990-1997. Am J Rhinol 1999;13:117–23.
38. Shah JP, Kraus DH, Bilsky MH, et al. Craniofacial resection for malignant tumors involving the anterior skull base. Arch Otolaryngol 1997;123:1312–7.

39. Raveh J, Turk JB, Ladrach K, et al. Extended anterior subcranial approach for skull base tumors: long-term results. J Neurosurg 1995;82:1002–10.
40. Ducic Y, Coimbra C. Minimally invasive transfrontal sinus approach to resection of large tumors of the subfrontal skull base. Laryngoscope 2011;121:2290–4.
41. Stammberger H, Anderhuber W, Walch C, et al. Possibilities and limitations of endoscopic management of nasal and paranasal sinus malignancies. Acta Otorhinolaryngol Belg 1999;53:199–205.
42. Hanna E, DeMonte F, Ibrahim S, et al. Endoscopic resection of sinonasal cancers with and without craniotomy. Arch Otolaryngol Head Neck Surg 2009;135(12):1219–24.
43. Devaiah AK, Andreoli MT. Treatment of esthesioneuroblastoma: a 16-yr meta-analysis of 361 patients. Laryngoscope 2009;199:1412–6.
44. Folbe A, Herzallah I, Duvvuri U, et al. Endoscopic endonasal resection of esthesioneuroblastoma: a multicenter study. Am J Rhinol Allergy 2009;23:91–4.
45. Snyderman CH, Gardner PA. "How much is enough?" endonasal surgery for olfactory neuroblastoma. Skull Base 2010;20(5):309–10.
46. Lund VJ, Howard D, Wei W, et al. Olfactory neuroblastoma: past present and future? Laryngoscope 2003;113(3):502–7.
47. Kim HJ, Kim CH, Lee BJ, et al. Surgical treatment versus concurrent chemoradiotherapy as an initial treatment modality in advanced olfactory neuroblastoma. Auris Nasus Larynx 2007;34:493–8.
48. Ozsahin M, Gruber G, Olszyk O, et al. Outcome and prognostic factors in olfactory neuroblastoma: a rare cancer network study. Int j Radiat Oncol Biol Phys 2010;78(4):992–7.
49. Smee RI, Broadley K, Williams JR, et al. Retained role of surgery for olfactory neuroblastoma. Head Neck 2011;33:1486–92.
50. Oskouian RJ Jr, Jane Sr JA, Dumont AS, et al. Esthesioneuroblastoma: clinical presentation, radiological and pathological features, treatment, review of the literature and the University of Virginia experience. Neurosurg Focus 2002;12(5):1–9.
51. Polin RS, Sheehan JP, Chenelle AG, et al. The role of preoperative adjuvant treatment in the management of esthesioneuroblastoma: the University of Virginia experience. Neurosurgery 1988;42(5):1029–37.
52. Demiroz C, Gutfeld O, Aboziada M, et al. Esthesioneuroblastoma: is there a need for elective neck dissection? Int J Radiat Oncol Biol Phys 2011;81(4):e255–61 [Epub 2011 Jun 15].
53. Fitzek MM, Thornton AF, Vavares M, et al. Neuroendocrine tumors of the sinonasal tract: results of a prospective study incorporating chemotherapy, surgery, and combined proton-photon radiotherapy. Cancer 2002;94:2623–34.
54. Loy AH, Reibel JF, Read PW, et al. Esthesioneuroblastoma: continued follow-up of a single institution's experience. Arch Otolaryngol Head Neck Surg 2006;132:134–8.
55. Bhattacharyya N, Thornton AF, Joseph MP, et al. Successful treatment of esthesioneuroblastoma and neuroendocrine carcinoma with combined chemotherapy and proton radiation. Arch Otolaryngol Head Neck Surg 1997;123:34–40.
56. Porter AB, Bernold DM, Giannini C, et al. Retrospective review of adjuvant chemotherapy for esthesioneuroblastoma. J Neurooncol 2008;90(2):201–4.
57. Aljumaily RM, Nystrom JS, Wein RO. Neoadjuvant chemotherapy in the setting of locally advanced olfactory neuroblastoma with intracranial extension. Rare Tumors 2011;3(1):e1.

58. Sohrabi S, Drabick JJ, Crist H, et al. Neoadjuvant concurrent chemoradiation for advanced esthesioneuroblastoma: a case series and review of the literature. J Clin Oncol 2011;29(13):e358–61 [Epub 2011 Jan 31].
59. Kim DW, Jo YH, Kim JH, et al. Neoadjuvant etoposide, ifosfamide, and cisplatin for the treatment of olfactory neuroblastoma. Cancer 2004;101(10):2257–60.
60. Simon JH, Zhen W, McCulloch TM, et al. Esthesioneuroblastoma: the University of Iowa experience 1978–1998. Laryngoscope 2001;111(3):488–93.
61. Mishima Y, Nagasaki E, Terui Y, et al. Combination chemotherapy (cyclophosphamide, doxorubicin, and vincristine with continuous-infusion cisplatin and etoposide) and radiotherapy with stem cell support can be beneficial for adolescents and adults with esthesioneuroblastoma. Cancer 2004;101:1437–44.
62. Gupta S, Husain N, Sundar S. Esthesioneuroblastoma chemotherapy and radiotherapy for extensive disease: a case report. World J Surg Oncol 2011;9:118.
63. Kiyota N, Tahara M, Fujii S, et al. Nonplatinum-based chemotherapy with irinotecan plus docetaxel for advanced or metastatic olfactory neuroblastoma. Cancer 2008;112:885–91.
64. Monroe AT, Hinerman RW, Amdur RJ, et al. Radiation therapy for esthesioneuroblastoma: rationale for elective neck irradiation. Head Neck 2003;25:529–34.
65. Park MC, Weaver CE, Donahue JE, et al. Intracavitary chemotherapy (Gliadel) for recurrent esthesioneuroblastoma: case report and review of the literature. J Neurooncol 2006;77:47–51.
66. Gore MR, Zanation AM. Salvage treatment of late neck metastasis in esthesioneuroblastoma. Arch Otolaryngol Head Neck Surg 2009;135(10):1030–4.
67. Zanation AM, Ferlito A, Rinaldo A, et al. When, how and why to treat in patients with esthesioneuroblastoma: a review. Eur Arch Otorhinolaryngol 2010;267(11): 1667–71.
68. Kim HJ, Cho HJ, Kim KS, et al. Results of salvage therapy after failure of initial treatment for advanced olfactory neuroblastoma. J Craniomaxillofac Surg 2008; 36(1):47–52.
69. McElroy EA Jr, Buckner JC, Lewis JE. Chemotherapy for advanced esthesioneuroblastoma: the Mayo Clinic experience. Neurosurgery 1998;42(5):1023–7.
70. Kryzanski JT, Annino DJ, Gopal H, et al. Low complication rates of cranial and craniofacial approaches to the midline anterior skull base lesions. Skull Base 2008;18(4):229–41.

Synovial Cell Sarcoma of the Larynx

Shruti Jayachandra, MBBS, BBioMedSc[a],
Ronald Y. Chin, Bsc(Med), MBBS, FRACS[b],*, Peter Walshe, FRCSI, ORL, MD[c]

KEYWORDS

- Synovial cell sarcoma • Ifosfamide • Larynx • Head neck

KEY POINTS

- Synovial sarcoma of the larynx represents a rare entity, with challenging diagnosis and management issues.
- A multidisciplinary therapeutic approach is essential for management of this malignancy.
- Long-term follow-up is essential to monitor for recurrence and improve disease-free survival.

INTRODUCTION

Synovial cell sarcomas are rare, aggressive, mesenchymal malignancies constituting a high-grade histologic variety of sarcomas. These tumors represent the fourth most common type of sarcoma after malignant fibrous histiocytomas, liposarcomas, and rhabdomyosarcomas.[1] Synovial cell sarcomas predominantly affect soft tissues of the extremities such as large joints, bursal structures, and tendon sheaths,[2] particularly in adolescents, among whom they account for 10% of all soft-tissue sarcomas.[3] This malignancy has preponderance in males with a male/female ratio of 1:2.[4] Approximately 3% of synovial cell sarcomas can also occur in the head and neck region, which is poor in synovioblastic tissue,[4] and fewer than 100 cases in this region have been described in the literature to date. It has been reported to occur in various sites within the head and neck, most commonly the hypopharynx.[5] Other sites include the oropharynx and soft tissues of the neck. However, synovial cell sarcomas of the larynx are extremely rare, with only a handful of cases reported to date.[6–14] As a result it is not often diagnosed until later in the course of the disease, which therefore affects management and prognosis. Being such a rare entity, the treatment of head and neck synovial cell sarcomas is not well researched and classified.

[a] Department of Otolaryngology Head and Neck Surgery, Nepean Hospital, Sydney, Australia; [b] Department of Otolaryngology Head and Neck Surgery, Nepean Hospital, The University of Sydney, Sydney, Australia; [c] Department of Otolaryngology Head and Neck Surgery, Beaumont Hospital, Royal College of Surgeons in Ireland, Dublin, Ireland
* Corresponding author.
E-mail address: drronaldchin@gmail.com

Hematol Oncol Clin N Am 26 (2012) 1209–1219
http://dx.doi.org/10.1016/j.hoc.2012.09.001
0889-8588/12/$ – see front matter © 2012 Elsevier Inc. All rights reserved.

EPIDEMIOLOGY

Synovial cell sarcoma is a rare malignancy with an incidence of 2.75 per 100,000.[15] The incidence in the head and neck is significantly lower, with approximately 80 cases of head and neck synovial sarcomas reported to date.[16] Laryngeal synovial cell sarcomas are extremely rare, with about 20 cases reported in the literature.[6–14,17–26]

Synovial cell sarcoma is primarily a malignancy affecting adults in the third to fifth decade of life. In the head and neck region, synovial cell sarcoma is noted to occur during this age range as well, although it can also occur outside of this range. Of the specific cases of laryngeal synovial cell sarcoma, the youngest known patient was 14[12] and the oldest 79 years old.[26] Furthermore, males are predisposed to this malignancy more than females, with a male/female ratio of 2:1.

ETIOLOGY

Synovial sarcomas are thought to arise from pluripotent mesenchymal cells that have the ability to differentiate into epithelial and mesenchymal lineages.[27] Despite the name, synovial cell sarcomas can arise from cells outside of the synovium as exemplified by synovial cell sarcomas arising in the parapharyngeal, hypopharyngeal, or laryngeal regions.[28]

The underlying defect in synovial cell sarcoma is primarily a specific chromosomal translocation t(X;18)(p11;q11). This translocation creates a so-called fusion gene *SYT-SSX1*, *SYT-SSX2*, or *SYT-SSX4*.[1] The SYT component arises from chromosome 18 and the SSX gene arises from chromosome X.

PATHOGENESIS

The pathogenesis of this tumor involves the creation of aberrant transcriptional regulators resulting in the inhibition of tumor suppressor genes or the activation of proto-oncogenes. The SYT component (chromosome 18) fuses with homologous genes at Xp11 with 1 of 3 sites: SSX1, SSX2, or SSX4.[1] Monophasic tumors may have any of the transcripts, but biphasic tumors predominantly express the SYT-SSX1 transcript.

PATHOLOGIC FINDINGS
Macroscopic Pathology

On gross appearance, no distinguishing characteristics have been described for synovial cell sarcomas. The tumors may have a gray-white almost ivory appearance with an oleaginous texture on palpation. In the head and neck, synovial cell sarcomas most commonly occur in the hypopharynx and very rarely in the larynx. Laryngeal synovial cell sarcomas have been known to occur in the supraglottis, glottis, and subglottis.[10,11,14] Macroscopically, synovial cell sarcomas may have a cystic, solid, or necrotic appearance.[29] In the upper airways, these cancers may appear as exophytic lesions with superficial ulceration.[25] **Fig. 1** depicts the gross appearance of a laryngeal synovial cell sarcoma encountered by the authors.

Histopathology

Up to 3 subtypes of synovial cell sarcomas have been described in the literature: monophasic, biphasic, and poorly differentiated.

The monophasic and biphasic subtypes are the 2 main histologic subtypes of synovial cell sarcomas. Histologically both subtypes have proliferating spindle cells and branching, dilated, thin-walled blood vessels (hemangiopericytomatous pattern)

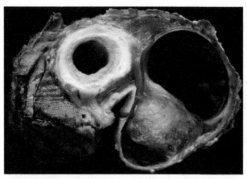

Fig. 1. Gross appearance of a laryngeal synovial cell sarcoma: a tan-pink colored, solid, well-circumscribed, smooth mass in the larynx.

within a heterogeneous collagenous stroma.[29] Tumor necrosis, cystic changes, and calcification are other features recognized in synovial cell sarcomas.[28]

The monophasic subtypes usually contain only spindle cells with a high nuclear to cytoplasm ratio, and tend to grow in a fascicular pattern. Alternatively, although this subtype does not have the tendency to develop epithelial-like cells, it may occasionally develop with solely an epithelioid component.[29,30] Owing to its appearance, this subtype poses a diagnostic problem and can be misdiagnosed as a spindle cell sarcoma or a hemangiopericytoma.[5,13]

The biphasic subtype varies, and contains glandular structures in addition to all the other histologic features.[3] Furthermore, it contains clustering epithelioid structures intermixed with spindle cells, giving it a biphasic appearance microscopically. **Figs. 2**A, B and **3** depict a biphasic laryngeal synovial cell sarcoma. Gland formation can be identified using reticulin staining and immunohistochemistry.

The third and more recently identified form is the poorly differentiated synovial sarcoma.[28] This subtype is composed of uniform, densely packed, small cells. Poorly differentiated synovial sarcoma histology may be interspersed with other histologic subtypes, therefore posing a diagnostic dilemma.[31]

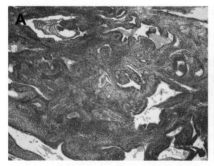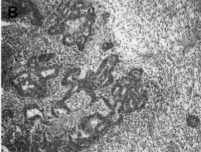

Fig. 2. (A) Low-power image depicting laryngeal synovial cell sarcoma consisting of both glandular components interspersed with spindle cell components, which is a histologic hallmark of diagnosis of the biphasic type of synovial cell sarcoma (hematoxylin and eosin [H&E] stain, original magnification ×40). (B) Medium-power image depicting biphasic synovial sarcoma with both glandular and spindle cell components (H&E stain, original magnification ×100).

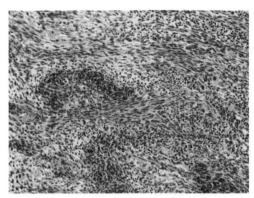

Fig. 3. Biphasic synovial cell sarcoma detailing the spindle cell component (H&E stain, original magnification ×200).

Molecular Pathology

Synovial cell sarcomas contain the (X; 18) (p11.2; q11.2) translocation, which is specific to this malignancy and is present in 99% of the cases. This translocation results in the fusion of SYT genes located on autosomal chromosome 18 with highly homologous SSX-1, SSX-2, and SSX-4 genes on the X chromosome.[1] Identification of this translocation plays an important role in diagnosing synovial cell sarcoma. The SYT-SSX-1 fusion gene occurs more commonly than the SYT-SSX-2 fusion gene, in a ratio of 3:2. The SYT-SSX4 combination is rare.[32] The SYT-SSX1 fusion gene is mainly found in the biphasic synovial cell sarcoma subtype, whereas monophasic and poorly differentiated forms contain a mixture of SYT-SSX1 and SYT-SSX-2 translocations.[33,34] Based on this observation, Eilber and Dry[28] suggest that SSX1 proteins promote epithelial cell differentiation whereas SSX2 proteins inhibit the same.

CLINICAL PRESENTATION

Synovial cell sarcomas tend to present with nonspecific symptoms and vary with location of the tumor.[25] Several studies have reported asymptomatic presentation of these cancers.[4,16,20] However, among symptomatic patients the most frequently reported symptoms include dysphagia, dyspnea, dysphonia, pain, and facial mass.[35]

DIAGNOSTIC WORKUP

Diagnosis of a suspected laryngeal synovial cell sarcoma involves obtaining a thorough history of presentation, clinical examination, and meticulous tumor staging. These investigations include radiologic imaging, biopsy of the lesion, immunohistochemistry to obtain a histologic diagnosis, and molecular testing.

Radiologic investigation of the suspected malignancy includes computed tomography (CT) and magnetic resonance imaging (MRI) to identify the exact size, location, and extent of the malignancy, as well as invasion of adjacent structures (**Figs. 4** and **5**).

A fine-needle aspiration (FNA) biopsy is considered suitable for diagnosing synovial cell sarcomas.[36] Features of malignancy such as high cellularity, poor degree of differentiation, high nucleus to cytoplasmic ratio, and high number of mitoses may be identified. The positive and negative predictive values of FNA biopsy in detecting malignant versus benign soft-tissue abnormality is high, with figures ranging between 85% and 100%.[37]

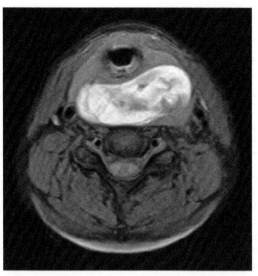

Fig. 4. Transverse-section magnetic resonance image of a biphasic laryngeal synovial cell sarcoma appearing as a mass with varying levels of attenuation.

Immunohistochemistry (IHC) is an important aspect in the diagnosis of laryngeal synovial cell sarcoma. These cancers express epithelial components such as cytokeratin and epithelial membrane antigen (EMA) as well as mesenchymal elements such as vimentin. This distinct immunophenotype noted in synovial cell sarcomas[3] is based on staining synovial sarcoma–specific markers within these cells such as CAM5.2, EMA, and pankeratin, which are particularly useful in the diagnosis of the epithelial component of the malignancy; CD 99, which is found in approximately two-thirds of synovial sarcomas; and S100, which although nonspecific for this cancer is found in approximately 40% of all cases.[28,38,39] **Fig. 6** depicts a laryngeal synovial cell sarcoma with positive staining of the glandular and stromal components with EMA.

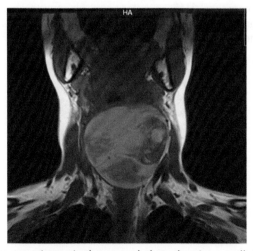

Fig. 5. Magnetic resonance image in the coronal plane showing a well-circumscribed round mass of varying density, depicting biphasic laryngeal synovial cell sarcoma.

Key Points: Diagnostic workup of laryngeal synovial cell sarcoma

- Radiological investigation with CT and MRI
- FNA biopsy of the suspicious lesion for cytology
- IHC to identify cellular components such as cytokeratin, EMA, vimentin
- Synovial sarcoma–specific markers include CAM 5.2, pankeratin, and CD 99, which are identified by IHC
- Molecular testing by FISH and real-time PCR to identify the synovial cell sarcoma–specific (X; 18) (p11.2; q11.2) translocation

---

Detection of the (X; 18) translocation on molecular testing is diagnostic of synovial cell sarcoma.[32,40] Molecular testing can be done via fluorescence in situ hybridization (FISH), real-time polymerase chain reaction (PCR), and cytogenetics.[40] The former 2 types of molecular testing are superior because they can be performed on specimens in formalin and the results may be obtained relatively quickly, in comparison with cytogenetic testing that requires cells in a fresh specimen to be cultured for weeks before results are obtained.[28]

STAGING

In general, staging of laryngeal cancers is based on initial workup beginning with laryngoscopy and biopsy, followed by a multidetector staging CT scan.[41] It may or may not be followed by an MRI of the larynx and neck to determine the most suitable management plan, and a positron emission tomography (PET) scan to detect malignant lymph nodes and distant metastases.

The Royal Marsden National Health Service Trust has identified tumor size as a useful staging feature and has developed a staging system based on it for synovial cell sarcomas.[42] In this system, low, intermediate, and high grades of synovial sarcomas have been described (**Table 1**). Similarly, the French Federation of Cancer Centers Sarcoma Group System has divided sarcomas into intermediate (Grade 2) and high-grade (Grade 3) sarcomas based on the mitotic count and tumor necrosis (expressed as a percentage).[43,44]

On the other hand, other groups such as Eilber and Dry[28] believe that synovial sarcomas are by definition high-grade sarcomas.

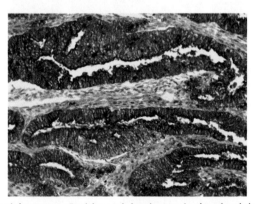

Fig. 6. Biphasic synovial sarcoma: Positive staining is seen in the glandular and stromal components with epithelial membrane antigen stain (original magnification ×200).

Table 1
The Royal Marsden National Health Service Trust staging system for synovial cell sarcomas

Stage	Grade
Stage IA	Low grade, <5 cm
Stage IB	Low grade, ≥5 cm to <10 cm; intermediate grade, <5 cm
Stage IIA	Low grade, ≥10 cm to <15 cm; intermediate grade, ≥5 cm to <10 cm; high grade, <5 cm
Stage IIB	Low grade, ≥15 cm; intermediate grade, ≥10 cm to <15 cm; high grade, ≥5 cm to <10 cm
Stage IIIA	Intermediate grade, ≥15 cm; high grade, ≥10 cm to <15 cm
Stage IIIB	High grade, ≥15 cm
Stage IVA	Any grade, any size, node metastases
Stage IVB	Any grade, any size, distant metastases IIA + B + C

It is apparent that a unified system for staging synovial sarcomas does not currently exist, and the authors recommend that all synovial sarcomas be treated as high-grade sarcomas for the present time.

PROGNOSTIC INDICATORS

Studies to date have revealed several prognostic indicators in synovial cell sarcoma of the head and neck, including patient's age, site and size of the malignancy greater than 5 cm, degree of necrosis, high level of mitotic activity, and neurovascular invasion.[25] Prognosis is worse and the likelihood of distant metastasis is high when the patient's age is older than 25 years, tumor size is larger than 5 cm, and the tumor has a high-grade histologic appearance with Ki-67 index over 10%.[25,45] In addition, a high Ki-67 proliferative index (>10%) implies the cancer is highly proliferative.[46] It is unclear whether the type of fusion genes and therefore the histologic subtype (STY-SSX1 vs STY-SSX2 translocations) affects prognosis in regard of having a more aggressive disease course. There is conflicting evidence in the literature, with some studies finding that the SYT-SSX1 biphasic subtype is associated with a poorer prognosis,[47] whereas others have not found an association between SYT-SSX translocation type and prognosis.[40]

MANAGEMENT
Surgery

Complete surgical resection with wide free margins and careful preservation of anatomic structures is considered the treatment of choice for synovial cell sarcoma of the head and neck, including the larynx, where a partial or total laryngectomy is indicated.[25] In the authors' experience, an appropriate margin may include a pharyngolaryngectomy with reconstruction. Complete surgical excisions with destruction of anatomic structures as indicated, as well as neoadjuvant chemotherapy are the mainstays of treatment for local, recurrent disease.[48] Surgery, however, is thought to have a limited role in metastatic disease.

The use of CO_2 lasers has been reported to be as effective as partial or total laryngectomy for the control of disease in localized synovial sarcomas. Disease-free survival periods of up to 3 years have been documented.[21,23] Laser therapy could thus potentially offer a less invasive approach for management of local disease in the future.

Key Points: Management of laryngeal synovial cell sarcoma

- Perform appropriate en bloc resection of all involved tumor with clear margins, which may involve laryngectomy/pharyngolaryngectomy/neck dissection with appropriate reconstruction.
- CO_2 lasers may offer an alternative to partial or total laryngectomy in future for excision of localized synovial cell sarcomas.
- Chemotherapy using ifosfamide ± other agents such as doxorubicin is mainly used as adjuvant or palliative therapy in treatment of these cancers.
- Adjuvant radiotherapy is used in local disease for tumors larger than 5 cm and in the postoperative period.
- Follow-up is recommended on a yearly basis for longer than 10 years to detect and treat late recurrences of the cancer.

Chemotherapy

The role of chemotherapy has traditionally been in the form of adjuvant treatment or when the tumors are larger than 5 cm. Chemotherapy is controversial, with several agents such as ifosfamide with or without liposomal daunorubicin, doxorubicin, and cyclophosphamide being used.[49,50] In addition, granulocyte colony–stimulating factor may be used for bone marrow stimulation. Recent studies have described the experimental use of a murine monoclonal antibody that targets the homologue FZD10, a surface receptor on synovial sarcoma cells.[51] Another experimental chemotherapeutic agent being researched is a peptide vaccine derived from SYT-SSX.[52]

In practical terms, however, chemotherapy may only be useful in the adjuvant or palliative setting, and no studies have shown a survival benefit from the use of chemotherapy.

Radiotherapy

Adjuvant radiotherapy is administered to all synovial sarcomas greater than 5 cm in size, as these are considered high-grade malignancies. Radiotherapy is reported to be of benefit in local disease management.[27] Postoperative adjuvant radiotherapy is found to be especially useful in the synovial sarcomas in the head and neck in comparison with other sites.[1,27]

Follow-Up

Synovial cell sarcomas are known to have a high rate of local recurrence and metastases 5 to 10 years after remission. Therefore, frequent follow-up for longer than 10 years is recommended, combined with patient education.[53] This approach would enable detection of cancer recurrence at a stage where they can still be treated.

SUMMARY

Synovial sarcoma of the larynx represents a rare entity, with challenging diagnosis and management issues. A multidisciplinary therapeutic approach is essential for the management of this malignancy, and long-term follow-up is essential to monitor for recurrence and improve disease-free survival.

REFERENCES

1. Rigante M, Visocchi M, Petrone G, et al. Synovial sarcoma of the parotid gland: a case report and review of the literature. Acta Otorhinolaryngol Ital 2011;31(1):43–6.

2. O'Sullivan PJ, Harris AC, Munk PL. Radiological features of synovial cell sarcoma. Br J Radiol 2008;81(964):346–56.
3. Dei Tos AP, Dal Cin P, Sciot R, et al. Synovial sarcoma of the larynx and hypopharynx. Ann Otol Rhinol Laryngol 1998;107:1080–5.
4. Amble FR, Olsen KD, Nascimento AG, et al. Head and neck synovial cell sarcoma. Otolaryngol Head Neck Surg 1992;107:631–7.
5. Carillo R, Rodriguez-Peralto JL, Bastakis JG. Synovial sarcoma of the head and neck. Ann Otol Rhinol Laryngol 1992;101:367–70.
6. Danninger R, Hurner U, Stammberger H. Das Synovialsarkom, einseltener Tumor des Larynx. Falldarstellung und differential diagnostische Überlegungen. Laryngorhinootologie 1994;73:442–4.
7. Ferlito A, Caruso G. Endolaryngeal synovial sarcoma: an update on diagnosis and treatment. ORL J Otorhinolaryngol Relat Spec 1991;53:116–9.
8. Gatti WM, Strom CG, Orfei E. Synovial sarcoma of the laryngopharynx. Arch Otolaryngol 1975;101:633–6.
9. Ianniello F, Ferri E, Armato E, et al. Carcinosarcoma of the larynx: immunohistochemical study, clinical considerations, therapeutic strategies. Acta Otorhinolaryngol Ital 2001;21:192–7 [in Italian].
10. Kitsmaniuk ZD, Volkov I, Demochko VB, et al. Synovial sarcoma of the larynx. Vestn Otorinolaringol 1985;2:61–2.
11. Miller LH, Santaella-Latimer L, Miller T. Synovial sarcoma of the larynx. Trans Sect Otolaryngol Am Acad Ophthalmol Otolaryngol 1975;80:448–51.
12. Morland B, Cox G, Randall C, et al. Synovial sarcoma of the larynx in a child: case report and histological appearances. Med Pediatr Oncol 1994;23:64–8.
13. Pruszczynski M, Manni JJ, Smedt F. Endolaryngeal synovial sarcoma: case report with immunohistochemical studies. Head Neck 1989;11:76–80.
14. Quinn HJ. Synovial sarcoma of the larynx treated by partial laryngectomy. Laryngoscope 1984;94:1158–61.
15. Deshmukh R, Mankin HJ, Singer S. Synovial sarcoma: the importance of size and location for survival. Clin Orthop Relat Res 2004;419:155–61.
16. Pai S, Chinoy RF, Pradhan SA, et al. Head and neck synovial sarcomas. J Surg Oncol 1993;54:82–6.
17. Bilgic B, Mete O, Ozturk AS, et al. Synovial sarcoma: a rare tumor of the larynx. Pathol Oncol Res 2003;9:242–5.
18. Jernstrom P. Synovial sarcoma of the pharynx; report of a case. Am J Clin Pathol 1954;24(8):957–61.
19. Pricolo V, Cenci N. Malignant synovioma of hypopharynx. Minerva Otorinolaringol 1957;7(4):218–22 [in Italian].
20. Shmookler BM, Enzinger FM, Brannon RB. Orofacial synovial sarcoma: a clinicopathologic study of 11 new cases and review of the literature. Cancer 1982;50: 269–76.
21. Papaspyrou S, Kyriakides G, Tapis M. Endoscopic CO_2 laser surgery for large synovial sarcoma of the larynx. Otolaryngol Head Neck Surg 2003;129(6):630–1.
22. Geahchan NE, Lambert J, Micheau C, et al. Malignant synovioma of the larynx. Ann Otolaryngol Chir Cervicofac 1983;100(1):61–5.
23. Boniver V, Moreau P, Lefebvre P. Synovial sarcoma of the larynx: case report and literature review. B-ENT 2005;1(1):47–51.
24. Mohr W, Pirsig W. Synovial sarcoma of the larynx. Case report and brief review of the literature. Laryngol Rhinol Otol (Stuttg) 1984;63(9):453–6 [in German].
25. Capelli M, Bertino G, Morbini P, et al. CO_2 laser in the treatment of laryngeal synovial sarcoma: a clinical case. Tumori 2007;93(3):296–9.

26. Mhawech-Fauceglia P, Ramzy P, Bshara W, et al. Synovial sarcoma of the larynx in a 79-year-old woman, confirmed by karyotyping and fluorescence in situ hybridization analysis. Ann Diagn Pathol 2007;11(3):223–7.

27. Leader M, Patel J, Collins M, et al. Synovial sarcomas. True carcinosarcomas? Cancer 1987;59(12):2096–8.

28. Eilber FC, Dry SM. Diagnosis and management of synovial sarcoma. J Surg Oncol 2008;97(4):314–20.

29. Kusuma S, Skarupa DJ, Ely KA, et al. Synovial sarcoma of the head and neck: a review of its diagnosis and management and a report of a rare case of orbital involvement. Ear Nose Throat J 2010;89(6):280–3.

30. Majeste RM, Beckman EN. Synovial sarcoma with an overwhelming epithelioid component. Cancer 1988;61:2527–31.

31. Fletcher CD, Unni KK, Mertens F, editors. Pathology and genetics of tumours of the soft tissues and bones. World Health Organization classification of tumours. Lyon (France): W.H. Organization; 2003.

32. dos Santos NR, de Bruijn DR, van Kessel AG. Molecular mechanisms underlying human synovial sarcoma development. Genes Chromosomes Cancer 2001;30: 1–14.

33. Antonescu CR, Kawai A, Leung DH, et al. Strong association of SYT-SSX fusion type and morphologic epithelial differentiation in synovial sarcoma. Diagn Mol Pathol 2000;9(1):1–8.

34. Yang K, Lui WO, Xie Y, et al. Co-existence of SYT-SSX1 and SYT-SSX2 fusions in synovial sarcomas. Oncogene 2002;21:4181–90.

35. Moore DM, Berke GS. Synovial sarcoma of the head and neck. Arch Otolaryngol Head Neck Surg 1987;113:311–3.

36. Ouansafi I, Klein M, Sugrue C, et al. Monophasic parapharyngeal synovial sarcoma diagnosed by cytology, immunocytochemistry, and molecular pathology: case report and review of the literature. Diagn Cytopathol 2010;38(11):822–7.

37. Ryan M. Cytology and mesenchymal pathology. How far will we go? Am J Clin Pathol 1996;106:561–4.

38. Heim-Hall J, Yohe SL. Application of immunohistochemistry to soft tissue neoplasms. Arch Pathol Lab Med 2008;132:476–89.

39. Akerman M, Willen H, Carlen B, et al. Fine needle aspiration (FNA) of synovial sarcoma a comparative histological-cytological study of 15 cases, including immunohisto-chemical, electron microscopic and cytogenetic examination and DNA-ploidy analysis. Cytopathology 1996;7:187–200.

40. Guillou L, Coindre JM, Gallagher G, et al. Detection of the synovial sarcoma translocation t(X;18) (SYT-SSX) in paraffin-embedded tissues using reverse transcriptase-polymerase chain reaction: a reliable and powerful diagnostic tool for pathologists—a molecular analysis of 221 mesenchymal tumors fixed in different fixatives. Hum Pathol 2001;32:105–12.

41. Curtin HD. Imaging of the larynx: current concepts. Radiology 1989;173:1–11.

42. Spillane AJ, A'Hern R, Judson IR, et al. Synovial sarcoma: a clinicopathologic, staging, and prognostic assessment. J Clin Oncol 2000;18:3794–803.

43. Guillou L, Coindre JM, Bonichon F, et al. Comparative study of the National Cancer Institute and French Federation of Cancer Centers Sarcoma Group grading systems in a population of 410patients with soft tissue sarcoma. J Clin Oncol 1997;15:350–62.

44. Hasegawa T, Yokoyama R, Matsuno Y, et al. Prognostic significance of histologic grade and nuclear expression of beta-catenin in synovial sarcoma. Hum Pathol 2001;32:257–63.

45. Kraus DH, Dubner S, Harrison LB, et al. Prognostic factors for recurrence and survival in head and neck soft tissue sarcomas. Cancer 1994;74:697–702.
46. Skytting BT, Bauer HC, Perfekt R, et al. Ki- 67 is strongly prognostic in synovial sarcoma: analysis based on 86 patients from the Scandinavian Sarcoma Group Register. Br J Cancer 1999;80:1809–14.
47. Kawai A, Naito N, Yoshida A, et al. Establishment and characterization of a biphasic synovial sarcoma cell line, SYO-1. Cancer Lett 2004;204(1):105–13.
48. Eilber FC, Brennan MF, Riedel E, et al. Prognostic factors for survival in patients with locally recurrent extremity soft tissue sarcomas. Ann Surg Oncol 2005;12: 228–36.
49. Ladenstein R, Treuner J, Koscielniak E, et al. Synovial sarcoma of childhood and adolescence. Report of the German CWS-81 study. Cancer 1993;71(11): 3647–55.
50. Siehl J, Thiel E, Schmittel A, et al. Ifosfamide/liposomal daunorubicin is a well tolerated and active first-line chemotherapy regimen in advanced soft tissue sarcoma cancer. Cancer 2005;104(3):611–7.
51. Fukukawa C, Hanaoka H, Nagayama S, et al. Radioimmunotherapy of human synovial sarcoma using a monoclonal antibody against FZD10. Cancer Sci 2008;99(2):432–40.
52. Kawaguchi S, Wada T, Ida K, et al. Phase I vaccination trial of SYT-SSX junction peptide in patients with disseminated synovial sarcoma. J Transl Med 2005;3:1.
53. Krieg1 AH, Hefti1 F, Speth BM, et al. Synovial sarcomas usually metastasize after >5 years: a multicenter retrospective analysis with minimum follow-up of 10 years for survivors. Ann Oncol 2011;22(2):458–67.

Parathyroid Carcinoma
Challenges in Diagnosis and Treatment

Arash Mohebati, MD, Ashok Shaha, MD, Jatin Shah, MD*

KEYWORDS

- Parathyroid carcinoma • Hypercalcemia • Hyperparathyroidism • Endocrine tumors

KEY POINTS

- Parathyroid carcinoma is a rare disease.
- Severe hypercalcemia, very high parathyroid hormone, and palpable mass are suspicious for parathyroid carcinoma.
- Intraoperative findings may reveal a hard and fixed mass adherent to the thyroid gland and occasionally lymph node suspicious for metastatic tumor.
- The pathologic diagnosis may be difficult, as atypical parathyroid adenoma may mimic carcinoma.
- The best treatment would be appropriate surgical resection with the ipsilateral thyroid node and excision of the lymph nodes if suspicious.
- Adjuvant therapy has very little impact but postoperative radiation therapy may be indicated in locally aggressive tumor or bulky nodal metastases.

INTRODUCTION

Parathyroid carcinoma is a rare endocrine neoplasm. Its incidence ranges from 0.5% to 5.0% of the cases with primary hyperparathyroidism.[1–3] Parathyroid carcinoma commonly has an indolent growth with a tendency for local invasion, and it occurs with equal frequency in men and women.[4,5] The age at presentation for parathyroid carcinoma compared with adenoma is reported to be a decade earlier.[6] It was first described by the Swiss surgeon Fritz De Quervain.[7] In 1904, he described a case of nonfunctioning metastatic parathyroid carcinoma, and 26 years later, Sainton and Millot described the first case of functioning metastatic parathyroid carcinoma.[8] Armstrong in 1938 described another patient with metastatic parathyroid carcinoma and hypercalcemia,[9] and in 1968, Holmes and colleagues[10] reviewed 50 cases of parathyroid carcinoma reported in the literature. Of those, 46 tumors were functioning

Department of Surgery, Memorial Sloan-Kettering Cancer Center, 1275 York Avenue, Room C-1061, New York, NY 10065, USA
* Corresponding author.
E-mail address: shahj@mskcc.org

Hematol Oncol Clin N Am 26 (2012) 1221–1238
http://dx.doi.org/10.1016/j.hoc.2012.08.009
0889-8588/12/$ – see front matter © 2012 Elsevier Inc. All rights reserved.

with a mean serum calcium level of 15.9 mg/dL. Fewer than 10% of parathyroid carcinoma cases present as nonfunctional tumors.[11–13] Although most patients with parathyroid carcinoma present with hyperparathyroidism, a diagnosis of hyperparathyroidism attributable to carcinoma may be difficult to arrive at preoperatively or even intraoperatively.[4] In many cases, because of the rarity of the disease and clinical features mimicking benign parathyroid pathology, preoperative diagnosis of parathyroid carcinoma is difficult. In addition, the pathologic diagnosis of malignancy is challenging; however, severe hypercalcemia combined with high parathyroid hormone levels and gross operative findings should arouse suspicion of parathyroid carcinoma. This article reviews the relevant literature on parathyroid carcinoma in an attempt to provide diagnostic and therapeutic strategies.

ANATOMY, ETIOLOGY, AND EPIDEMIOLOGY

The parathyroid glands are endodermal in origin and develop from the dorsal wing of the third and fourth pharyngeal pouches.[14,15] They produce parathyroid hormone (PTH), which regulates the circulating level of calcium through intestinal and renal absorption and bone remodeling. There are typically 4 parathyroid glands; however, supernumerary glands and fewer than 4 glands have been reported. The superior parathyroid glands originate from the fourth pharyngeal pouch, and they attach to the posterior surface of the inferiorly migrating thyroid.[14,16] They have a much shorter migration distance compared with the inferior parathyroid glands, accounting for their more predictable location. The dorsal wing of the third pharyngeal pouch gives rise to the inferior parathyroid glands, whereas the ventral wing gives rise to the thymus during the fifth week of gestation.[14] Both primitive glands join the thymus as it travels caudally and medially to its final position in the mediastinum.[14,17] This migration of the inferior parathyroid glands with the thymus results in the inferior parathyroid gland to be in a plane that is usually ventral to that of the superior parathyroid glands.[17] For this reason, ectopic inferior parathyroid glands can be found anywhere along this large area of descent up to the superior border of the pericardium.[18]

Etiology of parathyroid carcinoma is not known. There is an association between multiple endocrine neoplasia type 1, the autosomal dominant form of familial hyperparathyroidism and an increased risk of parathyroid carcinoma.[19] Additionally, there have been reports of carcinoma occurring in an adenoma, hyperplastic gland, or in patients with history of neck irradiation and end-stage renal disease.[20–24] In the report by Koea and Shaw,[19] 1.4% of the patients with parathyroid carcinoma had prior history of neck irradiation; however, robust causal relationship between parathyroid carcinoma and radiation or lifestyle factors has not been described.

Parathyroid carcinoma by all means is a rare disease with the reported incidence ranging from 0.5% to 5.0%.[1–3] There may be a geographic variation in the distribution of this disease, with reported incidence of about 1% in Europe and the United States and about 5% in Japan and Italy.[20,25–28] Hundahl and colleagues[4] in their review of the National Cancer Data Base (NCDB) between 1985 and 1995 identified 286 cases of parathyroid cancer, accounting for 0.005% of the total NCDB cancer cases. This variation may represent a discrepancy in histopathological and clinical criteria in recognition of malignancy. Parathyroid carcinoma occurs with equal frequency in men and women, whereas a higher female-to-male ratio (3–4:1) has been reported in parathyroid adenoma.[2,4,19] On average, it presents a decade earlier than parathyroid adenoma during the fourth and fifth decade of life; however, these demographic data have no value in diagnosing parathyroid carcinoma.[11] In the NCDB study, the investigators were unable to detect any disproportionate clustering by race, income level, or geographic region in their study population. The median age of this cohort at presentation was 55 years with equal gender distribution.[4]

Molecular Pathogenesis

Although the etiology of these tumors remains unclear, mutations of both oncogenes and tumor suppressor genes have been associated with the development of parathyroid tumors. Some of these genes include the oncogene cyclin DI, retinoblastoma, and the p53 tumor suppressor gene.[11,29] Oncogenes in locations 1q, 5q, 9q, 16p, 19p, and Xq and tumor suppressor genes in locations 1p, 3q, 4q, 13q, and 21q may be involved in the pathogenesis of parathyroid carcinoma.[11,30] Cyclin D1 or PRAD1 (*parathyroid adenoma 1*) is an oncogene that is located at chromosome 11q13 and is involved in cell cycle regulation.[31] A chromosomal rearrangement of the cyclin D1 gene with the regulatory region of the PTH gene has been reported in 5% of parathyroid adenomas with the cyclin D1 oncoprotein being overexpressed in 18% to 40% of adenomas.[32–35] Similarly, overexpression of the cyclin D1 oncogene is observed in up to 91% of the parathyroid carcinoma specimens as reported by Vasef and colleagues[36,37] and only in 39% and 61% of the adenoma and hyperplasia specimens, respectively. Although this association appears to be strong, direct causality between cyclin D1 and parathyroid carcinoma has not been established. It has been shown that altered expression of the Rb (retinoblastoma) gene is common in parathyroid carcinoma and is likely to be an important contributor to its molecular pathogenesis. In a study of 11 parathyroid carcinoma specimens, all lacked the Rb allele on chromosome 13.[38] In another study, by Pearce and colleagues,[39] allelic deletions of the 13q12–14 region involving both the Rb gene and the hereditary breast cancer susceptibility gene (BRCA2) was found in 3 of 19 parathyroid adenomas with aggressive clinical or histopathological features and 1 parathyroid carcinoma specimen. The significance of loss of heterozygosity (LOH) in parathyroid malignancy has been suggested by some studies. In one study, combined 1q and 11q LOH in parathyroid tumors was suggestive of malignant behavior.[40] Others have shown that LOH at BRCA2 and Rb protein is a common event in parathyroid tumorigenesis and retention of heterozygosity seems to exclude parathyroid malignancy.[41] This loss, which involves both the Rb gene and the BRCA2 locus on chromosome 13, suggests that tumor suppressor genes in this region other than Rb or BRCA2 may be involved in the development and progression of some endocrine tumors.

Another tumor suppressor gene that plays an important role in cell cycle regulation and its inactivation has been associated with human cancers is the p53 gene. This has also been studied in parathyroid carcinoma, but the frequency of p53 allelic loss or abnormal p53 protein expression is low in parathyroid carcinoma, and it does not appear to be a major contributor to the pathogenesis of parathyroid carcinoma.[42,43] HRPT2 gene, a tumor suppressor gene on chromosome 1q25 that encodes the protein parafibromin, has been implicated in the pathogenesis of parathyroid carcinoma.[44–47] The expression of parafibromin is shown to be decreased or absent in parathyroid carcinomas and the identification of inactivating germ-line mutations in HRPT2 may have significant implications for its diagnosis and management.[48–50] In a recent study, 26 tumor specimens from 18 patients with adenoma and 8 patients with carcinoma were immune-stained with an antibody against parafibromin (CDC 73).[49] Parafibromin immunostaining showed strong positivity in 17 of 18 adenomas and 2 of the carcinomas. Negative staining was noted in 3 of 8 carcinomas, and weak positivity was found in 3 of 8 carcinomas. The investigators concluded that the loss of parafibromin expression (negative or weak positivity) demonstrated 94.4% specificity in the diagnosis of parathyroid carcinoma. HPRT2 mutations are observed in 15% to 100% of the carcinomas and 0% to 4% of the adenomas.[45,51–54] Although tumor-specific chromosomal gains and losses have been shown in adenoma and carcinoma, the hypothesis that carcinoma may arise from adenoma has not been proven. Additionally, despite reports of carcinoma in cases of MEN1, loss of regions commonly lost in adenomas, such as the 11q region associated with MEN1, is not seen in the carcinomas.[30,55,56] Identification of the molecular markers associated with the pathogenesis of parathyroid carcinoma is essential in improving the diagnostic challenges and may serve as vital therapeutic targets in the management of this disease.

Histopathology

Two cardinal features for the diagnosis of any carcinoma are local invasion and metastasis. Some investigators believe that an unequivocal diagnosis of parathyroid carcinoma should be restricted to those tumors that invade adjacent soft tissues, thyroid gland, blood vessels, or perineural spaces or to those cases with documented metastases[57]; however, this may underestimate the diagnosis of carcinoma and histologic criteria may be useful in making this challenging diagnosis. Clinical and gross features of the parathyroid tumor at the time of surgical resection can significantly aid in the diagnosis of carcinoma. The size of tumor has been reported to range from 0.75 cm to larger than 6 cm.[2,4,6,58,59] Parathyroid carcinoma often appears adherent to the surrounding tissue and is poorly circumscribed.[2] Grossly, carcinomas are firm and grayish white compared with adenomas that are usually soft and tan colored.[60] In one series, extent of local invasion was reported with ipsilateral thyroid invasion being the most common in 89% of the cases followed by strap muscles (71%), ipsilateral recurrent laryngeal nerve (26%), esophagus (18%), and trachea (17%).[19]

Histologic features of lesions may be used in diagnosis of carcinoma before infiltration and metastasis has occurred. This approach has presented with difficulty in diagnosis of parathyroid carcinoma with no single feature being pathognomonic of malignancy.[61] In making the diagnosis of carcinoma, some investigators[27,60] adopt histologic criteria similar to those described by Schantz and Castleman in 1973.[2] In studying 67 cases, they observed certain histologic features that distinguished parathyroid carcinoma from adenoma. These features were fibrous capsule or fibrous trabeculae, or both, a trabecular or rosettelike cellular architecture, the presence of mitotic figures, and capsular or vascular invasion. Similar to other investigators, however, they emphasized the importance of considering the overall picture rather than any single criterion.[60,62] In one study, presence of vascular or capsular invasion and fibrous trabeculae were the most common indicators of malignancy.[63] Some investigators consider high mitotic rate as an important feature of the diagnosis,[64] whereas other investigators express reservation regarding the significance of vascular and capsular invasion, and feel that mitotic activity alone has limited value in diagnosis of malignancy because high mitotic rate is also observed in benign disease **(Fig. 1)**.[65,66]

Although ultrastructural features of parathyroid carcinoma have been described, in establishing the diagnosis of malignancy, electron microscopic investigation did not add significantly to light microscopy.[67–71] In almost all cases of carcinoma, the microscopic features were those of the chief cells.[71] Flow-cytometric analysis of parathyroid tumors using fresh material confirms that parathyroid carcinomas are more apt to be aneuploid than are adenomas, and determination of the DNA ploidy pattern is a valuable adjunct to the histologic diagnosis of parathyroid carcinoma.[72,73] Additionally, special staining, such as Ki-67, may be beneficial in diagnosis of parathyroid carcinoma.[74]

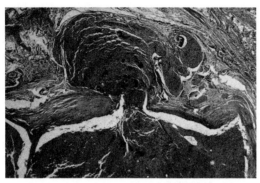

Fig. 1. Major capsular and vascular invasion with high mitotic activity confirming diagnosis of parathyroid carcinoma.

Staging

Because of the rarity of this disease, the American Joint Committee on Cancer has not yet developed a TNM staging for parathyroid carcinoma. Hundahl and colleagues,[4] in their review of 286 parathyroid carcinoma cases, reported an average tumor size of 3.3 cm and reported that lymph node status and tumor size did not appear to have a significant prognostic impact. These data have been questioned owing to lack of available information from the reviewed NCDB patient information; however, other reviews have found the presence of lymph node metastasis to be prognostically significant.[75] Shaha and Shah,[76] based on the information provided by the various reviews, proposed a staging system based on the size of the tumor, extent of local invasion, and presence of regional nodal disease and distant metastasis.

Clinical Presentation and Features

The observation that malignant parathyroid disease has a different presentation than the common benign forms of primary hyperparathyroidism has been made by many investigators.[10] The overwhelming majority of parathyroid cancers are functioning tumors. Thus, many clinical symptoms of parathyroid cancer are similar to the benign primary hyperparathyroidism, such as weakness, fatigue, nervousness, depression, weight loss, bone disease, abdominal pain, nephrolithiasis, pancreatitis, and peptic ulcer disease.[2,5,26,77,78] These symptoms usually manifest before local or regional invasion by the tumor. The challenge for the physician remains to differentiate between hyperparathyroidism attributable to benign disease, which is much more common than parathyroid carcinoma. Renal and skeletal involvement is a prominent manifestation of parathyroid carcinoma.[10] Skeletal involvement, such as bone pain, osteopenia, osteoporosis, osteofibrosis, and pathologic fractures, are observed in up to 90% of the patients, and renal involvement, such as nephrolithiasis and renal insufficiency, are seen in up to 80% of the patients.[10,26] The skeletal involvement is commonly observed in the spine or long bones, followed by diseases in the hands and skull and consisting mainly of subperiosteal erosions.[79] Concomitant renal and bone involvement is reported in nearly 50% of the patients.[58]

In most patients with parathyroid carcinoma, serum calcium and PTH are elevated, similar to benign primary hyperparathyroidism; however, the average serum calcium level for patients with parathyroid carcinoma is higher than that reported in patients with parathyroid adenoma.[10,12] The serum calcium levels in patients with parathyroid carcinoma are usually higher than 14 mg/dL, and mean serum calcium levels as high as 16 mg/dL and serum PTH levels as high as 10-fold to 15-fold higher than the normal range have been reported.[10,26,58,75,77,80,81] In a recent population study, a PTH level 10 times or more than the upper normal limit had a positive predictive value of 81% for parathyroid carcinoma.[12] For this reason, hypercalcemic crisis is not uncommon in parathyroid carcinoma and is observed in 8% to 12% of patients.[74,79] One should be cautious of using any single preoperative laboratory value in diagnosis of carcinoma, however. Additionally, levels of alkaline phosphatase and α and β subunits of human chorionic gonadotropin may be higher in patients with carcinoma than those with primary hyperparathyroidism.[82–84]

Physical findings of palpable neck mass and recurrent laryngeal nerve paralysis, which are rare in benign disease, have been associated with carcinoma. Presence of palpable neck mass has been observed in up to 70% of patients with parathyroid carcinoma at presentation[11,12,80,85] and in conjunction with hyperparathyroidism is suspicious for parathyroid carcinoma. Clinical presence of lymph node metastases, local invasion, and distant metastases are the sine qua non of parathyroid carcinoma.[76,86] Local invasion was observed in up to 67% of patients at the time of diagnosis in one study.[77] Nonfunctioning carcinomas are quite rare, and usually present with signs and symptoms of local growth and invasion, such as neck mass, hoarseness, and dysphagia, making this diagnosis even more challenging.[11,87] Selected differentiating clinical and histologic characteristics of primary hyperparathyroidism and parathyroid carcinoma are presented in **Table 1**.

Table 1
Differentiating characteristics of primary hyperparathyroidism and parathyroid carcinoma

	Primary Hyperparathyroidism	Parathyroid Carcinoma
Female: Male ratio	3–4:1	1:1
Average age	5th to 6th decades	4th to 5th decades
Serum calcium (mg/dL)	≤14	≥ 14
Parathyroid hormone	Mildly elevated	Markedly elevated
Local recurrence	Rare	Common
Nodal involvement	No	Common
Distant metastases	No	Occasional
Palpable neck mass	Uncommon	Frequent
Symptoms	Mostly asymptomatic	Commonly symptomatic
Renal involvement	Less common	More common
Skeletal involvement	Less common	More common
Concomitant renal and skeletal involvement	Rare	Common
Fibrosis	Variable	Common
Inflammation	Infrequent	Common
Necrosis	Rare	Common
Capsular invasion	Infrequent	Common
Vascular invasion	Infrequent	Common
Atypia	Infrequent	Common
Ploidy	Variable	Commonly aneuploid
Mitosis	Rare	Common
HRPT2 mutation	Infrequent	Common

IMAGING STUDIES AND DIAGNOSIS

The same noninvasive imaging studies used for the diagnosis of benign parathyroid disease may be used in aiding the initial diagnosis, and in identifying recurrence and extent of parathyroid carcinoma. Ultrasonography, sestamibi scanning, computed tomography (CT), single-photon emission CT, magnetic resonance imaging (MRI), and positron emission tomography have been used for the initial diagnosis and to detect the recurrence of parathyroid carcinoma (**Figs. 2** and **3**).[88–91] Ultrasound is a noninvasive and useful study to localize primary and locally recurrent disease. Typically, parathyroid carcinomas are lobulated, hypoechoic, and relatively large, with ill-defined borders compared with adenomas.[92–94] In a retrospective study, 69 patients with parathyroid lesions larger than 15 mm were evaluated by ultrasound. A high positive predictive value (PPV) for cancer was identified for infiltration (PPV 100%) and calcification (PPV 100%), and a high negative predictive value (NPV) was found for the absence of suspicious vascularity (NPV 97.6%), a thick capsule (NPV 96.7%), and inhomogeneity (NPV 100%). The investigators concluded that in parathyroid lesions larger than 15 mm, ultrasonography for specific features provides a valuable tool to identify parathyroid cancers before surgery.[88] Other investigators, however, have pointed out that it could be challenging to distinguish a large adenoma from a carcinoma by ultrasound.[93] Additionally, ultrasound may be used to guide fine-needle aspiration (FNA) biopsy when regional nodal metastasis is suspected. Technecium-99 m sestamibi scanning is widely used to localize parathyroid tumors. Sestamibi can also be used to detect primary parathyroid cancer or recurrent disease; however, no specific characteristics exist for distinguishing benign disease from parathyroid carcinoma.[95,96] Other anatomic studies, such as MRI and CT scan, could be used for localizing recurrence or metastasis, such as in bone and liver. In a retrospective review, the sensitivity of scintigraphy, CT, and ultrasonography in detecting recurrent disease was 86%, 79%, and 100%, respectively.[97] The addition of imaging studies to clinical presentation and the biochemical values as discussed previously may raise the suspicion of parathyroid carcinoma. Once this diagnosis is suspected, FNA biopsy of the primary lesion should be avoided, as it has been associated with tumor seeding of the biopsy tract.[98] Furthermore, FNA cytology will not be able to distinguish benign from malignant parathyroid tumor of the primary lesion.[79,99] FNA biopsy may be used to help distinguish thyroid from parathyroid tissue or identify metastatic parathyroid carcinoma.[100] Intraoperatively, in the absence of gross local

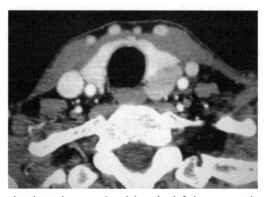

Fig. 2. CT scan showing irregular mass involving the left lower parathyroid, suggestive of parathyroid malignancy.

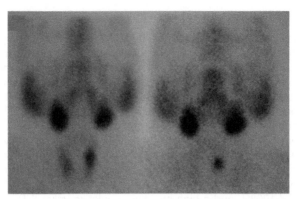

Fig. 3. Sestamibi scan showing intense activity in large left upper parathyroid.

invasion or regional metastasis, the diagnosis of carcinoma can be difficult. Frozen-section analysis is also of little value and unreliable, as the histopathological features of carcinoma may overlap with those of parathyroid adenoma.[11] In the study by Hundahl and colleagues,[4] 86% of patients did not receive the diagnosis of carcinoma intraoperatively, even with experienced parathyroid surgeons.

MANAGEMENT

Parathyroid carcinoma is a slow-growing but aggressive malignant tumor and most patients die of the metabolic complications of hypercalcemia. Thus, the goals of treatment of the primary lesion, local recurrence, or metastatic disease should be to eliminate all demonstrable disease when possible and to control the metabolic complications of hyperparathyroidism.[20,96,101] Other treatments, however, such as chemotherapy, embolization, and radio frequency ablation, have been attempted.[102–104]

SURGERY

The most effective treatment of parathyroid carcinoma remains surgical. Although the diagnosis of carcinoma can be difficult even at the time of initial surgical resection, intraoperatively, parathyroid tumors are usually large and firm, with a whitish capsule and are adherent to adjacent structures.[105] When suspected, en bloc resection of the carcinoma and the adjacent involved structures in the neck, including the ipsilateral thyroid lobe, with gross clear margins and avoidance of tumor spillage, is the gold standard treatment of parathyroid carcinoma.[19,76,100,101,106,107] Incomplete tumor extirpation will result in high rates of local recurrence. In such situations, although reoperation can be performed to palliate the symptoms of hypercalcemia, it rarely results in cure of the disease.[97] Patients with parathyroid carcinoma are at high risk of recurrent laryngeal nerve (RLN) invasion during their lifetime and if RLN is grossly involved by tumor, it needs to be sacrificed.[75,108] When cervical nodes are involved, a therapeutic modified neck dissection is necessary; however, prophylactic neck dissection has not shown to improve survival and is associated with increased morbidity.[109] The extensive surgical resection suggested by Holmes and colleagues[10] that includes removal of the strap muscles, skeletonization of the trachea, and sacrifice of the recurrent laryngeal nerve, in addition to removal of the tumor and ipsilateral thyroid lobe, is not usually undertaken. In the review by Koea and Shaw,[19] en bloc resection of the carcinoma and the adjacent structures in the neck was associated with an 8% local recurrence rate and a long-term overall survival rate of 89% (mean follow-up 69 months). In contrast, simple parathyroidectomy resulted in a 51% local recurrence rate and 53% long-term survival rate (mean follow-up 62 months). In another retrospective review of 13 patients, all of those who underwent local excision of the tumor developed recurrent disease compared with 33% who underwent en bloc resection.[110] Use of rapid PTH assay has been reported to be useful in the management of parathyroid carcinoma.[111] If the diagnosis of carcinoma is suspected before the operation, and the level of PTH falls into the normal range postoperatively, this can provide reassurance that the tumor is likely completely removed. If the PTH levels do not fall into the normal range or the diagnosis of carcinoma is not suspected until the postoperative pathologic evaluation, however, the management becomes controversial. When the tumor has low-grade features and the patient has normal calcium and PTH levels, close and lifelong monitoring and measurement of serum calcium and PTH at 3-month intervals is adequate.[112] However, if aggressive features, such as extensive capsular or vascular invasion, are seen and the patient remains hypercalcemic, additional investigational studies and reoperation may be warranted.[11,112] During the immediate postoperative period, patients should be closely monitored and treated for symptoms of hypocalcemia owing to hungry bone syndrome.[106] Serum calcium level should be maintained at lower limit of the normal range.[11]

Usually, parathyroid carcinoma recurs 2 to 5 years after initial surgery.[107,109] It is associated with a local recurrence rate of 33% to 82% within 5 years.[2,11,58,77,109] The high recurrence rate is likely because of incomplete resection of the tumor or tumor spillage. The rate of nodal metastasis is reported as high as 17% to 32%[10,20]; however, this is more commonly in the setting of local recurrence. The incidence of distant metastasis is difficult to determine owing to the rarity of this disease.[86] Metastases occur both via lymphatics and hematogenously, and the most common sites of distant metastases are the lung and liver, with the reported incidence of up to 40% and 10%, respectively.[2,11,100,113] Patients with recurrent disease or distant metastasis have recurrent progressive hypercalcemia along with high PTH level.[100] For this reason, medical management of hypercalcemia and appropriate imaging studies to locate the site of recurrence are essential.[25] Because these tumors are slow growing, repeated resection of local recurrences and/or distant metastases can result in significant palliation.[20,26,114,115] The goal of the operation is to remove all gross disease in the neck, mediastinum, and the distant sites with clear margins. In a retrospective review of 12 reoperations for locoregional control and 2 pulmonary metastatectomies, symptomatic relief in 86% of patients and a transient biochemical remission in 1 patient were achieved.[97] In a series of 6 patients who underwent pulmonary metastatectomies, 50% had biochemical resolution of their hypercalcemia, although some required multiple operations.[114] Patients with recurrent or metastatic parathyroid carcinoma may benefit from an aggressive surgical approach when feasible; however, in most cases, the symptomatic relief and biochemical normalization are temporary.

RADIOTHERAPY

Efficacy of radiotherapy in the management of parathyroid carcinoma has been difficult to prove because of the rarity of this condition; however, there is some evidence suggesting the benefit of postoperative radiotherapy (PORT).[77,78,116–118] There is no algorithm for adding PORT in parathyroid carcinoma, but in general, it is considered in patients who are at high risk of locoregional recurrence. In the M. D. Anderson experience, the local recurrence rate appeared to be lower if PORT was used after initial surgery, independent of the type of surgery and disease stage. Additionally, PORT seemed to increase the disease-free interval, but this difference was not statistically significant.[77] In the report from the Mayo Clinic, all patients who received PORT for aggressive features after the initial surgery achieved locoregional disease control; however, this is small and all patients had negative margins.[116] Similarly, in the Princess Margaret Hospital experience, all 6 patients at high risk of local relapse who received PORT did not have recurrence.[118] The investigators recommend adjuvant radiation with 40 to 50 Gy in patients at high risk of local relapse, such as patients with microscopic residual disease postoperatively.[118] The radiation dosage as high as 70 Gy has been used in other series.[116] The best chance of cure for a patient with parathyroid carcinoma is en bloc resection of the tumor with clear margins. The PORT results should be interpreted with caution, as they are all retrospective with a small number of patients in each group.

CHEMOTHERAPY

The experience with the role of chemotherapy in the management of parathyroid carcinoma is limited to case reports.[119–122] The overall attempts at controlling tumor burden have been disappointing, however, and no cytotoxic regimen with proven efficacy is currently available for patients with parathyroid carcinoma.[29,114,115] Complete objective response of pulmonary metastases from parathyroid carcinoma was seen in 1 patient following chemotherapy with fluorouracil, cyclophosphamide, and dacarbazine.[119] In another patient with mediastinal metastasis and left pleural effusion, treatment with a combination of methotrexate, doxorubicin, cyclophosphamide, and lomustine resulted in complete regression of the mediastinal mass and pleural effusion for a duration of 18 months.[121] In another report, treatment of a patient with nonfunctional metastatic parathyroid carcinoma with a combination of radiotherapy and chemotherapy resulted in good response and prolonged survival.[122] Use of synthetic estrogen has also been reported with some response.[58,123] The results of these case reports in efficacy of chemotherapy in the management of parathyroid carcinoma should be interpreted with extreme caution.

HYPERCALCEMIA

Surgical resection is not effective when parathyroid carcinoma has become widely disseminated. These patients have poor prognosis, with hypercalcemia being the most frequent cause of death rather than the tumor burden.[26,112,124] Prolonged survival at this point is still possible, however, with the therapeutic goal of controlling hypercalcemia. This is a challenging task owing to the associated intensity of bone resorption. Acute hypercalcemia caused by parathyroid carcinoma is treated in a similar fashion as hypercalcemia owing to any other cause. These patients become severely dehydrated because of nephrogenic diabetes insipidus and associated nausea and vomiting, so prompt aggressive hydration with normal saline is the first step of management.[96] Subsequently, loop diuretics may be administered to increase the excretion of calcium; however, addition of agents that interfere with osteoclast activity is often necessary. Usefulness of bisphosphonates, calcitonin, and calcimimetic agents (such as cinacalcet) in patients with parathyroid carcinoma and severe hypercalcemia has been suggested.[29] The bisphosphonates are a group of drugs that inhibit osteoclast-mediated bone resorption and lower serum calcium level. Several of these drugs, such as clodronate, etidronate, and pamidronate, have been shown to reduce serum calcium in patients with parathyroid cancer.[25,114,124–127] Bisphosphonates are poorly absorbed when administered orally and intravenous administration is required. Additionally, they are associated with acute renal failure when administered rapidly and avascular necrosis of the jaws has been reported.[128–130] Intravenous pamidronate is administered at a dose range of 60 to 90 mg with calcium levels falling in the following 2 to 4 days. Its response lasts for 1 to 3 weeks and the dosage can be repeated.[96] Even though long-term control of hypercalcemia can be achieved with bisphosphonates, the efficacy of these drugs reduces with time.

Calcimimetics are another class of drugs that bind to calcium-sensing receptor on the surface of parathyroid cells, increasing the receptor's sensitivity to extracellular calcium. This results in a decrease in PTH secretion and lowers the serum calcium level.[131] Cinacalcet, a calcimimetic, is administered orally at a dose range of 30 to 60 mg daily and is well tolerated.[132–134] Calcitonin inhibits both osteoclast-mediated bone resorption and increases urinary calcium excretion.[135,136] It has a rapid onset of 12 to 24 hours when administered at a dose range of 3 to 6 IU/kg, and the serum calcium level returns to pretreatment level at about 48 hours.[119,137] Corticosteroids alone or in combination with calcitonin have also been used in the management of hypercalcemia.[136] Plicamycin or mithramycin is another specific inhibitor of bone resorption that lowers serum calcium levels in parathyroid carcinoma that is seldom used. Its effectiveness is transient and decreases with repeated doses.[138] The toxic effects of plicamycin on liver, kidney, and bone marrow increase with repeated administration, and it should be reserved for therapy of life-threatening hypercalcemia, unresponsive to intravenous bisphosphonates.[11] Other agents, such as octreotide and gallium nitrate may also be used in the management of hypercalcemia caused by parathyroid cancer.[139–141]

PROGNOSIS

Variable survival after diagnosis ranging from 1 month to more than 20 years has been reported.[4,77,78] In a recent review by Harari and colleagues,[75] a median overall survival of 14.3 years was observed. The 5-year and 10-year survival rates from less than 50% to 85%,[58,77,78,116] and between 35% and 79% have been reported, respectively.[4,12,58,77,117] Early identification and complete resection of the tumor at the time of initial surgery offers the best prognosis. Koea and Shaw[19] observed that the adverse prognostic factors for survival were initial management with simple parathyroidectomy alone, the presence of nodal or distant metastatic disease at presentation, and nonfunctioning parathyroid carcinoma. In another study, factors associated with worse survival were lymph node or distant metastases, number of recurrences, higher calcium level at recurrence, and a high number of calcium-lowering medications.[75] Although prolonged survival is possible in patients with recurrent disease, cure is unlikely. A comprehensive multidisciplinary approach with appropriate initial surgery, selective use of radiation therapy, and medical treatment for hypercalcemia offers patients with parathyroid carcinoma the best chance of cure.

REFERENCES

1. Pyrah LN, Hodgkinson A, Anderson CK. Primary hyperparathyroidism. Br J Surg 1966;53(4):245–316.
2. Schantz A, Castleman B. Parathyroid carcinoma. A study of 70 cases. Cancer 1973;31(3):600–5.
3. Clark P, Wooldridge T, Kleinpeter K, et al. Providing optimal preoperative localization for recurrent parathyroid carcinoma: a combined parathyroid scintigraphy and computed tomography approach. Clin Nucl Med 2004;29(11):681–4.

4. Hundahl SA, Fleming ID, Fremgen AM, et al. Two hundred eighty-six cases of parathyroid carcinoma treated in the U.S. between 1985-1995: a National Cancer Data Base Report. The American College of Surgeons Commission on Cancer and the American Cancer Society. Cancer 1999;86(3):538–44.

5. Rao SR, Shaha AR, Singh B, et al. Management of cancer of the parathyroid. Acta Otolaryngol 2002;122(4):448–52.

6. Cohn K, Silverman M, Corrado J, et al. Parathyroid carcinoma: the Lahey Clinic experience. Surgery 1985;98(6):1095–100.

7. DeQuervain F. Parastruma maligna aberrata [Malignant aberrant parathyroid]. Deusche Zeitschr Chir 1904;100(1):334–52.

8. Sainton P, Millot J. Malegne dun adenoma parathyroidiene eosinophile [Malignant eosinophilic parathyroid]. Au cours dune de Recklinghausen. Ann Anat Pathol 1933;10(1):813–4.

9. Armstrong H. Primary carcinoma of parathyroid gland with report of case. Bull Acad Med Tor 1938;11:105–10.

10. Holmes EC, Morton DL, Ketcham AS. Parathyroid carcinoma: a collective review. Ann Surg 1969;169(4):631–40.

11. Shane E. Clinical review 122: parathyroid carcinoma. J Clin Endocrinol Metab 2001;86(2):485–93.

12. Schaapveld M, Jorna FH, Aben KK, et al. Incidence and prognosis of parathyroid gland carcinoma: a population-based study in The Netherlands estimating the preoperative diagnosis. Am J Surg 2011;202(5):590–7.

13. Wilkins BJ, Lewis JS Jr. Non-functional parathyroid carcinoma: a review of the literature and report of a case requiring extensive surgery. Head Neck Pathol 2009;3(2):140–9.

14. Sadler TW, Langman J. Langman's medical embryology. 10th edition. Philadelphia: Lippincott Williams & Wilkins; 2006. xiii, p. 371.

15. Larsen WJ, Sherman LS, Potter SS, et al. Human embryology. 3rd edition. New York: Churchill Livingstone; 2001. xix, p. 548.

16. Fancy T, Gallagher D 3rd, Hornig JD. Surgical anatomy of the thyroid and parathyroid glands. Otolaryngol Clin North Am 2010;43(2):221–7, vii.

17. Mansberger AR Jr, Wei JP. Surgical embryology and anatomy of the thyroid and parathyroid glands. Surg Clin North Am 1993;73(4):727–46.

18. Gray SW, Skandalakis JE, Akin JT Jr. Embryological considerations of thyroid surgery: developmental anatomy of the thyroid, parathyroids and the recurrent laryngeal nerve. Am Surg 1976;42(9):621–8.

19. Koea JB, Shaw JH. Parathyroid cancer: biology and management. Surg Oncol 1999;8(3):155–65.

20. Obara T, Fujimoto Y. Diagnosis and treatment of patients with parathyroid carcinoma: an update and review. World J Surg 1991;15(6):738–44.

21. Ashkenazi D, Elmalah I, Rakover Y, et al. Concurrent nonfunctioning parathyroid carcinoma and parathyroid adenoma. Am J Otolaryngol 2006;27(3):204–6.

22. Shapiro DM, Recant W, Hemmati M, et al. Synchronous occurrence of parathyroid carcinoma and adenoma in an elderly woman. Surgery 1989;106(5):929–33.

23. Walls J, Lauder I, Ellis HA. Chronic renal failure in a patient with parathyroid carcinoma and hyperplasia. Beitr Pathol 1972;147(1):45–50.

24. Jayawardene S, Owen WJ, Goldsmith DJ. Parathyroid carcinoma in a dialysis patient. Am J Kidney Dis 2000;36(4):E26.

25. Sandelin K, Thompson NW, Bondeson L. Metastatic parathyroid carcinoma: dilemmas in management. Surgery 1991;110(6):978–86 [discussion: 986–8].

26. Wynne AG, van Heerden J, Carney JA, et al. Parathyroid carcinoma: clinical and pathologic features in 43 patients. Medicine (Baltimore) 1992;71(4):197–205.
27. Fujimoto Y, Obara T. How to recognize and treat parathyroid carcinoma. Surg Clin North Am 1987;67(2):343–57.
28. Favia G, Lumachi F, Polistina F, et al. Parathyroid carcinoma: sixteen new cases and suggestions for correct management. World J Surg 1998;22(12):1225–30.
29. Lumachi F, Basso SM, Basso U. Parathyroid cancer: etiology, clinical presentation and treatment. Anticancer Res 2006;26(6C):4803–7.
30. Kytola S, Farnebo F, Obara T, et al. Patterns of chromosomal imbalances in parathyroid carcinomas. Am J Pathol 2000;157(2):579–86.
31. Arnold A, Kim HG, Gaz RD, et al. Molecular cloning and chromosomal mapping of DNA rearranged with the parathyroid hormone gene in a parathyroid adenoma. J Clin Invest 1989;83(6):2034–40.
32. Arnold A, Motokura T, Bloom T, et al. PRAD1 (cyclin D1): a parathyroid neoplasia gene on 11q13. Henry Ford Hosp Med J 1992;40(3–4):177–80.
33. Arnold A. Molecular mechanisms of parathyroid neoplasia. Endocrinol Metab Clin North Am 1994;23(1):93–107.
34. Mallya SM, Arnold A. Cyclin D1 in parathyroid disease. Front Biosci 2000;5: D367–71.
35. Hemmer S, Wasenius VM, Haglund C, et al. Deletion of 11q23 and cyclin D1 overexpression are frequent aberrations in parathyroid adenomas. Am J Pathol 2001;158(4):1355–62.
36. Vasef MA, Brynes RK, Sturm M, et al. Expression of cyclin D1 in parathyroid carcinomas, adenomas, and hyperplasias: a paraffin immunohistochemical study. Mod Pathol 1999;12(4):412–6.
37. Hsi ED, Zukerberg LR, Yang WI, et al. Cyclin D1/PRAD1 expression in parathyroid adenomas: an immunohistochemical study. J Clin Endocrinol Metab 1996; 81(5):1736–9.
38. Cryns VL, Thor A, Xu HJ, et al. Loss of the retinoblastoma tumor-suppressor gene in parathyroid carcinoma. N Engl J Med 1994;330(11):757–61.
39. Pearce SH, Trump D, Wooding C, et al. Loss of heterozygosity studies at the retinoblastoma and breast cancer susceptibility (BRCA2) loci in pituitary, parathyroid, pancreatic and carcinoid tumours. Clin Endocrinol (Oxf) 1996;45(2): 195–200.
40. Haven CJ, van Puijenbroek M, Karperien M, et al. Differential expression of the calcium sensing receptor and combined loss of chromosomes 1q and 11q in parathyroid carcinoma. J Pathol 2004;202(1):86–94.
41. Cetani F, Pardi E, Viacava P, et al. A reappraisal of the Rb1 gene abnormalities in the diagnosis of parathyroid cancer. Clin Endocrinol (Oxf) 2004;60(1):99–106.
42. Cryns VL, Rubio MP, Thor AD, et al. p53 abnormalities in human parathyroid carcinoma. J Clin Endocrinol Metab 1994;78(6):1320–4.
43. Hakim JP, Levine MA. Absence of p53 point mutations in parathyroid adenoma and carcinoma. J Clin Endocrinol Metab 1994;78(1):103–6.
44. Shattuck TM, Valimaki S, Obara T, et al. Somatic and germ-line mutations of the HRPT2 gene in sporadic parathyroid carcinoma. N Engl J Med 2003;349(18): 1722–9.
45. Carpten JD, Robbins CM, Villablanca A, et al. HRPT2, encoding parafibromin, is mutated in hyperparathyroidism-jaw tumor syndrome. Nat Genet 2002;32(4): 676–80.
46. Weinstein LS, Simonds WF. HRPT2, a marker of parathyroid cancer. N Engl J Med 2003;349(18):1691–2.

47. Caron P, Simonds WF, Maiza JC, et al. Nontruncated amino-terminal parathyroid hormone overproduction in two patients with parathyroid carcinoma: a possible link to HRPT2 gene inactivation. Clin Endocrinol (Oxf) 2011;74(6):694–8.

48. Mittendorf EA, McHenry CR. Parathyroid carcinoma. J Surg Oncol 2005;89(3): 136–42.

49. Kim HK, Oh YL, Kim SH, et al. Parafibromin immunohistochemical staining to differentiate parathyroid carcinoma from parathyroid adenoma. Head Neck 2012;34(2):201–6.

50. Senior K. Vital gene linked to parathyroid carcinoma. Lancet Oncol 2003;4(12): 713.

51. Howell VM, Gill A, Clarkson A, et al. Accuracy of combined protein gene product 9.5 and parafibromin markers for immunohistochemical diagnosis of parathyroid carcinoma. J Clin Endocrinol Metab 2009;94(2):434–41.

52. Howell VM, Haven CJ, Kahnoski K, et al. HRPT2 mutations are associated with malignancy in sporadic parathyroid tumours. J Med Genet 2003;40(9):657–63.

53. Krebs LJ, Shattuck TM, Arnold A. HRPT2 mutational analysis of typical sporadic parathyroid adenomas. J Clin Endocrinol Metab 2005;90(9):5015–7.

54. Cetani F, Pardi E, Borsari S, et al. Genetic analyses of the HRPT2 gene in primary hyperparathyroidism: germline and somatic mutations in familial and sporadic parathyroid tumors. J Clin Endocrinol Metab 2004;89(11):5583–91.

55. Dionisi S, Minisola S, Pepe J, et al. Concurrent parathyroid adenomas and carcinoma in the setting of multiple endocrine neoplasia type 1: presentation as hypercalcemic crisis. Mayo Clin Proc 2002;77(8):866–9.

56. Agha A, Carpenter R, Bhattacharya S, et al. Parathyroid carcinoma in multiple endocrine neoplasia type 1 (MEN1) syndrome: two case reports of an unrecognised entity. J Endocrinol Invest 2007;30(2):145–9.

57. Delellis RA. Challenging lesions in the differential diagnosis of endocrine tumors: parathyroid carcinoma. Endocr Pathol 2008;19(4):221–5.

58. Shane E, Bilezikian JP. Parathyroid carcinoma: a review of 62 patients. Endocr Rev 1982;3(2):218–26.

59. DeLellis RA. Parathyroid carcinoma: an overview. Adv Anat Pathol 2005;12(2): 53–61.

60. Smith JF, Coombs RR. Histological diagnosis of carcinoma of the parathyroid gland. J Clin Pathol 1984;37(12):1370–8.

61. Sandelin K, Auer G, Bondeson L, et al. Prognostic factors in parathyroid cancer: a review of 95 cases. World J Surg 1992;16(4):724–31.

62. Thompson LD. Parathyroid carcinoma. Ear Nose Throat J 2009;88(1):722–4.

63. Chang YJ, Mittal V, Remine S, et al. Correlation between clinical and histological findings in parathyroid tumors suspicious for carcinoma. Am Surg 2006;72(5): 419–26.

64. Obara T, Okamoto T, Kanbe M, et al. Functioning parathyroid carcinoma: clinico-pathologic features and rational treatment. Semin Surg Oncol 1997;13(2):134–41.

65. Bondeson L, Sandelin K, Grimelius L. Histopathological variables and DNA cytometry in parathyroid carcinoma. Am J Surg Pathol 1993;17(8):820–9.

66. McKeown PP, McGarity WC, Sewell CW. Carcinoma of the parathyroid gland: is it overdiagnosed? A report of three cases. Am J Surg 1984;147(2):292–8.

67. Faccini JM. The ultrastructure of parathyroid glands removed from patients with primary hyperparathyroidism: a report of 40 cases, including four carcinomata. J Pathol 1970;102(4):189–99.

68. Holck S, Pedersen NT. Carcinoma of the parathyroid gland. A light and electron microscopic study. Acta Pathol Microbiol Scand A 1981;89(4):297–302.

69. Yamashita H, Noguchi S, Nakayama I, et al. Light and electron microscopic study of nonfunctioning parathyroid carcinoma. Report of a case with a review of the literature. Acta Pathol Jpn 1984;34(1):123–32.

70. Altenahr E, Saeger W. Light and electron microscopy of parathyroid carcinoma. Report of three cases. Virchows Arch A Pathol Pathol Anat 1973;360(2):107–22.

71. Bichel P, Thomsen OF, Askjaer SA, et al. Light and electron microscopic investigation of parathyroid carcinoma during dedifferentiation. Survey and study of a case. Virchows Arch A Pathol Anat Histol 1980;386(3):363–70.

72. Obara T, Fujimoto Y, Hirayama A, et al. Flow cytometric DNA analysis of parathyroid tumors with special reference to its diagnostic and prognostic value in parathyroid carcinoma. Cancer 1990;65(8):1789–93.

73. August DA, Flynn SD, Jones MA, et al. Parathyroid carcinoma: the relationship of nuclear DNA content to clinical outcome. Surgery 1993;113(3):290–6.

74. Iihara M, Okamoto T, Suzuki R, et al. Functional parathyroid carcinoma: long-term treatment outcome and risk factor analysis. Surgery 2007;142(6):936–43 [discussion: 943.e1].

75. Harari A, Waring A, Fernandez-Ranvier G, et al. Parathyroid carcinoma: a 43-year outcome and survival analysis. J Clin Endocrinol Metab 2011;96(12): 3679–86.

76. Shaha AR, Shah JP. Parathyroid carcinoma: a diagnostic and therapeutic challenge. Cancer 1999;86(3):378–80.

77. Busaidy NL, Jimenez C, Habra MA, et al. Parathyroid carcinoma: a 22-year experience. Head Neck 2004;26(8):716–26.

78. Hakaim AG, Esselstyn CB Jr. Parathyroid carcinoma: 50-year experience at The Cleveland Clinic Foundation. Cleve Clin J Med 1993;60(4):331–5.

79. Thompson SD, Prichard AJ. The management of parathyroid carcinoma. Curr Opin Otolaryngol Head Neck Surg 2004;12(2):93–7.

80. Kleinpeter KP, Lovato JF, Clark PB, et al. Is parathyroid carcinoma indeed a lethal disease? Ann Surg Oncol 2005;12(3):260–6.

81. Robert JH, Trombetti A, Garcia A, et al. Primary hyperparathyroidism: can parathyroid carcinoma be anticipated on clinical and biochemical grounds? Report of nine cases and review of the literature. Ann Surg Oncol 2005;12(7):526–32.

82. Silverberg SJ, Shane E, Jacobs TP, et al. Nephrolithiasis and bone involvement in primary hyperparathyroidism. Am J Med 1990;89(3):327–34.

83. Rubin MR, Bilezikian JP, Birken S, et al. Human chorionic gonadotropin measurements in parathyroid carcinoma. Eur J Endocrinol 2008;159(4):469–74.

84. Stock JL, Weintraub BD, Rosen SW, et al. Human chorionic gonadotropin subunit measurement in primary hyperparathyroidism. J Clin Endocrinol Metab 1982;54(1):57–63.

85. Levin KE, Galante M, Clark OH. Parathyroid carcinoma versus parathyroid adenoma in patients with profound hypercalcemia. Surgery 1987;101(6):649–60.

86. Shaha AR, Ferlito A, Rinaldo A. Distant metastases from thyroid and parathyroid cancer. ORL J Otorhinolaryngol Relat Spec 2001;63(4):243–9.

87. Shattuck TM, Kim TS, Costa J, et al. Mutational analyses of RB and BRCA2 as candidate tumour suppressor genes in parathyroid carcinoma. Clin Endocrinol (Oxf) 2003;59(2):180–9.

88. Sidhu PS, Talat N, Patel P, et al. Ultrasound features of malignancy in the preoperative diagnosis of parathyroid cancer: a retrospective analysis of parathyroid tumours larger than 15 mm. Eur Radiol 2011;21(9):1865–73.

89. Kitapci MT, Tastekin G, Turgut M, et al. Preoperative localization of parathyroid carcinoma using Tc-99m MIBI. Clin Nucl Med 1993;18(3):217–9.

90. Evangelista L, Sorgato N, Torresan F, et al. FDG-PET/CT and parathyroid carcinoma: review of literature and illustrative case series. World J Clin Oncol 2011; 2(10):348–54.

91. Neumann DR, Esselstyn CB, Kim EY. Recurrent postoperative parathyroid carcinoma: FDG-PET and sestamibi-SPECT findings. J Nucl Med 1996;37(12): 2000–1.

92. Hara H, Igarashi A, Yano Y, et al. Ultrasonographic features of parathyroid carcinoma. Endocr J 2001;48(2):213–7.

93. Edmonson GR, Charboneau JW, James EM, et al. Parathyroid carcinoma: high-frequency sonographic features. Radiology 1986;161(1):65–7.

94. Tamler R, Lewis MS, LiVolsi VA, et al. Parathyroid carcinoma: ultrasonographic and histologic features. Thyroid 2005;15(7):744–5.

95. Al-Sobhi S, Ashari LH, Ingemansson S. Detection of metastatic parathyroid carcinoma with Tc-99m sestamibi imaging. Clin Nucl Med 1999;24(1):21–3.

96. Rodgers SE, Perrier ND. Parathyroid carcinoma. Curr Opin Oncol 2006;18(1): 16–22.

97. Iacobone M, Ruffolo C, Lumachi F, et al. Results of iterative surgery for persistent and recurrent parathyroid carcinoma. Langenbecks Arch Surg 2005;390(5): 385–90.

98. Spinelli C, Bonadio AG, Berti P, et al. Cutaneous spreading of parathyroid carcinoma after fine needle aspiration cytology. J Endocrinol Invest 2000;23(4): 255–7.

99. Kassahun WT, Jonas S. Focus on parathyroid carcinoma. Int J Surg 2011;9(1): 13–9.

100. Owen RP, Silver CE, Pellitteri PK, et al. Parathyroid carcinoma: a review. Head Neck 2011;33(3):429–36.

101. Fujimoto Y, Obara T, Ito Y, et al. Surgical treatment of ten cases of parathyroid carcinoma: importance of an initial en bloc tumor resection. World J Surg 1984;8(3):392–400.

102. Artinyan A, Guzman E, Maghami E, et al. Metastatic parathyroid carcinoma to the liver treated with radiofrequency ablation and transcatheter arterial embolization. J Clin Oncol 2008;26(24):4039–41.

103. Iguchi T, Yasui K, Hiraki T, et al. Radiofrequency ablation of functioning lung metastases from parathyroid carcinoma. J Vasc Interv Radiol 2008;19(3):462–4.

104. Tochio M, Takaki H, Yamakado K, et al. A case report of 20 lung radiofrequency ablation sessions for 50 lung metastases from parathyroid carcinoma causing hyperparathyroidism. Cardiovasc Intervent Radiol 2010;33(3):657–9.

105. Kebebew E, Clark OH. Parathyroid adenoma, hyperplasia, and carcinoma: localization, technical details of primary neck exploration, and treatment of hypercalcemic crisis. Surg Oncol Clin N Am 1998;7(4):721–48.

106. Rawat N, Khetan N, Williams DW, et al. Parathyroid carcinoma. Br J Surg 2005; 92(11):1345–53.

107. Givi B, Shah JP. Parathyroid carcinoma. Clin Oncol (R Coll Radiol) 2010;22(6): 498–507.

108. Kebebew E, Arici C, Duh QY, et al. Localization and reoperation results for persistent and recurrent parathyroid carcinoma. Arch Surg 2001;136(8):878–85.

109. Kebebew E. Parathyroid carcinoma. Curr Treat Options Oncol 2001;2(4): 347–54.

110. Wiseman SM, Rigual NR, Hicks WL Jr, et al. Parathyroid carcinoma: a multicenter review of clinicopathologic features and treatment outcomes. Ear Nose Throat J 2004;83(7):491–4.

111. Cavalier E, Daly AF, Betea D, et al. The ratio of parathyroid hormone as measured by third- and second-generation assays as a marker for parathyroid carcinoma. J Clin Endocrinol Metab 2010;95(8):3745–9.

112. Fujimoto Y, Obara T, Ito Y, et al. Localization and surgical resection of metastatic parathyroid carcinoma. World J Surg 1986;10(4):539–47.

113. Witteveen JE, Haak HR, Kievit J, et al. Challenges and pitfalls in the management of parathyroid carcinoma: 17-year follow-up of a case and review of the literature. Horm Cancer 2010;1(4):205–14.

114. Obara T, Okamoto T, Ito Y, et al. Surgical and medical management of patients with pulmonary metastasis from parathyroid carcinoma. Surgery 1993;114(6): 1040–8 [discussion: 1048–9].

115. Anderson BJ, Samaan NA, Vassilopoulou-Sellin R, et al. Parathyroid carcinoma: features and difficulties in diagnosis and management. Surgery 1983;94(6): 906–15.

116. Munson ND, Foote RL, Northcutt RC, et al. Parathyroid carcinoma: is there a role for adjuvant radiation therapy? Cancer 2003;98(11):2378–84.

117. Clayman GL, Gonzalez HE, El-Naggar A, et al. Parathyroid carcinoma: evaluation and interdisciplinary management. Cancer 2004;100(5):900–5.

118. Chow E, Tsang RW, Brierley JD, et al. Parathyroid carcinoma—the Princess Margaret Hospital experience. Int J Radiat Oncol Biol Phys 1998;41(3):569–72.

119. Bukowski RM, Sheeler L, Cunningham J, et al. Successful combination chemotherapy for metastatic parathyroid carcinoma. Arch Intern Med 1984;144(2): 399–400.

120. Chahinian AP. Chemotherapy for metastatic parathyroid carcinoma. Arch Intern Med 1984;144(9):1889.

121. Chahinian AP, Holland JF, Nieburgs HE, et al. Metastatic nonfunctioning parathyroid carcinoma: ultrastructural evidence of secretory granules and response to chemotherapy. Am J Med Sci 1981;282(2):80–4.

122. Eurelings M, Frijns CJ, Jeurissen FJ. Painful ophthalmoplegia from metastatic nonproducing parathyroid carcinoma: case study and review of the literature. Neuro Oncol 2002;4(1):44–8.

123. Goepfert H, Smart CR, Rochlin DB. Metastatic parathyroid carcinoma and hormonal chemotherapy. Case report and response to hexestrol. Ann Surg 1966;164(5):917–20.

124. Jungst D. Disodium clodronate effective in management of severe hypercalcaemia caused by parathyroid carcinoma. Lancet 1984;2(8410):1043.

125. Jacobs TP, Siris ES, Bilezikian JP, et al. Hypercalcemia of malignancy: treatment with intravenous dichloromethylene diphosphonate. Ann Intern Med 1981;94(3): 312–6.

126. Mann K. Oral bisphosphonate therapy in metastatic parathyroid carcinoma. Lancet 1985;1(8420):101–2.

127. Jacobs TP, Gordon AC, Silverberg SJ, et al. Neoplastic hypercalcemia: physiologic response to intravenous etidronate disodium. Am J Med 1987;82(2A):42–50.

128. Marx RE. Pamidronate (Aredia) and zoledronate (Zometa) induced avascular necrosis of the jaws: a growing epidemic. J Oral Maxillofac Surg 2003;61(9): 1115–7.

129. Bounameaux HM, Schifferli J, Montani JP, et al. Renal failure associated with intravenous diphosphonates. Lancet 1983;1(8322):471.

130. Gevorgyan A, Enepekides DJ. Bisphosphonate-induced necrosis of the jaws: a reconstructive nightmare. Curr Opin Otolaryngol Head Neck Surg 2008; 16(4):325–30.

131. Nemeth EF, Steffey ME, Hammerland LG, et al. Calcimimetics with potent and selective activity on the parathyroid calcium receptor. Proc Natl Acad Sci U S A 1998;95(7):4040–5.

132. Silverberg SJ, Rubin MR, Faiman C, et al. Cinacalcet hydrochloride reduces the serum calcium concentration in inoperable parathyroid carcinoma. J Clin Endocrinol Metab 2007;92(10):3803–8.

133. Peacock M, Bilezikian JP, Bolognese MA, et al. Cinacalcet HCl reduces hypercalcemia in primary hyperparathyroidism across a wide spectrum of disease severity. J Clin Endocrinol Metab 2011;96(1):E9–18.

134. Peacock M, Bilezikian JP, Klassen PS, et al. Cinacalcet hydrochloride maintains long-term normocalcemia in patients with primary hyperparathyroidism. J Clin Endocrinol Metab 2005;90(1):135–41.

135. Trigonis C, Cedermark B, Willems J, et al. Parathyroid carcinoma—problems in diagnosis and treatment. Clin Oncol 1984;10(1):11–9.

136. Au WY. Calcitonin treatment of hypercalcemia due to parathyroid carcinoma. Synergistic effect of prednisone on long-term treatment of hypercalcemia. Arch Intern Med 1975;135(12):1594–7.

137. Pecherstorfer M, Brenner K, Zojer N. Current management strategies for hypercalcemia. Treat Endocrinol 2003;2(4):273–92.

138. Singer FR, Neer RM, Murray TM, et al. Mithramycin treatment of intractable hypercalcemia due to parathyroid carcinoma. N Engl J Med 1970;283(12): 634–6.

139. Koyano H, Shishiba Y, Shimizu T, et al. Successful treatment by surgical removal of bone metastasis producing PTH: new approach to the management of metastatic parathyroid carcinoma. Intern Med 1994;33(11):697–702.

140. Denney AM, Watts NB. The effect of octreotide on parathyroid carcinoma. J Clin Endocrinol Metab 2004;89(2):1016.

141. Warrell RP Jr, Issacs M, Alcock NW, et al. Gallium nitrate for treatment of refractory hypercalcemia from parathyroid carcinoma. Ann Intern Med 1987;107(5): 683–6.

Gastrointestinal Stromal Tumor— Background, Pathology, Treatment

Burton L. Eisenberg, MD[a],*, J. Marc Pipas, MD[b]

KEYWORDS

- Gastrointestinal stromal tumor • Imatinib • KIT mutation

KEY POINTS

- The discovery of KIT mutations as a driver of GIST malignant transformation has resulted in an effective therapy with Imatinib KIT Tyrosine Kinase inhibitor.
- The adjuvant use of Imatinib has now been shown to improve both progression free and overall survival for high risk GIST.
- Neoadjuvant Imatinib in high risk GIST can be useful for tumor downstaging and subsequent organ sparing and less morbid surgical resection.

INTRODUCTION

Gastrointestinal stromal tumor (GIST) has emerged as the most commonly reported mesenchymal tumor of the gastrointestinal (GI) tract.[1] This is due partly to the distinct defining characteristics of this tumor recognized by pathologists as a singular entity as well as an increase in reporting due to the unprecedented role of GIST as a model for the development of solid tumor targeted therapy. Although historically a purely surgical disease, this sarcoma is now managed through multimodality treatment considerations that often include a combination of surgical and systemic schemes to enhance disease control. This article reviews the background, prognostic factors, and current treatment recommendations for this rare but increasingly referenced malignancy.

Incidence

GISTs are the most common and prevalent sarcomas of the GI tract, accounting for at least 5% of all sarcomas and 80% of all GI mesenchymal tumors. The diagnosis of GIST

[a] Surgical Oncology, Geisel School of Medicine at Dartmouth, Norris Cotton Cancer Center, Dartmouth-Hitchcock Medical Center, One Medical Center Drive, Lebanon, NH 03756, USA;
[b] Gastrointestinal Oncology Program, Norris Cotton Cancer Center, Gastrointestinal Department, Dartmouth-Hitchcock Medical Center, One Medical Center Drive, Lebanon, NH 03756, USA
* Corresponding author.
E-mail address: Burton.L.Eisenberg@Dartmouth.edu

Hematol Oncol Clin N Am 26 (2012) 1239–1259
http://dx.doi.org/10.1016/j.hoc.2012.08.003
0889-8588/12/$ – see front matter © 2012 Elsevier Inc. All rights reserved.

has increased 25-fold over the past 20 years partly due to a reclassification of most GI smooth muscle tumors as GISTs.[1] Within the Surveillance, Epidemiology and End Results patient registry, age-adjusted incidence of GIST diagnosis increased from 0.028 per 100,000 in 1992 to 0.688 in 2002. This is confirmatory to other studies that report an incidence of 7 to 14 GIST cases per 1 million in the general population.[2–5]

Pathobiology

The novel observation and seminal article by Hirota and colleagues[6] provided the basis for the subsequent expansive discoveries regarding the therapeutic targeting of the KIT oncoprotein in GISTs. This group first reported the link between activating mutations in the C-KIT proto-oncogene and its tyrosine kinase protein and the occurrence of GISTs. The hypothesis was initially based on observations that the interstitial cells of Cajal (ICC) found in the GI myenteric plexus express the KIT protein. They deduced that GIST seemed to have similar staining and ulrastructural characteristics to the ICC and found that GISTs almost universally demonstrate KIT gain-of-function mutations, suggesting that these tumors are a malignant variant of an ICC developmental cell. Subsequent to this discovery, gain-of-function mutations were found in platelet-derived growth factor receptor, alpha polypeptide (PDGFRA) in KIT-negative GISTs.[7,8] It has been reported that approximately 80% of GISTs have an activating mutation in the KIT proto-oncogene and 5% to 8% have a mutually exclusive activating mutation in PDGFRA.[9] These data have provided for advancements in both the diagnosis and therapy for GIST. These tumors can present a biologic continuum representing a spectrum from essentially benign small incidentally found bowel associated nodules to large highly metastatic tumors. Their prognosis and predictable clinical activity depend on presentation of size, mitotic activity, and molecular features.

GIST—Clinical Presentation

GISTs are most commonly diagnosed in adults between 50 to 80 years of age with a male-to-female ratio of 1:1. The majority of patients with GIST are symptomatic, with the most likely symptoms of pain and bloating related to an abdominal space–occupying mass. GI bleeding and anemia are less common and related to tumor mucosal erosion, which in itself is considered a negative prognostic factor. Because GISTs are generally extrinsic and exophytic (**Fig. 1**), a large tumor can lead to intra-abdominal

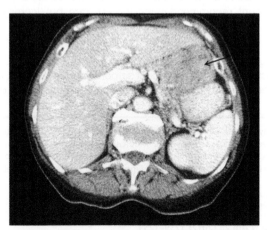

Fig. 1. Arrow indicates large exophytic gastric GIST on abdominal CT scan. The majority of the mass is movable and only attached to a small segment of stomach.

rupture or bleeding, signaling a poor prognostic event associated with an increased risk of tumor peritoneal implantation. The most common locations for GISTs are gastric (60%–70%), small bowel (20%–25%), colorectal (5%), esophagus (5%), and, rarely, omental, retroperitoneal, or mesenteric. Approximately 20% of GISTs are asymptomatic, small, and discovered incidentally on imaging or endoscopy. Endoscopic ultrasound indicates a typical appearance of a submucosal noncystic homogeneous mass and has proved useful in the evaluation of these visualized submucosal abnormalities. Although surgical resection is the standard therapy for localized GIST, and this is true for those tumors 2 cm and larger, there is some controversy regarding small incidental and asymptomatic gastric GISTs. Current recommendations suggest that gastric GISTs under 2 cm with low risk for malignant potential can be managed by active surveillance.[10,11] Several pathology-based studies evaluating micro-GISTs (0.2–10 mm) found that they are widespread within specific populations and likely most do not progress to overt malignant disease. A study in Japan identified unsuspected GISTs less than 5 mm in 35% of 100 consecutive gastrectomy specimens and a study from Germany found GISTs less than 10 mm in size in 22.5% of autopsies in those greater than 50 years old.[12,13] Although there is evidence that micro-GISTs frequently display an activating mutation in the C-KIT oncogene, it seems that multiple genetic alterations are necessary after the transforming KIT mutation before the malignant phenotype is fully expressed.[14]

The clinical work-up of a suspected GIST should be similar to the evaluation of an undiagnosed intra-abdominal mass in any patient. Most are clinically apparent because of size and related symptoms of an intestinal associated mass with the occasional presentation of occult blood loss and anemia. Generally a cross-sectional imaging study is indicated to determine size, location, and associated organ involvement. A contrast-enhanced CT scan of the chest, abdomen, and pelvis is recommended to allow assessment of primary tumor extent and the possible presence of metastatic disease. A typical primary GIST images as an intestinal-based mass with the tumor bulk extrinsic to the bowel (unlike mucosal-based malignancies.) (**Fig. 2**). In many instances, the primary tumor, although bulky, may be pedunculated, particularly if originating from the stomach, allowing for wedge resection rather than a formal gastrectomy. It is unnecessary to obtain a percutaneous image-guided biopsy of a suspected operable GIST because any potential tumor spillage from this procedure can increase the recurrence risk and the tumor can be pathologically characterized

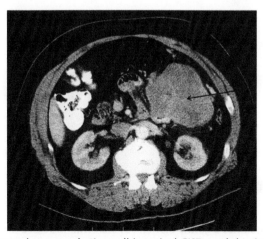

Fig. 2. Arrow indicates large exophytic small intestinal GIST on abdominal CT scan.

after surgical resection. Endoscopic biopsy of accessible tumors can provide for preoperative tissue diagnosis when clinically indicated.

Functional imaging[15] with fludeoxyglucose F 18 position emission tomography (PET) can be an important component to CT, because GISTs tend to be metabolically active and PET avid. Assessment of early metabolic changes, particularly in response to targeted KIT kinase inhibition, may be particularly helpful in a neoadjuvant treatment regimen (**Fig. 3**) or as a diagnostic modality to detect recurrence or complement an ambiguous CT scan. In these specific instances, it is preferable to obtain a baseline PET scan as a comparison before initiation of specific therapy. Because of the added expense and varied interpretation of serial PET imaging, however, the CT evaluation of tumor density changes can often serve as a surrogate for PET evaluative measure of tumor response to kinase targeted therapy in either a primary GIST or in the metastatic setting.[16]

Diagnosis

Elucidation of the pathology of GIST has been closely paralleled by therapeutic advancements. The specific diagnosis of GISTs is defined by morphology, ultrastructure, and immunohistochemistry. These tumors have common immunospecific lineage markers with ICC because both GISTs and ICC stain positive for KIT (CD117).[17] Approximately 95% of GISTs stain for KIT; however, other immunomarkers can also be demonstrated, the most common of which is CD34. Some of the KIT-negative GISTs belong to a small subset oncologically driven by PDGFRA.[10] In a clinically and morphologically suspected GIST that is KIT negative, a diagnosis can sometimes be confirmed by PDGFRA mutational analysis. These GISTs are more likely, however, to be clinically indolent, located within the stomach, and have epithelioid morphology.[18]

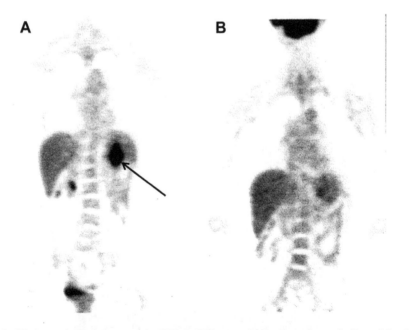

Fig. 3. (A) Arrow indicates a gastric GIST on PET scan with increased metabolic activity. (B) Same patient after induction KIT kinase inhibition before surgery.

The majority of GISTs are composed of a uniform population of spindle cells (70%), epitheloid cells (20%), or a mixed type (10%). GISTs generally have uniform cytologic features, because marked pleomorphism is uncommon, suggesting the expected biology cannot always be predicted by routine hematoxylin-eosin histology alone. KIT staining intensity is not related to either prognosis or response to therapeutic KIT specific inhibitors.

Molecular Classification

The molecular characterization of malignant solid tumors has become increasingly important for both diagnostic and therapeutic considerations. Along with the success of KIT kinase targeted therapy has come a considerable amount of data in GIST related to studies in genotype/phenotype relationships that have led to a molecular classification that is useful for treatment optimization. It is established that 70% to 80% of GISTs harbor a KIT gene mutation and that these mutations lead to constitutive activation of the transmembrane tyrosine kinase, which is an important therapeutic target. Approximately two-thirds of the mutations in KIT affect the juxtamembrane domain encoded by exon 11.[15,19] These mutations disrupt the juxtamembrane scaffolding that normally prevents the kinase activation loop from alternating into an active configuration.[20] These mutations can manifest as in-frame deletions, insertions, substitutions, or a combination.[15] The deletions, in particular codon 557 or 558, are associated with a decrease in progression-free survival (PFS) and overall survival when compared with the other mutations in exon 11.[21] Exon 11 mutated GISTs as a group, however, have the most favorable response as a drugable target for KIT kinase inhibition. The next most common KIT mutation (10%) occurs in the extracellular domain encoded by exon 9. These mutations recapitulate the structural change associated with the binding of the KIT natural ligand stem cell factor. This provides for a downstream signaling mechanism similar to that of a wild-type (lacking KIT or PDGFRA mutation) KIT and this has an effect on inhibitor sensitivity requiring dose escalation of imatinib mesylate, a first-line approved drug for KIT kinase inhibition. The GISTs harboring an exon 9 mutation are more commonly seen in the small and large intestines and are rarely seen in a gastric location.[22] Mutations are uncommonly found (1%) in KIT exon 17 (activation loop) and in (1%) exon 13 (ATP binding site) (**Table 1**).

A minority of GISTs (8%) that lack a detectable gene mutation in KIT have a mutually exclusive activating mutation in PDGFRA, a transmembrane tyrosine kinase homolog of KIT. These mutations can occur within the juxtamembrane domain (exon 12), the ATP binding site (exon 14), or the activation loop (exon 18) and are characterized by a predilection for the stomach with variable and occasionally negative KIT expression. The most common PDGFRA mutation located in exon 18 (D842V) is resistant to present clinically available drugs for targeted tyrosine kinase inhibition (TKI).

Approximately 15% of GISTs do not display a definable KIT or PDGFRA mutation. These are classified by convention as wild-type GISTs. They represent a variety of different genomic changes but are not clinically distinct from mutant KIT or PDGFRA GISTs and generally have identical morphology, express KIT protein on IHC, and can occur anywhere in the GI tract. Although phosphorylated KIT is found in these GISTs, the mechanism of activation is unclear. BRAF, HRAS, and NRAS mutations have been identified as well as defects in succinate dehydrogenase. Approximately 50% of wild-type GISTs also show high expression levels of insulinlike growth factor.[15]

Phase III clinical trials using imatinib and sunitinib (potent inhibitors of KIT and PDGFRA) have confirmed the relationship in metastatic GIST between tumor response and kinase genotype.[22–24] The probabilities of initial exposure resistance to imatinib

Table 1
Molecular classification of GISTs

Genetic Type	Relative Frequency	Anatomic Distribution	Germline Examples
KIT mutation (relative frequency 75%–80%)			
Exon 8	Rare	Small bowel	One kindred
Exon 9 insertion AY502-503	10%	Small bowel and colon	None
Exon 11 (deletions, single nucleotide substitutions and insertions)	67%	All sites	Several kindreds
Exon 13 K642E	1%	All sites	Two kindreds
Exon 17 D820Y, N822K, and Y823D	1%	All sites	Five kindreds
PDGFRA mutation (relative frequency 5%–8%)			
Exon 12 (such as V561D)	1%	All sites	Two kindreds
Exon 14 N659K	<1%	Stomach	None
Exon 18 D842V	5%	Stomach, mesentery and omentum	None
Exon 18 (such as deletion of amino acids IMHD 842–846)	1%	All sites	One kindred
KIT and PDGFRA wild type (relative frequency 12%–15%)			
BRAF V600E	~7%–15%		
SDHA, SDHB, SDHC, and SDHD mutations	~2%	Stomach and small bowel	Carney–Stratakis
HRAS and NRAS mutation	<1%		
Sporadic pediatric GISTs	~1%	Stomach	Not heritable
GISTs as part of the Carney triad	~1%	Stomach	Not heritable
NF1 related	Rare	Small bowel	Numerous

Abbreviations: NF1, neurofibromatosis type I; SDH, succinate dehydrogenase.

for KIT exon 11, KIT exon 9, and wild-type are 5%, 16%, and 23%, respectively. Of clinical relevance, the relationship between response and genotype indicates that the majority of GISTs (exon 11) are sensitive to standard-dose imatinib. Exon 9 mutations may require dose escalation of imatinib or a preference for sunitinib. Rare KIT mutations in the ATP binding domain are more sensitive to sunitinib whereas KIT activation loop mutations are generally resistant to either drug.

Recurrence Risk Factors

Based on histologic criteria alone, it is difficult to classify GISTs with reference to malignant potential and subsequent recurrence risk. The necessity of having a standardized classification for recurrence risk and metastatic potential is crucial to patient discussions regarding prognosis and potential for adjuvant therapy. Although surgical resection remains the cornerstone for the management of primary GIST, complete resection does not always lead to disease eradication. In an attempt to define the variables associated with surgical outcomes, several surgical, tumor, and pathologic related factors have been retrospectively analyzed for their correlation to recurrence **(Table 2)**. Completeness of surgical resection is a technical factor of prognostic importance as is tumor rupture. Patients with operable primary GIST who undergo R0 (complete gross and microscopic) resection have significantly longer survival than those who have incomplete resection. Tumor size, mitotic rate (as a surrogate for tumor grade), and tumor location have become the most significant variables for estimates of malignant potential and recurrence risk.

In 2001, a consensus conference attempted to correlate standards for recurrence risk based on tumor size and mitotic rate, which, by convention, was calculated as number of mitoses/50 high-power fields (HPF).[25] An additional retrospective large database review reported tumor grade as a variable for risk stratification with low-grade GIST 5-year disease-free survival at 100% and high-grade disease-free survival at 15%.[26] Tumor location has also been correlated to recurrence risk with small intestine and colorectal GISTs displaying the worst prognosis.[19] The most comprehensive data collection was published in a review of more than 1900 patients from the Armed Forces Institute of Pathology where risk was evaluated according to tumor size,

Table 2	
Prognostic factors for recurrence after primary surgery for GIST	
Factors	**Increased Risk[a]**

Tumor size, mitotic rate, and tumor site	Gastric GIST
	• Very low risk: 2–5 cm, ≤5/50 HPF
	• Low risk: 5–10 cm, ≤5/50 HPF
	• Moderate risk: >10 cm, ≤5/50 HPF: 2–5 cm, >5/50 HPF
	• High risk: 5–10 cm, >5/50 HPF; >10 cm, >5/50 HPF
	Small intestinal GIST
	• Low risk: 2–5 cm, ≤5/50 HPF
	• Moderate risk: 5–10 cm, ≤5/50 HPF
	• High risk: >10 cm, ≤5/50 HPF; 2–5 cm, >5/50 HPF;
	  5–10 cm, >5/50 HPF; >10 cm, >5/50 HPF
	Duodenal GIST
	• Low risk: 2–5 cm, ≤5/50 HPF
	• High risk: >10 cm, ≤5/50 HPF; 2–5 cm, >5/50 HPF; >10 cm,
	  >5/50 HPF, 5–10 cm > or <5/50 HPF
	Rectal GIST
	• Low risk: 2–5 cm, ≤5/50 HPF
	• High risk: >10 cm, ≤5/50 HPF; ≤2 cm, >5/50 HPF; 2–5 cm,
	  >5/50 HPF; >10 cm, >5/50 HPF, 5–10 cm < or >5/50 HPF

Tumor size and mitotic rate	• Very low risk: <2 cm, <5/50 HPF • Low risk: 2–5 cm, <5/50 HPF • Intermediate risk: <5 cm, 6–10/50 HPF; 5–10 cm, <5/50 HPF • High risk: >5 cm, >5/50 HPF; >10 cm, any mitotic rate; any size >10/50 HPF
KIT mutations	• Deletions in KIT exon 11 at codons 557 to 559
Location of primary GIST	• Small bowel, colon, rectum
Intraoperative factors	• Mucosal invasion • Spontaneous or iatrogenic tumor rupture
Completeness of resection	• R1 (microscopic residual tumor) • R2 (macroscropic residual tumor)
Tumor bulk	• Greater versus lesser tumor bulk

[a] Approximate collective risk: very low—0%, low—3%–9%, moderate—12%–24%, high—55%–90%.

location, and mitotic rate, indicating a spectrum of what constitutes very low recurrence risk to high risk (see **Table 2**).[27–29] Based on these data, nomograms have been developed to provide a more accurate individual patient risk assessment.[30] GIST represents a continual spectrum of biologic potential from essentially benign tumors to aggressive malignancy. Even low-risk GISTs can result, however, in metastatic disease recurrence many years after initial resection and, therefore, patients need long-term and continued follow-up. It is recommended for those patients with resected intermediate-risk/high-risk primary GIST that an abdominal-pelvic imaging study be performed every 3 to 6 months for 3 years, then every 6 months until year 5, followed by yearly imaging. For low-risk patients, every 6 to 12 months for 5 years followed by yearly imaging is recommended. For very low risk GISTs, there is no recommended standard follow-up regimen.

TREATMENT
Surgical Treatment

The surgical management of primary GIST follows those guidelines that apply to the management of sarcomas in general. Complete surgical resection with negative microscopic margins provides the best long-term results. Despite aggressive surgical management, however, historical data suggest a recurrence probability of 50% with an overall survival rate of less than 50% at 5 years. The median time to recurrence after R0 surgical resection has been calculated to be between 19 and 25 months. Recurrences are generally abdominal, involving peritoneum and/or liver, and often not amendable to repeat surgical resection.[31–33] Because GIST develops from stroma of the intestinal wall, lymphatics are rarely involved and, unlike GI mucosal cancers, formal lymph node dissection is rarely indicated. The goal of resection is to provide for negative margins and a segmental resection with a 2 to 3 cm gross margin should suffice for small bowel GIST. For gastric GISTs, a resection margin of several microscopically free millimeters is acceptable and this can usually be accomplished with a wedge resection particularly if the GIST is located on the greater curvature. Segmental or total gastrectomy is reserved for large GISTs that require that extent of surgical resection because of size or location.[34] Careful intraoperative handling of the tumor is essential because rupture can lead to implanted recurrence. Rectal GISTs are rare but can often present as an extraluminal extrinsic mass better defined by endoscopic ultrasound. Small rectal GISTs can be resected by transanal or transsphincteric methods if feasible. Various limited series of laparoscopic resection of small GISTs (generally 5 cm or less and gastric in location) have been reported.[35,36]

The recommended surgical considerations for a microscopically positive margin after surgical resection are controversial. Re-excision may be an option when the original site of the margin can be located and the expected surgical morbidity is low. This is especially relevant to low-risk GISTs where there is a lack of data to demonstrate that redo surgery is associated with better outcome.

Surgery Combined with Tyrosine Kinase Inhibitor for Primary GIST

The surgical management of locally advanced but operable GISTs continues to evolve. Both European Society for Medical Oncology[11] and National Comprehensive Cancer Network[37] guidelines acknowledge the consideration of use of cytoreductive preoperative KIT kinase inhibition as a means of obtaining optimal surgical margins while also promoting potential organ sparing to decrease postoperative morbidity in those patients in whom R0 resection may be difficult to achieve. In addition, this type of cytoreduction may be considered when there is a significant perceived risk of tumor bleeding or rupture during surgical manipulation because of the extensive nature of the tumor.

The prognosis for patients with advanced GIST, whether primary or recurrent/metastatic, was historically poor, with median survival ranging from 9 to 23 months. Surgical resection of large GISTs with high-risk features was generally followed by short disease-free duration. Surgical metasectomy rarely resulted in long-term favorable outcome and standard sarcoma-based chemotherapy or radiation had only marginal benefit if at all. During the past decade, with the better definition of GIST biology, came the nearly simultaneous discovery of oncogenic kinase mutations and the introduction of kinase inhibitor therapy. Based on preclinical activity against KIT-mutated GIST cell lines, imatinib mesylate (Gleevec; Novartis Pharmaceuticals Corporation, One Health Plaza, East Hanover, NJ), a selective oral inhibitor against KIT signaling, was used in a single-drug metastatic GIST phase II trial. The clinical benefit, seen in 85% of the patients in this trial, lead to the first-line indication Food and Drug Administration (FDA) approval of this drug for metastatic GIST in 2001. The study was closely followed by larger phase III trials proving the efficacy of imatinib in metastatic GISTs, with resulting median survival of 5 years with 34% of patients surviving more than 9 years.[38–40]

Based on favorable efficacy and safety data for imatinib in the metastatic disease trials, interest turned to its potential use in the adjuvant setting for primary GISTs to prevent recurrence and improve survival. Initially, small institutional nonrandomized studies suggested the potential for imatinib as a surgical adjuvant in GIST.[41,42] The American College of Surgeons Oncology Group (ACOSOG) Z9000 study established the efficacy for 1 year of adjuvant imatinib in patients with large resected GISTs. This was a single-arm phase II trial for patients with R0 resection of GISTs greater than or equal to 10 cm. With a median follow-up of 4 years, the relapse-free survival (RFS) rates were 94% at 1 year, 73% at 2 years, and 61% at 3 years comparing favorably to historical control of 50% recurrence rate at 5 years for surgery alone.[43] This study was closely followed by ACOSOG Z9001, which was designed as a double-blinded phase III trial randomizing imatinib (400 mg/d) versus placebo for 1 year after R0 surgical resection of primary GISTs ($\geq$3 cm). The clinical endpoint of RFS was reached at a median follow-up of 20 months, with a significant difference favoring the treated group (98% vs 83%). Patients with the larger tumors ($\geq$10 cm) had the greatest statistical benefit. This study with RFS serving as a surrogate for overall survival was the basis for FDA approval of imatinib as an adjuvant therapy after resection of GISTs greater than or equal to 3 cm.[44] This study included a crossover design, which allowed for placebo patients with recurrence to receive imatinib and, therefore, there was not an impact on overall survival by report of the last follow-up. Subgroup analysis from this phase III trial was recently reported at the ACOSOG meeting. Multivariate analysis identified several tumor-related factors for recurrence risk in the placebo group, including large tumor size, small intestine location, high mitotic count, and the presence of exon 11 mutations. The placebo group with tumors indicating mitotic count greater than or equal to 5/50 HPF had a 17-fold higher recurrence risk than those tumors with less than 5/50 HPF. Genotype review revealed that tumors with exon 11 mutations or mutations in PDGFRA were significantly less likely to recur by 2 years when treated with imatinib. It seemed that tumors with exon 9 mutations did not benefit in RFS from imatinib (400 mg/d) although the numbers were too small for statistical relevance. There was a suggestion that 1 year of adjuvant imatinib can delay recurrence in this group; however, there was a steep recurrence rate immediately after imatinib was discontinued. Patients with a wild-type GIST signature showed no benefit from adjuvant treatment.[45] This is suggestive of the importance of GIST genotype and accurate reporting of mitotic counts in discussion of adjuvant therapy benefit.

One of the most compelling questions that remains unanswered from the Z9001 study relates to the optimal duration of adjuvant therapy. It seems that overall RFS in the treated group decreased sharply beginning 6 months after 1 year of imatinib. Although, based on this trial, imatinib was FDA approved for adjuvant use and recommended duration of adjuvant therapy was specifically left as an open consideration, suggesting that perhaps longer drug administration should be a consideration for high-risk GIST patients. Recent data from a European trial addresses the efficacy of 3 years of postoperative imatinib. This study Scandinavian Sarcoma Group XVIII/ Arbeitsgemeinschaft Internistische Onkologie (SSGXVIII/A10) randomized 400 patients with intermediate-risk/high-risk primary GISTs defined as risk of recurrence greater than or equal to 50% (tumor >10 cm or mitotic rate >10/per 50 HPF or tumor >5 and mitotic rate >5/50 HPF), into 2 groups given adjuvant imatinib (400 mg/d) (1 year vs 3 years). After 54 months of median follow-up, GIST patients who received 3 years of imatinib were 54% less likely to recur compared with patients receiving adjuvant therapy for 1 year. This advantage was found irrespective of site or tumor size, although the small subset of patients with exon 9 mutation or wild type did not benefit in terms of RFS compared with the 1-year adjuvant group. In addition, patients receiving extended treatment were 55% less likely to die of progressive disease (92% alive 3-year cohort vs 82% 1-year cohort). This is the first GIST adjuvant study to publish statistical evidence of a survival advantage to prolong treatment duration and should establish 36 months as the new standard duration of adjuvant imatinib for high-risk patients.[46] The duration question will be further examined in a US phase II study designed as a nonrandomized multicenter trial evaluating RFS after 5 years of adjuvant imatinib. Accrual has been completed and the results from this study should add to the accumulating evidence regarding the necessity for long-term adjuvant imatinib coverage.

In those instances of primary GIST where there is concern about the feasibility of achieving a reasonable R0 resection, therapy with neoadjuvant imatinib can be considered. Locally, extensive GISTs can be friable and hypervascular, creating concern for intraoperative tumor fracture. The usefulness of solid tumor downstaging has been a subject of clinical research. The advantage of size and extent of reduction of a duodenal, rectal, or esophageal GIST has the potential of decreasing the morbidity or mortality of a large surgical resection (**Figs. 4** and **5**).[10,47,48] Additionally, neoadjuvant application can potentially combine the cytostatic effect of imatinib

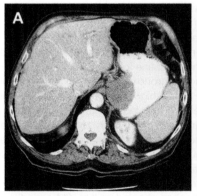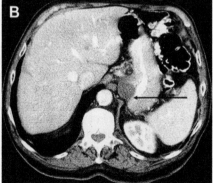

Fig. 4. (*A*) Arrow indicates a large GE junction GIST on CT scan. Without neoadjuvant KIT inhibition, the extent of the tumor would require esophagogastric resection. (*B*) Arrow indicates CT scan evidence of size reduction (6 cm to 2.5 cm) after 3 months of imatinib.

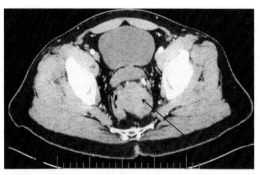

Fig. 5. Arrow indicates a large rectal GIST on CT scan.

with complete resection for a large GIST in an attempt to obviate the subsequent development of imatinib-resistant GIST clones, which have been shown to confound the long-term administration of imatinib in metastatic disease. Several retrospective small patient series support these conceptual advantages.[49,50] In a retrospective subset analysis of the BFR14 phase III trial, the benefits of combining surgical resection and neoadjuvant imatinib were evaluated. Nine of 25 patients had complete resection after a median of 7.3 months of imatinib. All patients who underwent a surgical resection had significantly longer RFS compared with those who did not.[51] The only prospective multi-institutional neoadjuvant GIST trial to date was the Radiation Therapy Oncology Group 0132 study.[52,53] Patients eligible for this trial were required to have greater than or equal to 5-cm primary GISTs or a resectable metastatic GIST index lesion of greater than or equal to 2 cm. Imatinib was given at 600 mg/d for 8 to 12 weeks preoperative and continued for 24 months postoperative. This trial established the safety profile of preoperative imatinib and the potential for down-staging large operable GISTs. Response to neoadjuvant imatinib in resectable GISTs should be evaluated early and continuously and surgical resection should be offered within a 3-month to 12-month time frame because of concern for tumor progression due to development of imatinib resistance and potential loss of operability. The ideal surgical intervention should probably occur within the 6-month to 12-month window depending on clinical objective and subjective response. Adjuvant imatinib should be continued postoperatively in high-risk patients. The advantages of neoadjuvant versus standard postoperative adjuvant for primary GISTs in terms of recurrence or survival have not been well delineated and are largely theoretic. Individual patient clinical information is necessary to consider the optimal recommendations, which should be made in the context of multidisciplinary management.

Historically, surgical treatment for metastatic/recurrent GIST has not been either a viable option or a solution for long-term disease management. This is mostly because recurrent GIST tends to be multifocal within the peritoneal cavity and organ specific to multiple hepatic sites. The median survival for a series of 94 GIST patients in a retrospective review was 19 months, with only 30% able to undergo complete surgical resection.[32] With the successful clinical trials of KIT, TKI surgical resection of metastatic/recurrent GIST has become an increasingly considered adjunct for continued disease control. The expected median time for disease progression on imatinib is approximately 2 years and in selected cases surgical resection of residual stable or limited progressive disease may provide additional patient benefit. There is at least a theoretic potential for the consideration of surgical intervention after initial downsizing of metastatic disease. Reports evaluating specimens retrieved from patients where even complete clinical response to imatinib was anticipated based on preoperative imaging was often noted on final pathology to have residual tumor harboring viable GIST cells.[54] This supports surgical consideration in a patient on imatinib or sunitinib with advanced GIST, indicating stable or responding disease within a 24-month time frame. Perhaps the best window of opportunity is for surgical resection within a 6-month to 12-month drug treatment interval. It has also been shown to be critically important to continue drug postsurgery, perhaps indefinitely, to maintain PFS. There have been several published retrospective studies suggesting an important role for surgical intervention in patients with global stable or responding recurrent GIST. Even those patients with limited progression taking place in 1 or 2 sites with stable disease elsewhere have reported benefit from surgical resection. There is generally no benefit, however, from surgical management of progressive disease at multiple sites not responding to drug therapy. A recent retrospective study of recurrent GIST patients correlated imatinib disease response to surgical outcomes and survival with 12-month overall survival rates of 95%, 86%, and 0% in patients after surgical resection of stable, limited disease progression, and generalized progression.[50] This is consistent with other small institutional retrospective series of similar type. The indications for surgery in recurrent GIST for patients on TKI are the anticipation for complete gross resection in responding patients with measurable disease, the surgical eradication of potentially resistant clones in limited disease progression sites, and the emergent situations of obstruction, perforation, or hemorrhage.

Metastatic Gastrointestinal Stromal Tumors—Treatment

Before an improved understanding of GIST pathobiology, nearly all GI mesechymal tumors were considered in the broad category of leiomyosarcoma. Even at that point, the majority of these tumors had a particularly poor response to sarcoma-based chemotherapy.[55,56] Once the entity of GIST was defined and separable from GI leiomyosarcoma, application of chemotherapy to metastatic GIST was definitively unsuccessful and radiation had limited application for these widespread abdominal tumors. The clinical use of imatinib in GIST followed several significant preclinical studies and was preceded by its successful clinical application for BCR-ABL chronic myeloid leukemia (CML).[57–59]

Imatinib mesylate is an oral potent selective small molecule inhibitor of a family of structurally related tyrosine kinase signaling enzymes. These include KIT, the ABL family of kinases, and PDGFR.[60] Imatinib has a proliferation inhibiting effect on leukemic cell lines expressing BCR-ABL as well as GIST cell lines harboring activated KIT. In 2001, the New England Journal of Medicine reported a rapid and durable regression to imatinib in a single heavily pretreated patient with metastatic GIST.[61] This single patient report was quickly followed by a phase II open-label trial of imatinib for advanced GIST based partially on dosing and toxicity experience from the CML patient trials.[38] This phase II trial assigned 147 patients with heavily pretreated metastatic or unresectable GIST to either 400 mg/d or 600 mg/d of imatinib. Early results from this study indicated a partial response in 54% with reduction in tumor bulk ranging from 50% to 94%. Additionally, 14% had stable disease for a clinical benefit of nearly 70% (Fig. 6). With a median time of 3 months to partial response, it became clear that in some cases, a therapeutic effect could take several months to manifest. There were no reported complete responses, however, in this advanced disease group. Long-term follow-up in these patients indicated a median survival of 57 months with 28% of the patients remaining on imatinib after 71 months.[40] Equivalent response rates were demonstrated in both treatment arms but the study was not powered to address a dosing question.

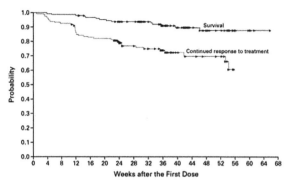

Fig. 6. Kaplan-Meier estimates of overall survival and time to treatment failure. (*From* Demetri GD, von Mehren M, Blanke CD, et al. Efficacy and safety of imatinib mesylate in advanced gastrointestinal stromal tumors. N Engl J Med 2002;347:472–80; with permission.)

Early data with imatinib scheduling indicated a minimum effective dose of 400 mg/d and dose-limiting toxicities at 1000 mg/d, with a dose of 400 mg twice daily (800 mg/d) as a tolerable dose for phase III evaluation.[62] Two large trials (European-Australian Study 62,005 and North American Sarcoma Intergroup Study S0033) studied imatinib (800 mg/d vs 400 mg/d) as initial therapy or as crossover in patients with advanced disease.[39,63] Together, these trials enrolled nearly 1700 patients. Response rates in the European trial were 54% and 50% for the high-dose and low-dose arms, respectively, and 48% in both arms of the North American trial. PFS and overall survival were no different between the 2 arms of the North American study. In the European trial, PFS was prolonged by high-dose therapy. After 3 years of follow-up, however, the PFS advantage seen in the European trial was no longer significant.[64] Together, these data confirmed the 400-mg/d dose as an appropriate starting dose for most patients. For patients with progression of disease at standard dose, approximately 1 in 3 benefited from dose escalation to 400 mg twice daily (800 mg/d). Toxicity data suggested that most patients were able to tolerate the higher dosing after initial dose at 400 mg/d. Clinical benefit of higher dose therapy seemed to result most often from disease stabilization.

Tumor analysis in both trials suggested that patients whose tumors exhibited KIT exon 11 mutations had significantly longer PFS than did patients whose tumors showed exon 9 mutations. Furthermore, patients showing exon 9 mutations in their tumors experienced increased PFS when treated with 800 mg/d initially. Unfortunately, this PFS advantage did not translate into improved overall survival. Controversy remains as to whether exon 9 mutant GIST patients should be started at 800 mg/d or dose escalated when optimal clinical response is lacking.

For patients who experience drug-related side effects, symptom management should be considered before dose reduction, because dose intensity is important for continued maintenance of tumor response.[10] Continuation of therapy is of great importance in responding patients. In a reported prospective study, 50 metastatic GIST patients who were free of progression after 3 years of imatinib were randomized to continuation or interruption of treatment.[65] At a median follow-up of 35 months, 2-year PFS was 80% in the continuation group but only 16% in those who went off therapy. These data confirmed that most patients, even with complete radiographic response, have residual, biologically active, disseminated disease that recurs off treatment. Additionally, when patients experience focal or limited progression on a TKI after dose escalation and in the absence of a clinical trial, there should be consideration that the discontinuation of the TKI may lead to accelerated tumor growth because of withdrawal control of sensitive tumor clones.[66]

Assessing Response to TKI

Objective assessment of response to therapy is critical in all areas of oncology. This has been complicated by use of TKI small molecules where, unlike standard chemotherapy, biologic response may not directly correlate with CT scan response. PET scan has proved a dynamic tool for evaluation of response of GISTs to imatinib. Response to imatinib can be seen on PET within weeks of initiating therapy and may be detected after a single dose of imatinib.[67] Early response to PET correlates with time to progression and allows physician and patient to continue treatment with confidence. Typical dramatic, early response by PET of advanced GISTs to imatinib with only minor response by CT is illustrated in **Fig. 7** (see **Fig. 7**).

It has long been recognized that classic Response Evaluation Criteria in Solid Tumors (RECIST) criteria (30% decrease in measurable disease) significantly underestimate response of GIST to imatinib therapy. Strict use of RECIST criteria is probably only useful in identifying imatinib-resistant disease.[68] Evidence suggests that tumor size (10% decrease) or tumor density (15% decrease) after 2 months of imatinib therapy are predictive of time to progression and correlate extremely well with biologic response by PET scan.[69] This is a useful standard when following patient response by CT.

CT is recommended within 3 months of initiating TKI therapy. Response at this point may manifest by the index GIST tumors becoming more homogeneous and hypoattenuating with disappearance of tumor vasculature and enhancing nodules rather than tumor size difference. In some cases, tumor size might actually increase mainly due to intratumoral hemorrhage or myxoid degeneration and notably maximum tumor downsizing may not be achieved until 6 to 12 months on imatinib. Conversely, tumor progression may initially manifest as a new small intratumoral nodule without change

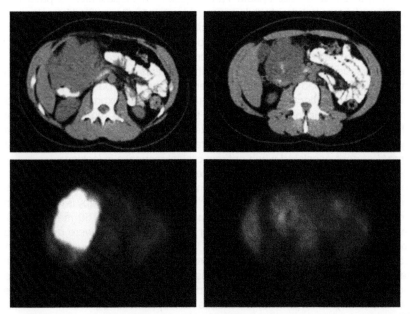

Fig. 7. CT/PET before (*left*) and 3 weeks after (*right*) imatinib in advanced duodenal GIST.

in overall tumor size or as an increase in size of an existing tumor nodule.[70] When findings are suggestive of progression on CT but are inconclusive, PET scan may be of benefit if early therapeutic decisions, such as surgical intervention, need to be considered.

Sunitinib After Imatinib Failure

Sunitinib malate (SU11248, Sutent; Pfizer Pharmaceuticals Corporate Office, New York, YK) is an oral multitargeted receptor TKI. Sunitinib differs from imatinib in its binding characteristics for KIT and PDGFR. In addition, it is an inhibitor of vascular endothelial growth factor receptors (VEGFR-1, VEGFR-2, and VEGFR-3). Preliminary activity led to a randomized, placebo-controlled, multicenter phase III trial of sunitinib in patients with confirmed failure to imatinib therapy.[71] Efficacy was judged by RECIST criteria; 312 patients were enrolled into the study in a 2:1 fashion of sunitinib (50 mg/d 4 weeks on and 2 weeks off [6-week cycle]) versus placebo. There was a crossover option on the trial for patients with progression on placebo. The trial was stopped early after a dramatic time to progression increase was noted for sunitinib (27.3 weeks vs 6.4 weeks) (**Fig. 8**). Time to progression was increased for all subgroups, and response rate was significantly higher than placebo (7% vs 0%). Thus, the vast majority of the sunitinib group had a clinical benefit defined by disease stabilization rather than partial response. Improvement in overall survival, compared with placebo, was also suggested in this trial.

Fatigue was the most common observed side effect with treatment but was similar to placebo, indicating that fatigue was largely due to disease and not treatment. Overall, clinically meaningful tumor control of imatinib-resistant GIST has established sunitinib as the preferred second-line therapy for imatinib failure to standard dose and dose escalation or intolerance.

Other Systemic Therapeutic Options

Salvage therapies for imatinib and sunitinib–resistant GIST have, to date, focused mostly on trials of oral kinase inhibitors. Several of these agents have activity in other diseases and have been studied in GISTs in phase II trials.

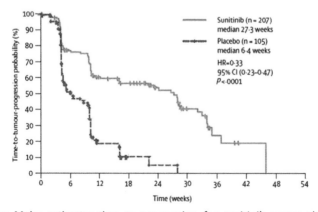

Fig. 8. Kaplan-Meier estimates time to progression for sunitinib versus placebo. (*From* Demetri G, van Oosterom AT, Garrett CR, et al. Efficacy and safety of sunitinib in patients with advanced gastrointestinal stromal tumor after failure of imatinib: a randomized controlled trial. Lancet 2006;368:1329–38; with permission.)

Sorafenib (BAY-43-9006, Nexavar) is an oral, multikinase inhibitor approved for hepatocellular carcinoma. A University of Chicago trial of sorafenib (400 mg twice daily) in patients with imatinib and sunitinib–resistant GIST yielded a disease control rate of 68%, PFS of 5.2 months, and overall survival of 11.6 months.[72] The investigators note that some patients experienced prolonged disease control. Dose reductions were often required in this group of patients, with grade 3 to 4 hand-foot syndrome occurring in 45% of patients.

Nilotinib (Tasigna) is an oral TKI approved for CML. A multicenter phase II trial of nilotinib (400 mg twice daily) as third-line therapy in GISTs showed the drug well tolerated with a median PFS of 113 days and an overall survival of 130 days.[73] Most common side effects were nausea/vomiting, elevated bilirubin, and decreased appetite.

Dasatinib is an oral, multikinase inhibitor with activity in CML. A multicenter trial of dasatinib (70 mg twice daily) in imatinib and sunitinib refractory GISTs showed a partial response rate of 32% by Choi criteria.[74] Overall survival in this group of patients was 19 months. The trial failed to meet, however, its primary target of PFS rate of 30% at 6 months.

Regorafenib is a novel oral kinase inhibitor with a broad spectrum of antitumor activity in preclinical and early phase trials. A multicenter phase II trial of 34 patients with imatinib and sunitinib refractory disease was conducted using regorafenib (160 mg/d) for 21 days on an every-28-day cycle.[75] The drug seemed active, with 19 of 22 patients without disease progression after 4 cycles of therapy on trial. Treatment seemed well tolerated, with hypertension, hand-foot syndrome, and low phosphorus the most common toxicities. A phase III trial is being conducted.

SUMMARY

Management of GISTs has changed dramatically in the past decade as a result of insights into the molecular biology of these tumors. Surgery remains the mainstay for primary GISTs with consideration for adjuvant imatinib to improve both PFS and overall survival in high-risk patients. A combination of imatinib and surgical resection can also be considered for patients with locally advanced or metastatic disease or in primary GISTs where surgical morbidity is potentially significant. Dramatic and clinically meaningful responses are common in patients with metastatic or unresectable disease with first-line imatinib (400 mg/d) therapy. Responding patients should be continued indefinitely on therapy because of the rapid recurrence of disease when drug is withdrawn. High-dose imatinib can be considered for patients with exon 9 mutations and those with progression at standard dose. For patients who are intolerant of or progress on imatinib, treatment with sunitinib 50 mg/d on a 4-week-on–2-week-off schedule can result in improved disease control and overall survival. For patients failing both agents, therapy with a novel kinase inhibitor, ideally on a clinical trial, offers the best option. Therapeutic recommendations for advanced GISTs will certainly change over the next few years as drugs with enhanced TKI and those with novel mechanisms of action are developed. This represents an important and exciting advance in solid tumor oncology and has implications for advances with other tumor types as well.

REFERENCES

1. Perez EA, Livingstone AS, Franceschi D, et al. Current incidence and outcomes of gastrointestinal mesenchymal tumors including gastrointestinal stromal tumors. J Am Coll Surg 2006;202:623–9.

2. Goettsch WG, Bos SD, Breekveldt-Postma N, et al. Incidence of gastrointestinal stromal tumours is underestimated: results of a nation-wide study. Eur J Cancer 2005;41:2868–72.
3. Mucciarini C, Rossi G, Bertolini F, et al. Incidence and clinicopathologic features of gastrointestinal stromal tumors. A population-based study. BMC Cancer 2007; 7:230.
4. Nilsson B, Bumming P, Meis-Kindblom JM, et al. Gastrointestinal stromal tumors: the incidence prevalence, clinical course, and prognostication in the preimatinib mesylate era—a population-based study in western Sweden. Cancer 2005;103: 821–9.
5. Tran T, Davila JA, El Serag HB. The epidemiology of malignant gastrointestinal stromal tumors: an analysis of 1,458 cases from 1992 to 2000. Am J Gastroenterol 2005;100:162–8.
6. Hirota S, Isozaki K, Moriyama Y, et al. Gain-of-function mutations of c-kit in human gastrointestinal stromal tumors. Science 1998;279:577–80.
7. Heinrich MC, Corless CL, Duensing A, et al. PDGFRA activating mutations in gastrointestinal stromal tumors. Science 2003;299:708–10.
8. Hirota S, Ohashi A, Nishida T, et al. Gain-of-function mutations of platelet-derived growth factor receptor alpha gene in gastrointestinal stromal tumors. Gastroenterology 2003;125:660–7.
9. Corless CL, Heinrich MC. Molecular pathobiology of gastrointestinal stromal sarcomas. Annu Rev Pathol 2008;3:557–86.
10. Hohenberger P, Eisenberg B. Role of surgery combined with Kinase inhibition in the management of Gastrointestinal Stromal Tumor (GIST). Ann Surg Oncol 2010; 17:2585–600.
11. Casali PG, Jost L, Reichardt P, et al. Gastrointestinal stromal tumours: ESMO clinical recommendations for diagnosis, treatment and follow-up. Ann Oncol 2009; 20(Suppl 4):64–7.
12. Kawanowa K, Sakuma Y, Sakurai S, et al. High incidence of microscopic gastrointestinal stromal tumors in the stomach. Hum Pathol 2006;37:1527–35.
13. Agaimy A, Wunsch PH, Hofstaedter F, et al. Minute gastric sclerosing stromal tumors (GIST tumorlets) are common in adults and frequently show c-KIT mutations. Am J Surg Pathol 2007;31(1):113–20.
14. Corless CL, McGreevey L, Haley A, et al. C-Kit mutations are common in incidental gastrointestinal stromal tumors one centimeter or less in size. Am J Pathol 2002;160:1567–72.
15. Corless CL, Barnett C, Heinrich M. Gastrointestinal stromal tumors: origin and molecular oncology. Nat Rev Cancer 2011;11:865–78.
16. Choi H. Response evaluation of gastrointestinal stromal tumors. Oncologist 2008; 13(2):4–7.
17. Miettinen M, Sobin LH, Sarlomo-Rikala M. Immunohistochemical spectrum of GIST's at different sites and their differential diagnosis with a reference to CD117 (KIT). Mod Pathol 2000;13:1134–42.
18. Lasota J, Dansonka-Mieszkowska A, Sobin L, et al. A great majority of GIST's with PDGFRA mutations represents gastric tumors of low or no malignant potential. Lab Invest 2004;84:874–83.
19. Wardelmann E, Buttner R, Merkelback-Bruse S, et al. Mutation analysis of gastrointestinal stromal tumors: increasing significance for risk assessment and effective targeted therapy. Virchows Arch 2007;451:743–9.
20. Mol CD, Dougan DR, Schneider TR, et al. Structural basis for the autoinhitibion and STI-571 inhibition of c-kit tyrosine kinase. J Biol Chem 2004;279:31655–63.

21. Wardelmann E, Losen I, Hans V, et al. Deletion of Trp-557 and Lys-558 in the juxtamembrane domain of the c-kit protooncogene is associated with metastatic behavior of gastrointestinal stromal tumors. Int J Cancer 2003;106:887–95.

22. Heinrich M, Corless CL, Demetri GD, et al. Kinase mutations and imatinib response in patients with metastatic gastrointestinal stromal tumor. J Clin Oncol 2003;21: 4342–9.

23. Gajiwala K, Wu JC, Christensen J, et al. KIT kinase mutants show unique mechanisms of drug resistence to imatinib and sunitinib in gastrointestinal tumors. Proc Natl Acad Sci U S A 2009;106:1542–7.

24. Heinrich M, Maki RG, Corless CL, et al. Primary and secondary kinase genotypes correlate with the biological and clinical activity of sunitinib in imatinib resistant gastrointestinal stromal tumor. Clin Oncol 2008;26:5352–9.

25. Fletcher CD, Berman JJ, Corless C, et al. Diagnosis of gastrointestinal stromal tumors: a consensus approach. Hum Pathol 2002;33(5):459–65.

26. Singer S, Rubin BP, Lux ML, et al. Prognostic value of KIT mutation type, mitotic activity, and histologic subtype in gastrointestinal stromal tumors. J Clin Oncol 2002;20:3898–905.

27. Emory TS, Sobin LH, Lukes L, et al. Prognosis of gastrointestinal stromal smooth-muscle (stromal) tumors: dependence on anatomic site. Am J Surg Pathol 1999; 23:82–7.

28. Miettinen M, Lasota J. Gastrointestinal stromal tumors: pathology and prognosis at different sites. Semin Diagn Pathol 2006;23:70–83.

29. Takahashi T, Nakajima K, Nishitani A, et al. An enhanced risk-group stratification system for more practical prognostication of clinically malignant gastrointestinal stromal tumors. Int J Clin Oncol 2007;12:369–74.

30. Gold JS, Gonen M, Gutierez A, et al. Development and validation of a prognostic nomogram for recurrence free survival after complete surgical resection of localized primary gastrointestinal stromal tumor: a retrospective analysis. Lancet Oncol 2009;10:1045–52.

31. NG EH, Pollock E, Munssell MF, et al. Prognostic factors influencing survival in gastrointestinal leiomyosarcomas. Implications for surgical management and staging. Ann Surg 1992;215:68–77.

32. DeMatteo RP. Two hundred gastrointestinal stromal tumors: recurrence patterns and prognostic factors for survival. Ann Surg 2000;231:51–8.

33. Pierie JP, Choudry U, Muzikanski A, et al. The effect of surgery and grade on outcome of gastrointestinal stromal tumors. Arch Surg 2001;136:383–9.

34. Roberts P, Eisenberg B. Clinical presentation of gastrointestinal stromal tumors and treatment of operable disease. Eur J Cancer 2002;38:S37–8.

35. Hindmarsh A, Koo B, Lewis MP, et al. Laparoscopic resection of gastric gastrointestinal stromal tumors. Surg Endosc 2005;19:1109–12.

36. Choi Sm, Kim MC, Jung GJ, et al. Laporscopic wedge resection for gastric GIST: long term follow-up results. Eur J Surg Oncol 2007;33:444–7.

37. NCCN (version 1.2009). The NCCN soft tissue sarcoma clinical practice guidelines in oncology. © National Comprehensive Cancer Network, Inc. Hollywood (FL) 2009;1(15).

38. Demetri GD, von Mehren M, Blanke CD, et al. Efficacy and safety of imatinib mesylate in advanced gastrointestinal stromal tumors. N Engl J Med 2002;347:472–80.

39. Blanke CD, Rankin C, Demetri GD, et al. Phase III randomized intergroup trial assessing imatinib meslyate at two dose levels in patients with unresectable or metastatic gastrointestinal stromal tumors expressing the Kit receptor tyrosine kinase. S0033. J Clin Oncol 2008;26:626–32.

40. von Mehren M. Follow-up results after 9 years of the on-going phase II B2222 trial of imatinib mesylate in patients with metastatic or unresectable KIT positive gastrointestinal stromal tumors [abstract 10016]. J Clin Oncol 2011;29.
41. Nilsson B, Sjolund K, Kindblom LG, et al. Adjuvant imatinib treatment improves recurrence-free survival in patients with high risk gastrointestinal stromal tumors. Br J Cancer 2007;96:1656–8.
42. Brumming P, Andersson J, Meis-Kindblom JM, et al. Neoadjuvant, adjuvant and palliative treatment of gastrointestinal stromal tumors with imatinib: a center based study of 17 patients. Br J Cancer 2003;89:460–4.
43. Dematteo RP, Owzar K, Antonescu C, et al. Efficacy of adjuvant imatinib mesylate following complete resection of localized primary GIST at high risk of recurrence [abstract 8]. ASCO 2008 Gastrointestinal Cancers Symposium, Chicago (IL). 2008.
44. Dematteo RP, Ballman KV, Antonescu CR, et al. Adjuvant imatinib meslyate after resection of localized primary gastrointestinal stromal tumor: a randomized, double-blind, placebo-controlled trial. Lancet 2009;373:1097–104.
45. Corless CL, Ballman KV, Antonescu C, et al. Relation of tumor pathologic and molecular features to outcome after surgical resection of localized primary GIST. Results of the intergroup phase III trial ASOSOG Z9001 [abstracts]. J Clin Oncol 2010;28:10006.
46. Joensuu H, Eriksson M, Sundby Hall K, et al. One vs. three years of adjuvant imatinib for operable gastrointestinal stromal tumor: a randomized trial. JAMA 2012;307(12):1265–72.
47. Eisenberg B, Smith K. Adjuvant and neoadjuvant therapy for primary GIST. Cancer Chemother Pharmacol 2011;67:S3–8.
48. Eisenberg B, Judson I. Surgery and imatinib in the management of GIST. Emerging approaches to adjuvant and neoadjuvant therapy. Ann Surg Oncol 2004;5:465–75.
49. Andtbacka R, Ng DS, Scaife CL, et al. Surgical resection of gastrointestinal stromal tumor after treatment with imatinib. Ann Surg Oncol 2007;14:14–24.
50. Raut C, Posner M, Desai J, et al. Surgical management of advanced gastrointestinal stromal tumors after treatment with targeted systemic therapy using kinase inhibitors. J Clin Oncol 2006;24:2325–31.
51. Blesius A, Cassier PA, Bertucci F, et al. Neoadjuvant imatinib in patients with locally advanced non-metastatic GIST in the prospective BFR14 trial. BMC Cancer 2011;11:72–9.
52. Eisenberg B, Harris J, Blanke CD, et al. Phase II trial of neoadjuvant/adjuvant imatinib mesylate for advanced primary, metastatic/recurrent operable GIST—early results of RTOG 0132. J Surg Oncol 2009;99:42–7.
53. Wang D, Zhang Q, Blanke CD, et al. Phase II trial of neoadjuvant/adjuvant imatinib mesylate for advanced primary and metastatic/recurrent operable gastrointestinal stromal tumors: long term follow-up results of Radiation Therapy Oncology Group 0132. Ann Surg Oncol 2012;19(4):1074–80.
54. Bauer S, Hartmann JT, de Wit M, et al. Resection of residual disease in patients with metastatic gastrointestinal stromal tumors responding to treatment with imatinib. Int J Cancer 2005;117:316–25.
55. Ryan DP, Puchalski T, Supko JG, et al. A phase II and pharmacokinetic study of ecteinascidin 743 in patients with gastrointestinal stromal tumors. Oncologist 2002;7:531–8.
56. Edmonson JH, Marks RS, Buckner JC, et al. Contrast of response to dacarbazine, metomycin, docorubicin, and cisplatin (DMAP) plus GM-CSF between patients with advanced malignant gastrointestinal stromal tumors and patients with other advanced leiomuyosarcomas. Cancer Invest 2002;20:605–12.

57. Heinrich MC, Griffith DJ, Druker BJ, et al. Inhibition of c-kit receptor tyrosine kinase activity by STI 571, a selective tyrosine kinase inhibitor. Blood 2000;96: 925–32.

58. Tuveson DA, Willis NA, Jacks T, et al. STI 571 inactivation of the gastrointestinal stromal tumor c-Kit oncoprotein: biological and clinical implications. Oncogene 2001;20:5054–8.

59. Druker BJ, Tamura S, Buchdunger E, et al. Effects of a selective inhibitor of the Abl tyrosine kinase on the growth of Bcr-Abl positive cells. Nat Med 1996;2(5): 561–6.

60. Buchdunger E, Cioffi CL, Law N. Abl protein tyrosine kinase inhibitor STI 571inhibits in vitro signal transduction mediated by c-Kit and platelet-derived growth factor receptors. J Pharmacol Exp Ther 2000;295:139–45.

61. Joensuu H, Roberts PJ, Sarlomo-Rikala M, et al. Effect of the tyrosine kinase inhibitor ST1571 in a patient with a metastatic gastrointestinal stromal tumor. N Engl J Med 2001;344:1052–6.

62. van Oosterom AT, Judson I, Verweij J, et al. Safety and efficacy of imatinib (ST1571) in metastatic gastrointestinal stromal tumors: a phase I study. Lancet 2001;358:1421–3.

63. Verweij J, Casali PG, Zalcberg J, et al. Progression-free survival in gastrointestintal stromal tumours with high-dose imatinib: randomised trial. Lancet 2004;364: 1127–34.

64. Casali P, Verweij J, Kotasek D. Imatinib mesylate in advanced gastrointestinal stromal tumors (GIST): survival analysis of the EORTC ISG AGITG randomized trial in 946 patients [abstract 711]. Eur J Cancer Suppl 2005;2:201.

65. Le Cesne A, Ray-Coquard I, Bui BN, et al. Discontinuation of imatinib in patients with advanced gastrointestinal stromal tumours after 3 years of treatment: an open-label multicenter randomized phase 3 trial. Lancet Oncol 2010;11(10): 942–9.

66. Van den Abbeele AD, Badawi RD, Manola J, et al. Effects of cessation of imatinib mesylate (IM) therapy in patients with IM refractory gastrointestinal stromal tumors as visualized by FDG-PET scanning [abstract 3012]. J Clin Oncol 2004; 22(Suppl 14).

67. Choi H, Charnsangavej C, de Castro Faria S, et al. CT evaluation of the response of gastrointestinal stromal tumors after imatinib mesylate treatment: a quantitative analysis correlated with FDG PET findings. AJR Am J Roentgenol 2004;183: 1619–28.

68. Benjamin RS, Choi H, Macapinlac HA, et al. We should desist using RECIST, at least in GIST. J Clin Oncol 2007;25:1760–4.

69. Choi H, Charnsangavej C, Faria SC, et al. Correlation of computed tomography and positron emission tomography in patients with metastatic gastrointestinal stromal tumor treated at a single institution with imatinib mesylate: proposal of new computed tomography response criteria. J Clin Oncol 2007;25(13):1753–9.

70. Shankar S, vanSoonenberg E, Desai J, et al. Gastrointestinal stromal tumor: new nodule within a mass pattern of recurrence after partial response to imatinib mesylate. Radiology 2005;235:892–8.

71. Demetri G, van Oosterom AT, Garrett CR, et al. Efficacy and safety of sunitinib in patients with advanced gastrointestinal stromal tumour after failure of imatinib: a randomized controlled trial. Lancet 2006;368:1329–38.

72. Kindler H. Sorafenib in patients with imatinib and sunitinib resistant gastrointestinal stromal tumor: final results of a University of Chicago phase II consortium trial [abstract 10009]. J Clin Oncol 2011;29(Suppl).

73. Nishida T, Sawaki A, Doi T. Phase II trial of nilotinib as third-line therapy for gastrointestinal stromal tumor (GIST) patients in Japan [abstract 10015]. J Clin Oncol 2010;15(Suppl).

74. Trent JC. A phase II study of dasatinib for patients with imatinib resistant gastrointestinal stromal tumor [abstract 10006]. J Clin Oncol 2011;29(Suppl).

75. George S. A multicenter phase II study of regorafenib in patients with advanced gastrointestinal stromal tumor, after therapy with imatinib and sunitinib [abstract 10007]. J Clin Oncol 2011;29(Suppl).

Neoplasms of the Appendix
Current Treatment Guidelines

Suven Shankar, MBBS[a], Panayotis Ledakis, MD[b],
Hatem El Halabi, MD[a], Vadim Gushchin, MD[a],
Armando Sardi, MD[a],*

KEYWORDS

- Appendix cancer • Disseminated peritoneal adenomucinosis (DPAM)
- Peritoneal mucinous carcinoma appendix (PMCA) • Cytoreductive surgery (CRS)
- Hyperthermic intraperitoneal chemotherapy (HIPEC) • Peritoneal carcinomatosis

KEY POINTS

- Appendix tumors are rare and biologically diverse.
- Early referral after appendectomy results in improved outcomes.
- When confined to the abdominal cavity, peritoneal carcinomatosis from appendiceal origin is effectively treated with cytoreductive surgery (CRS) and hyperthermic intraperitoneal chemotherapy (HIPEC).
- Lymph node involvement is associated with poor prognosis.
- Patients with peritoneal carcinomatosis from appendiceal tumors should be referred and treated at a specialized center.

INTRODUCTION

Appendiceal cancers are found in less than 1% of appendectomy specimens.[1] A population-based study from the Surveillance, Epidemiology and End Results program (SEER), from 1973 to 1998, reported the incidence of cancer of the appendix was 0.12 cases per 100,000 people per year and that the most common histology was mucinous adenocarcinoma.[2]

Neoplasms of the appendix are not often suspected before surgery and are found either intraoperatively or on pathologic examination. The increasing awareness of the disease and its pathophysiology and presentation has sparked an increased interest in the surgical and medical oncology fields with respect to the treatment of diseases

Disclosure: None.
Conflict of Interest: None.
[a] Department of Surgical Oncology, Institute for Cancer Care, Mercy Medical Center, 227 Saint Paul Place, Baltimore, MD 21202, USA; [b] Department of Medical Oncology and Hematology, Institute for Cancer Care, Mercy Medical Center, 227 Saint Paul Place, Baltimore, MD 21202, USA
* Corresponding author.
E-mail address: asardi@mdmercy.com

Hematol Oncol Clin N Am 26 (2012) 1261–1290
http://dx.doi.org/10.1016/j.hoc.2012.08.010
0889-8588/12/$ – see front matter © 2012 Elsevier Inc. All rights reserved.

with peritoneal dissemination. The first reference to carcinoma of the appendix was a case reported by Merling in 1838.[3] In 1903 Elting reported a review and case series from 1838 to 1903. Forty-three cases of neoplasms of the appendix were reported of which only 23 were true carcinoma of the appendix. Awareness of neoplasms of the appendix is increasing. They were previously diagnosed as mucinous neoplasms of the ovary. Recent immunohistochemical, molecular, and genetic evidence support an origin in the appendix in most cases with secondary involvement of the peritoneum and/or ovaries. More recently, the classification of the appendiceal carcinomas has been separated from the colorectal tumors in the seventh edition of the American Joint Committee on Cancer *Cancer Staging Manual*.[4]

The appendix first appears at the eighth week of gestation as an out-pouching of the cecum and gradually rotates to a more medial location. Its length varies from 2 cm to 15 cm and is located at the convergence of the taeniae along inferior aspect of the cecum. The tip of the appendix is most commonly retrocecal, but it is pelvic in 30% and retroperitoneal in 7% of the population.[5] The lymphatic drainage is into the anterior ileocolic lymph nodes and histologic examination shows goblet cells that are scattered throughout the mucosa.

An analysis from the SEER 1973 to 2004[6] database of appendiceal cancers (n = 2791) showed that adenocarcinoma accounted for 65.4% of appendiceal cancers, followed by neuroendocrine neoplasms (0.1%–0.2% over 30 years). The incidence of neuroendocrine neoplasms seemed stable whereas that of adenocarcinoma increased 2.6-fold during that time. The overall 5-year survival of appendiceal adenocarcinomas was reported in the SEER database as 46.2%. The reported 5-year survival for subgroups was adenocarcinoma 47.9%, mucinous adenocarcinoma 47.7%, mucinous cystadenocarcinoma 59.0%, signet ring cell carcinoma 20.3%, and lymphomas were 1.7%.[6]

PATHOLOGY

Appendiceal tumors can be broadly classified as epithelial and nonepithelial tumors.[7]

Epithelial Tumors

There are many existing classifications of epithelial appendiceal neoplasms and this reflects the lack of consensus among the pathologists. The limitations of all classification systems are well recognized and even a benign-appearing tumor may exhibit aggressive clinical course.

In 1940, Woodruff and McDonald classified cystic mucinous tumors of the appendix as mucoceles and cystadenocarcinoma grade 1 but by the 1960s to 1970s they were reclassified as mucinous cystadenomas or villous adenomas of the appendix. Higa and colleagues[8] in 1973 classified appendiceal mucinous tumors as cystadenocarcinomas if associated with pseudomyxoma peritonei and cystadenomas if not. Over the past decades there has been controversy among pathologists regarding the classification of some appendiceal tumors due to lack of consensus on the invasive potential of the appendiceal epithelial cells. Some pathologists require destructive invasion of the appendix with infiltrating glands to make the diagnosis of adenocarcinoma and others require the presence of a broad front with neoplastic epithelium directly abutting the hyalinized cyst wall thinning out the muscularis mucosae.[7]

In 1995, Carr and colleagues[9] reviewed 184 tumors at the Armed Forces Institute of Pathology and proposed the following classification:

1. Adenoma: dysplastic epithelium with mucin dissecting into wall with intact muscularis mucosae

2. Mucinous tumors of uncertain malignant potential: well-differentiated mucinous epithelium without invasion or with mucin in the wall or outside the appendix with loss of muscularis mucosae
3. Adenocarcinoma: invasive neoplastic cells beyond muscularis mucosae

In 2003 Misdraji and colleagues[10] classified them as low-grade mucinous neoplasms and mucinous adenocarcinoma.

Pai and Longacre[11] in 2005 also proposed a classification:

1. Adenoma: mild-to-moderate atypia, mitosis, no stromal invasion, perforation with mucin
2. Mucinous tumor of uncertain potential: adenoma with positive margin, mucin present within the wall
3. Mucinous tumor–low malignant potential: adenoma with neoplastic cells in peritoneum
4. Adenocarcinoma: invasive mucinous tumor

In 1995, Ronnett and colleagues[12] analyzed the clinicopathologic features of 109 cases of multifocal peritoneal mucinous tumors and classified these as

1. Diffuse peritoneal adenomucinosis (DPAM): mucin with fibrosis and scant simple to focally proliferative mucinous epithelium with minimal cytologic atypia and mitotic figures. The primary appendiceal tumor was an adenoma in all these cases.
2. Peritoneal mucinous carcinoma (PMCA): the primary tumor is appendiceal adenocarcinoma with peritoneal tumors having more proliferative epithelium with signet ring cells and marked cytologic atypia.

There were 14 of 109 cases that were classified as PMCA–I (intermediate) because they showed features of DPAM with carcinoma in the peritoneal lesions, whether or not the primary site demonstrated carcinoma. In a follow-up study, Ronnett[12] clarified that PMCA–I should be included into the PMCA group because they behaved similarly.

The authors' group uses the modified Ronnett classification for peritoneal dissemination of appendiceal neoplasms.[12] Its advantage is that it approximately divides the tumors into less-aggressive DPAM and more-aggressive PMCA, the latter having a potential to develop nodal, liver, and other metastases.

Every team specializing in treatment of appendiceal malignancies should establish a clear communication with a pathologist to have a common language when classifying the appendix tumors. Also, a critical review of the oncological outcomes should be conducted periodically to realign the pathologic classification used and the clinical practice. Further efforts should be undertaken by the collaboration of all centers treating these conditions to try to standardize the pathology of appendiceal neoplasms.

Nonepithelial Tumors

1. Endocrine tumors
   a. Classic appendiceal endocrine tumors
   b. Goblet cell carcinomas
2. Lymphoma
3. Sarcoma

Endocrine tumors are classified according to the World Health Organization and TNM classifications.[13,14]

WHO classification

a. Well-differentiated endocrine tumor (benign behavior and uncertain behavior)
b. Well-differentiated endocrine carcinoma, low grade, malignant
c. Mixed exocrine-endocrine, malignant, goblet cell carcinoid (GCC)

A TNM classification and grading scheme was proposed by the European Neuroendocrine Tumor Society in 2007 (**Table 1**).

GCC tumors of appendix are rare endocrine tumors that have various names, such as adenocarcinoid, mucinous carcinoid, crypt cell carcinoma, and mucin-producing neuroendocrine tumor, but first coined, *goblet cell carcinoid*, in 1974 by Subbuswamy and colleagues.[15] Current understanding of GCC's origin states that it is an amphicrine tumor, which originates from a single undifferentiated pluripotent intestinal epithelial crypt base progenitor stem cell that has dual neuroendocrine and mucinous differentiation. The natural history of these tumors is intermediate between carcinoids and classical adenocarcinomas of the appendix[16]; hence, a proposed name is mucin-producing neuroendocrine tumor (or carcinoma) of the appendix. Unlike adenocarcinomas, K-ras and β-catenin expression is absent in these tumors. These tumors show allelic loss of chromosomes 11q, 16q, and 18q, similar to ileal carcinoids.

Classification
    Group A: typical low-grade GCC
    Group B: adenocarcinoma ex GCC with signet ring cell type
    Group C: adenocarcinomas ex GCC, poorly differentiated

CLINICAL PRESENTATION OF NONEPITHELIAL AND EPITHELIAL NEOPLASMS OF THE APPENDIX
Carcinoids

Carcinoids are most commonly located at the tip of the appendix and they present most of the time with appendicitis. They are divided into 2 types. The insular type resembles enterochromaffin cell and produces serotonin. Lymph node and liver metastasis are rare. The tubular variant of carcinoid arises from the L-cell, which produces enteroglucagons and peptide YY. Immunohistochemistry can distinguish an adenocarcinoma from a tubular carcinoid because the latter is positive for chromogranin and/or synaptophysin. Tumors less than or equal to 1 cm require only an appendectomy. If 1 cm to 2 cm in size without involvement of the base of appendix, they are managed with appendectomy and the question of adding a right hemicolectomy depends on grade, mitotic activity, invasion of mesoappendix, or lymphovascular invasion. These patients should be discussed at a multidisciplinary conference. Tumors 2 cm or larger are at risk for lymph node or distant metastasis and a right hemicolectomy is indicated. Also, for tumors with invasion into the

Table 1		
European Neuroendocrine Tumor Society grading of endocrine tumors		
Grade	**Mitotic Count (10/HPF)[a]**	**Ki -67 Index (%)[b]**
G1	<2	<2%
G2	2–20	3%–20%
G3	>20	>20%

[a] 10 high power field (HPF) = 2 mm², at least 40 fields (at 40 × magnification) evaluated in areas of highest mitotic density.
[b] MIB1 antibody; % of 2000 tumor cells in areas of highest nuclear labeling.

mesoappendix, lymphovascular invasion, or increased mitotic activity (Ki index >3%), a right hemicolectomy should be considered.[17]

Goblet Cell Carcinoids

The most common presentation is appendicitis but could also be a bowel obstruction, intussuception, gastrointestinal bleeding, and chronic lower abdominal pain. More than 50% of patients present with metastatic disease and frequently an appendiceal primary is not considered. This is more common in women, who have ovarian metastasis and are misdiagnosed as having ovarian primary. None of the patients presents with carcinoid syndrome, and urinary 5-hydroxyindoleacetic acid levels and other neuroendocrine markers are usually within normal limits. The clinical outcome of GCC is more favorable than stage-matched adenocarcinoma of the appendix. The most common route of metastasis is transcoelomic but metastasis to lymph nodes, ribs, and vertebra are also reported. Stage and grade of the tumor are important prognostic factors. High mitotic activity, high Ki index greater than 3%, nodal involvement, angioinvasion, and increased mucin production indicate aggressive behavior.[16]

Epithelial Tumors

Patterns of presentation vary widely, which adds to the inability of initial care providers to diagnose correctly the cause of appendiceal neoplasms. The tumors present as an incidental finding in the appendectomy specimen, for appendicitis, as a pelvic mass or as peritoneal carcinomatosis with or without ascites. Appendicitis is a common presentation in men and woman combined[18] but peritoneal dissemination of mucinous appendiceal neoplasm is an important initial presentation. Patients also present to primary care physicians with abdominal distension, increasing abdominal girth, fatigue, weight gain, shortness of breath, and early satiety. Women are usually referred to a gynecologist for possible ovarian cancer. A high percentage of patients are referred to general surgeons after debulking gynecologic surgery for pelvic masses presumed of ovarian origin. Umbilical, inguinal, and incisional hernias filled with mucin, discovered at the time of hernia surgery, is another mode of presentation.

When the mucin extrudes through the appendicular wall due to increased intraluminal pressure, the mucin-producing tumor cells are released into the free peritoneal cavity (**Fig. 1**). The flow of mucin follows that of peritoneal fluid and circulates in a clockwise direction from the right paracolic sulcus, right subdiaphragmatic area, retrohepatic vena cava, left diaphragm, splenic hilum, and ligament of Treitz. The

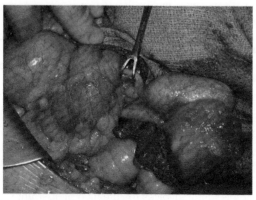

Fig. 1. Appendiceal neoplasm with mucin extrusion.

falciform ligament directs flow to the pelvis, the cul de sac, left paracolic sulcus, and ovaries. The small bowel due to peristalsis is generally initially not involved with the mucinous implants.[18]

DIAGNOSIS

The goals of the work-up include staging of the appendiceal tumor, characterizing the biologic behavior by its histology, clinical history, physical examination, and radiologic studies and deciding if surgery should be a part of the treatment plan. The authors recommend summarizing the final work-up and pretreatment diagnosis by a team familiar with treatment of appendiceal neoplasms and patients with peritoneal carcinomatosis. The reason for this recommendation is that patients could be denied surgical treatment and a chance for long-term survival based on widespread belief that peritoneal carcinomatosis is a contraindication for aggressive surgery. Only an experienced cytoreduction surgeon could determine if complete removal of all visible tumor is possible or if debulking surgery for palliation could help improve the quality of life (QOL) in patients with large accumulation of mucin. As discussed previously, the clinical presentation should be a clue to the physician about a potential appendiceal neoplasm. The physical examination of such patients should also include a digital rectal and pelvic examination to assess for masses in the pelvis and the mobility of these structures to the surrounding anatomy. It is confirmed by preoperative imaging studies, intraoperative findings, or postoperative pathology results. Delay in diagnosis is a common problem due to lack of understanding of the pathophysiology of this condition. The authors' group presented data that the time from diagnosis to treatment with CRS and HIPEC of more than 6 months correlated with worse outcome.

Preoperative Studies

CT
Most patients have a CT scan of the abdomen and pelvis before being referred to a peritoneal surface malignancy program. Findings suggestive of an appendiceal neoplasm are appendiceal dilation or mass and gross ascites with a mucinous component. The mucin maybe seen distributed as discussed previously or in hernia sacs when present. There is nodularity of the lining of the diaphragm and potential indentations on the surface of the liver from the solid component of mucin. The mesentery of the small bowel could be foreshortened from the fibrotic reaction of the tumor in the mesentery leading to a mushroom-shaped image on CT scan (**Fig. 2**). Rarely, hydroureter (**Fig. 3**) is seen when tumor involves the vesicoureteral junction, which may have compromised renal function **Fig. 4** shows extensive involvement of all areas of the peritoneal cavity. PET scan have not shown promise in the case of DPAM or PMCA.[19] The use of MRI is attractive due to reduced radiation exposure but its use should be determined based on the expertise of a radiologist to read abdominal MRI.

Tumor markers
Carcinoembryonic antigen (CEA), CA19-9, and CA-125 are potential tumor markers in epithelial appendiceal neoplasms. One or any combination of them can be elevated in 60% of patients. A preoperative level is routinely done. Their use is primarily for follow-up and as a response to therapy. After CRS and HIPEC, they are helpful in following a patient's clinical status and are indicative of recurrence. The elevation can precede the CT findings by several months. None of them is specific to either DPAM or PMCA. Multiple abnormal tumor markers were not useful as an exclusion criterion for

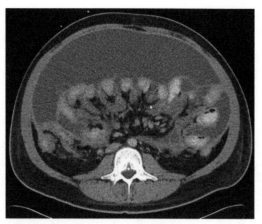

Fig. 2. Foreshortened mesentery on preoperative CT scan.

patients undergoing CRS. The 3-year survival rates in patients with elevated versus nonelevated CA-125 levels were 83% versus 52% (*P* = .003); hence, an elevation in CA-125 is an important indicator of survival in these patients.[20]

Preoperative Evaluation for Cytoreductive Surgery and Hyperthermic Intraperitoneal Chemotherapy

A thorough history and physical examination is important. Laboratory studies, including complete blood cell count and complete metabolic panel with tumor markers, CEA, cancer antigen (CA) 19-9, and CA-125, are obtained. A CT scan of the chest abdomen and pelvis with oral and intravenous (IV) contrast is important in assessment. Preoperative clearance studies in the form of ECG or chest radiograph (if no CT scan) are obtained. Cardiac stress test is indicated when patients are older than 65 years or have

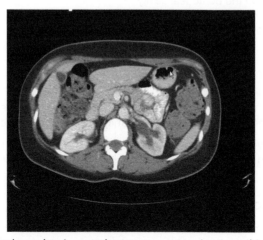

Fig. 3. Left-sided hydronephrosis secondary to tumor at vesicoureteral junction.

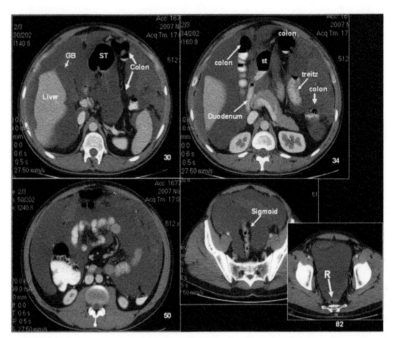

Fig. 4. Depiction of extensive involvement of tumor in all areas of the peritoneal cavity. GB, gallbladder; R, rectum; ST, stomach.

a positive cardiac history. The patients are also required to have a colonoscopy to assess for any polyps or masses. Split renal function studies are indicated only in a rare situation where a nephrectomy maybe considered necessary.

Contraindications to CRS/HIPEC

Absolute
1. Extension outside the peritoneal cavity
2. Biliary obstruction
3. Multiple small bowel obstructions

Relative
1. Poor functional status of patient
2. Cardiac contraindication
3. Foreshortened mesentery that would result in postoperative short bowel syndrome. Although the CT scan can suggest it, it is not always a reliable sign.

Parenchymal involvement of the liver, which is rare in appendiceal neoplasms, is not a contraindication to CRS and HIPEC but should be amenable to a complete resection.

SURGICAL TECHNIQUE AND POSTOPERATIVE CARE

Laparoscopy can be utilised to access the extent of small bowel involvement, but in patients with extensive disease in the omentum and previous surgeries, it is difficult to evaluate completely the extent of small bowel involvement. It is imperative to place all laparoscopic ports in the midline in an effort to reduce port site recurrences that could complicate further surgery. The authors' group has demonstrated a postsite recurrence of 34% of port sites resected. The extent of small bowel resection determines the QOL after cytoreduction. Every effort should be made to minimize bowel resection even if it requires multiple anastomosis or wedge resections to accomplish that goal.

Under general anesthesia, a midline xiphopubic incision is used to gain access to the abdominal cavity. Tumor burden is calculated using the peritoneal cancer index (PCI), as reported by Sugarbaker (**Fig. 5**).[20]

Lesion size score is applied to each of the 9 abdominopelvic regions, the jejunum, and the ileum. Summation of the lesion size score gives the PCI (range = 1–39).[18] Surgical resection of the primary tumor is done followed by peritonectomy procedures originally described by Sugarbaker.[20] The extent of surgery is determined by the size and location of the tumor. The objective is to remove all visible tumor (complete cytoreduction). Complete resection is defined as completeness of cytoreduction score, CC-0 or CC-1 (**Box 1**).

Findings at surgery could be consistent with appendiceal mass, mucin in the abdomen, bowel obstruction from mucinous component, foreshortened mesentery, peritoneal implants, diaphragmatic implants, masses, or nodules at previous laparoscopic port sites.

Peritonectomy procedures are done as needed to achieve a good cytoreduction and may include anterior abdominal wall peritonectomy, greater omentectomy and splenectomy; left and right upper quadrant peritonectomies with stripping of the respective hemidiaphragms, which requires the placement of chest tubes; lesser omentectomy with cholecystectomy and striping of the omental bursa and porta hepatis; or pelvic peritonectomy with total abdominal hysterectomy and bilateral salpingo-oophorectomy with/without anterior resection of the rectum. Visceral peritonectomy and resection is frequently needed to accomplish this goal. Final assessment of cytoreduction is recorded based on the CC score (see **Box 1**).

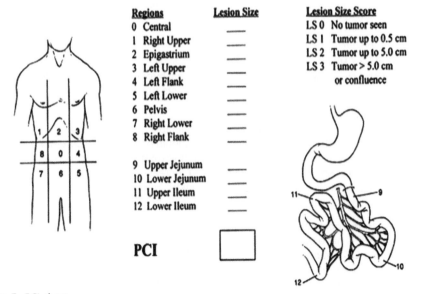

Regions	Lesion Size	Lesion Size Score
0 Central	——	LS 0 No tumor seen
1 Right Upper	——	LS 1 Tumor up to 0.5 cm
2 Epigastrium	——	LS 2 Tumor up to 5.0 cm
3 Left Upper	——	LS 3 Tumor > 5.0 cm
4 Left Flank	——	or confluence
5 Left Lower	——	
6 Pelvis	——	
7 Right Lower	——	
8 Right Flank	——	
9 Upper Jejunum	——	
10 Lower Jejunum	——	
11 Upper Ileum	——	
12 Lower Ileum	——	

PCI ☐

Fig. 5. PCI chart.

> **Box 1**
> **Estimating the CC score with respect to residual tumor size after cytoreduction**
>
> CC-0 = No visible tumor
>
> CC-1 = 0–0.25 cm
>
> CC-2 = 0.25–2.5 cm
>
> CC-3 = >2.5 cm

After the cytoreduction and before any anastomosis is made, HIPEC is performed intraoperatively with mitomycin C for 90 minutes at a total dose of 40 mg (30 mg given initially and 10 mg added after half an hour of perfusion) using a closed technique. The outflow temperature is maintained at 41°C to 42°C. Urine output is maintained (250–400 mL/h) by using crystalloids and albumin to prevent renal toxicity. During the perfusion the patient is shaken manually and the operating table is positioned in different directions every 15 minutes. On completion of perfusion, the abdomen is opened and gastrointestinal reconstruction is done as appropriate.

Patients are transferred to an ICU where hemodynamic parameters and fluid status are carefully monitored. The authors' practice is to place chest tubes bilaterally immediately postoperatively when diaphragmatic peritonectomy is performed. The Jackson-Pratt drains that are placed in the Morison pouch, pelvis, and near the tail of pancreas are also monitored. Patients are subsequently transferred to the surgical floor when stable. Usually the following morning, physical therapy is started on postoperative day 1 and early mobilization is encouraged. Deep vein thrombosis prophylaxis is implemented during and after using compression stockings, low-molecular-weight heparin, and early mobilization. Patients are discharged from hospital when clinically stable. Patients from out of town are requested to stay in town to make sure they can maintain good hydration and nutrition. It important to be proactive because patients become dehydrated and consult late, leading to increased rate of readmissions. Baseline clinical assessment with complete physical examination; CT scan or MRI of chest, abdomen, and pelvis; and tumor markers is done at 2 months postoperatively, then every 6 months for the first 5 years, and then yearly until year 10.

Important Technical Considerations

Open or closed HIPEC

The open and closed techniques for intraperitoneal hyperthermic chemotherapy have been used.[21] To date, no conclusive evidence exists that one is superior to another.[22]

Initial entrance into abdominal cavity

Most patients present to the authors with multiple previous surgeries and with advanced disease. Entrance into the abdomen should be performed carefully because frequently adhesions to the small bowel can lead to multiple enterotomies and consequently increased small bowel resections and increased complications. If possible, the abdominal cavity is entered high in the epigastric region where the liver or stomach can be found easily with less incidence of bowel adhesions.

Approach to the porta hepaticus during CRS

CRS and HIPEC have become important options for patients with peritoneal carcinomatosis. The CC determines survival. Frequently, the porta hepaticus and the lesser sac are massively involved by tumor (**Fig. 6**). Encasement of portal triad, lesser omentum, retrohepatic vena cava, duodenum, and stomach is frequently seen. The proximity to major portal structures and retrohepatic vena cava makes this dissection

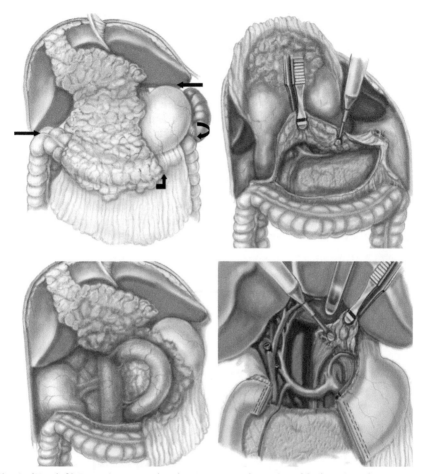

Fig. 6. (*Top left*) Extensive tumor burden over porta hepaticus; black arrows show routes of access to porta hepaticus. (*Top right*) Mobilization of tumor over pancreas to expose common hepatic artery. (*Bottom left*) Kocherization of duodenum. (*Bottom right*) Dissection of retrohepatic IVC and crus of diaphragm.

challenging. In the authors' experience, this is the area where meticulous surgical technique and expertise are necessary to obtain complete removal of all tumor. Some specific technical considerations are important to assure that all tumor is safely removed. These are

- Determining the extent of resection of other areas of the abdomen to assure the level of cytoreduction that can be accomplished
- Determining the extent of bowel resection needed to evaluate if a partial gastrectomy will significantly worsen QOL
- Performing right and left diaphragmatic peritonectomies and mobilizing all ligaments of the liver to obtain adequate liver mobility with the dissection of the round ligament at the end
- Completing mobilization of the greater curvature of stomach to evaluate the extent of involvement of the lesser sac

- Performing cholecystectomy and peritonectomy over the infrahepatic vena cava to gain access to the foramen of Winslow and portal triad. Peritonectomy at this level needs to be extended as far as possible to the retrohepatic vena cava and segment 1 of the liver, including the posterior aspect of the portal triad. This maneuver makes the dissection from the lesser sac easier.
- If the portal triad is not accessible anteriorly, as is frequently the case, it should be approached through the gastrocolic space (see **Fig. 6**). Performing the peritonectomy over the pancreas, where there is frequently large tumor bulk, facilitates the exposure to the celiac trunk and hepatic artery. Once the hepatic artery is identified and protected, the dissection can be carried anteriorly to the portal trial (**Fig. 7**) by transecting the tumor and separating stomach and duodenum from the porta hepaticus (see **Fig. 6**). The dissection is continued along the anterior aspect of the portal triad toward the base of the round ligament.
- Separating the lesser omentum by incising the peritoneum close to the liver down to the anterior portion of segment 1. An accessory left hepatic artery from the left gastric artery if present can be ligated. Extend the dissection over segment 1

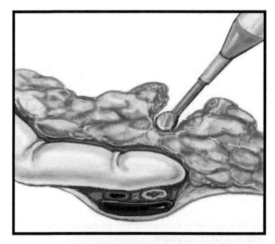

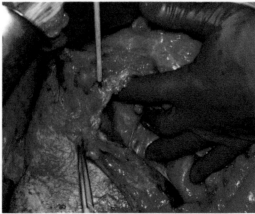

Fig. 7. Anterior approach to portal structures.

toward the foramen of Winslow to meet the previous dissection from the infrahepatic vena cava.

- Starting the dissection of the retrohepatic vena cava superiorly at the level of the esophagogastric junction and right crux of the diaphragm. By elevating this peritoneum, the left hepatic vein and inferior vena cava (IVC) can be approached safely. A Heywood-Smith clamp facilitates the traction and the peritoneum over the IVC and it can be dissected anteriorly at its junction to the liver. Dissection is extended inferiorly to meet the previous dissection from the foramen of Winslow. Once the portal area has been cleared (**Fig. 8**), the authors proceed to clear the round ligament. In this area, the tumor is frequently deeply imbedded into the fissure.
- To obtain complete cytoreduction in these cases, a partial gastrectomy is frequently required. If this is the case, the transsection of the antrum can be done first to facilitate the exposure of the porta hepaticus, but this should only be done once it is clear that the portal triad can be cleared and the first or second portion of duodenum is free of tumor for appropriate closure.

This meticulous surgical technique may allow complete cytoreduction in patients with high volume disease who otherwise would not be considered surgical candidates. The authors prefer low current electrocautery for dissection of the porta hepaticus,[23–33] allowing good hemostasis while minimizing the possibility of injury to the portal structures.

Bowel Resection and Anastomoses

It has been suggested that approximately 150 cm of small bowel should be left behind and 200 cm if a total colectomy is performed to avoid a short gut syndrome. This may require multiple anastomoses. All anastomosis are performed after the completion of the hyperthermic chemotherapy. The only exception is the esophageal anastomosis, due to the difficulty in performing the esohagojeunostomy when post-HIPEC edema is present. There are multiple ways to perform an anastomosis. The authors' preference is as follows.

Anastomosis of the stomach to small bowel is performed with an interrupted hand sewn single layer technique using 3.0 silk (Billroth II type end-to-side retrocolic gastrojejunostomy). The stomach is sutured to the transverse mesocolon to keep the anastomosis in the infracolonic position and avoid constriction of the bowel loop. If resection of the lesser omentum without gastrectomy compromised the vagus nerve,

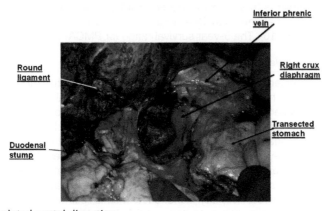

Fig. 8. Completed portal dissection.

an interrupted single layer pyloroplasty using 3.0 silk sutures (Heineke-Mikulicz type) is performed. For total gastrectomy, an end to side esophagojejunostomy (roux-en-Y) is done using a 28-mm EEA stapler. A total gastrectomy is rarely required even in patients with bulky disease.

The small bowel to small bowel, small bowel to colon, and colon to colon anastomoses are done with stapled side-to-side functional anastomosis using a linear cutter GIA-55, 3.2 mm, and a TA-55. The crossover of the staple lines is reinforced by 3.0 silk sutures.

Colorectal anastomosis is done with EEA 31-mm, 4.2-mm stapler. After the anastomosis is performed, the anastomotic rings are inspected and the anastomosis tested for leaks by insufflating air into the rectum while the pelvis is filled with normal saline. Protective ileostomies are not routinely performed. Commonly the rectal stump is at the level of the seminal vesicles or midvagina.

Occasionally, the authors perform a protective ileostomy in cases of extensive dissection of the distal rectum in patients with previous low anterior resections.

PROGNOSTICS INDICATORS OF TREATMENT OF APPENDICEAL NEOPLASM USING CRS AND HIPEC
Completeness of Cytoreduction

This is a major quantitative prognostic indicator for mucinous appendiceal neoplasms that is performed after CRS has been completed (**Fig. 9**). A complete cytoreduction is defined as CC-0 or CC-1.

The optimal cytoreduction of 2.5 mm has been adopted because it is the size of tumor that correlates with the level of penetration of the different agents used intraperitoneal hyperthermic chemotherapy.[18] CC score is an important prognostic indicator discussed by different investigators.[34-36] It is the only prognostic variable that is affected by the surgeon. It is important that every effort be made to accomplish a complete cytoreduction regardless the time required for it.

Omohwo and colleagues[37] have reported 60% overall 3-year survival for patients with high-grade appendiceal neoplasm. Survival by CC was 78% for patients with a low CC score (0–1) and 28% in patients with a high CC score (2–3; $P = .01$). Survival analysis by tumor histology was 80% for patients with low-grade tumors and 52% for patients with high-grade tumors ($P = .024$).

Histopathology

The survival of patients treated with CRS and HIPEC is affected significantly by the histopathology and patients with DPAM have better long-term survival than those with PMCA (see **Fig. 10**). The 5-year survival range for PMCA ranges 40% to 45%.[19]

Peritoneal Cancer Index

The PCI is determined at the time of surgical exploration of the abdomen/pelvis.[21] Higher levels of PCI have been associated with lower survival. This significance is more notable in patients with PMCA. Even though PCI has prognostic significance, it should not be considered an exclusion criteria.

El Halabi and colleagues[35] showed that with PMCA patients who had complete cytoreduction, the 5-year overall survival with PCI greater than 20 was 45% and PCI less than 20 was 66%. Patients who underwent a complete cytoreduction, excluding PCI data, had a 5-year overall survival of 40%.[35] Sugarbaker[18] (**Fig. 11**) reported that in appendiceal neoplasms that show adenomucinosis (DPAM) histology, PCI is an important prognostic indicator and PCI less than 20 has a prognosis of

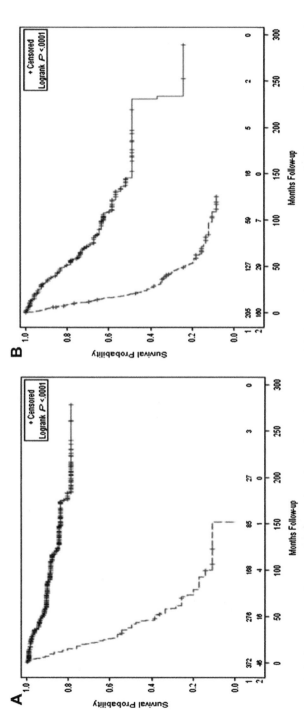

Fig. 9. Survival of patients with mucinous appendiceal neoplasms by CC score. (A) Shows adenomucinosis patients; the blue top line (N = 372) indicates patients with complete cytoreduction, and the red bottom line (N = 46) indicates incomplete cytoreduction. (B) The impact of complete versus incomplete cytoreduction for mucinous carcinoma patients. The blue top line indicates complete cytoreduction (N = 205), and the red bottom line indicates incomplete cytoreduction (N = 160). (*Data from* Sugarbaker PH. Epithelial appendiceal neoplasms. Cancer J 2009;15(3):225–35.)

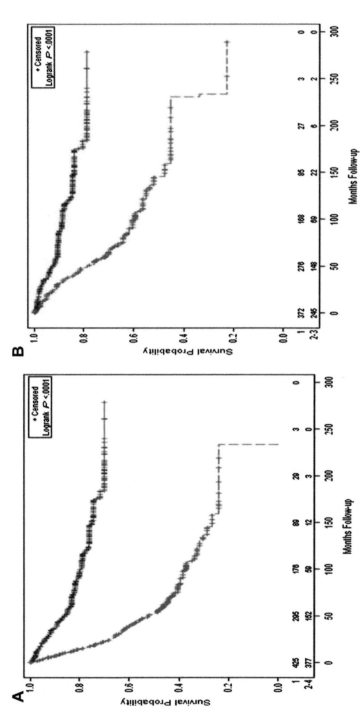

Fig. 10. Survival of patients with mucinous appendiceal neoplasms by histopathology. (*A*) The blue top line (N = 425) indicates patients with adenomucinosis. The red bottom line (N = 377) indicates patients with mucinous adenocarcinoma and includes patients with intermediate type histology. (*B*) Limited to patients with a complete cytoreduction. There were 372 adenomucinosis patients (*blue top line*) and 245 patients (*red bottom line*) with mucinous adenocarcinoma. (*Data from* Sugarbaker PH. Epithelial appendiceal neoplasms. Cancer J 2009;15(3):225–35.)

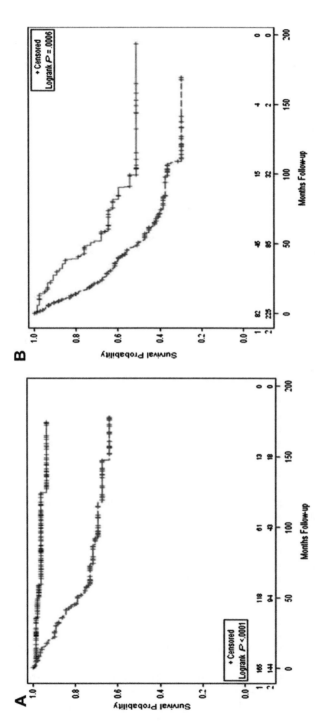

Fig. 11. Survival by PCI for mucinous appendiceal neoplasms. (A) Adenomucinous patients with PCI 1 to 20 (*blue top line*) (N = 165) versus 21 to 39 (*red bottom line*) (N = 144). (*B*) Mucinous carcinoma patients with PCI 1–20 (*blue top line*) (N = 82) versus 21–39 (*red bottom line*) (N = 225).

94% at 20 years. In patients who have histologically an invasive component, the PCI continues to show statistical difference on survival.[18]

Prior Surgical Score

Prior surgical score (PSS) quantitates the extent of surgery performed before the definitive CRS and HIPEC. The previous PCI diagram is used with the exclusion of sites 9 through 12.

PSS = 0, indicates that only a biopsy was performed
PSS = 1, one region with prior surgery
PSS = 2, indicates 2 to 5 regions previously dissected
PSS = 3, indicates more than 5 regions were dissected

PSS of 0 to 2 versus PSS 3 has been shown to have a statistically significant impact on survival in patients with DPAM, with improved survival with lower PSS (**Fig. 12**).[18] PSS does not correlate with significant survival advantage in PMCA patients.[18] The importance of PSS is that multiple and extent of previous surgeries make CRS more difficult and more extensive with prolonged operative time. This translates to higher number of patients having an incomplete CRS.

Lymph Node Involvement

In a study by Gonzalez-Moreno and colleagues,[38] lymph node metastases were shown not to affect survival after CRS and HIPEC in patients with appendiceal cancer. In a more recent publication, the same group reported minimal significance of lymph node metastases on overall survival.[18] Lymph node involvement is rarely found in adenomucinosis.

Halabi and colleagues[19] showed, in 77 patients who underwent CRS/HIPEC for PMCA, a 5-year survival status for lymph node–positive versus lymph node–negative of 21% and 73%, respectively (*P*<.001) (**Fig. 13**). All patients had complete cytoreduction. Their data also indicated that patient selection for CRS/HIPEC should take into consideration lymph node status, but it should not be a contraindication if preoperative evaluation revealed a high likelihood of complete cytoreduction.

SYSTEMIC CHEMOTHERAPY IN APPENDICEAL TUMORS

Systemic chemotherapy may have a role in the management of these tumors in 4 different settings:

1. Preoperative (neoadjuvant)
2. Postoperative (adjuvant)
3. Postoperative after suboptimal cytoreduction with residual bulky disease
4. Palliative in unresectable or progressive and metastatic disease

Unfortunately, the role of systemic chemotherapy has not been clarified or defined in any of the clinical settings listed. One main reason is the lack of prospective, randomized studies. Because this is a rare malignancy, a majority of data are from single-institution retrospective reviews. Another reason is the diversity of histologies and the lack of a clear consensus in reporting and describing them. In addition, because the appendix has been considered part of the colon, appendiceal tumors have historically been treated with regimens similar to colorectal adenocarcinomas, although their natural history, biology, and outcomes are different.[36]

One of the often-quoted retrospective analyses described 34 patients with pseudo-myxoma peritonei, diagnosed and treated at Memorial Sloan–Kettering Cancer Center

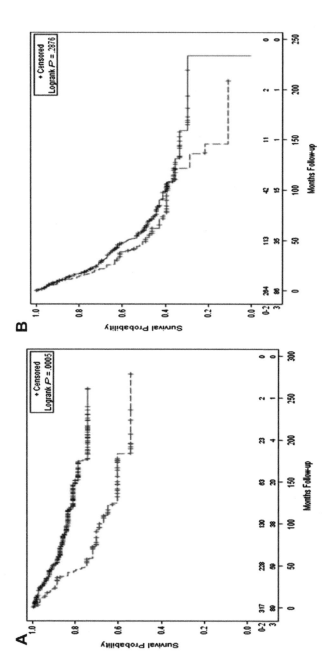

Fig. 12. (A) Survival of patients with mucinous appendiceal neoplasms by PSS. (A) Survival in patients with adenomucinosis of PSS 0 to 2 (*blue top line*) (N = 317) versus PSS of 3 (*red bottom line*) (N = 89). (B) PSS does not have a significant impact on survival of mucinous peritoneal carcinomatosis patients. PSS 0 to 2 (*blue top line*) (N = 264) versus PSS of 3 (*red bottom line*) (N = 86).

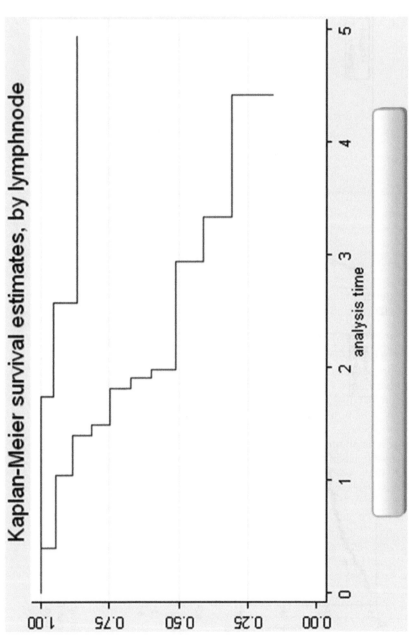

Fig. 13. OS with complete cytoreduction by lymph node status in years (lymph node negative—top line: 76%, lymph node positive—bottom line: 21%).

from 1952 to 1989. Of these, only 17 were of appendiceal origin and only 6 of them received IV chemotherapy with various agents, including 5-fluorouracil (5-FU). This analysis concluded that long-term survival could be obtained by cytoreduction alone, even if gross disease were present at the end of the procedure. No significant difference in survival was noted and chemotherapy should be administered only when there is clinical tumor recurrence."[39] Gough and colleagues[40] reported on 56 patients with pseudomyxoma peritonei treated at the Mayo Clinic between 1957 and 1983. Archival pathology was available in 37 patients and only 20 had appendiceal carcinoma. A majority of tumors were classified as adenocarcinomas grade 1. Adjuvant systemic chemotherapy with agents, such as 5-FU, cyclophosphamide, and doxorubicin, was administered in 27% of the patients after the initial surgery and in 53% after disease recurrence. A univariate analysis indicated that postoperative systemic chemotherapy was associated with shorter survival time. In a more recent study, the Milan group noticed that preoperative systemic chemotherapy had an adverse prognostic value in their series of 104 patients with pseudomyxoma peritonei.[41] Although most of those tumors were of appendiceal origin, 78 were DPAM and only 26 were characterized as PMCA. Twenty-six patients received preoperative chemotherapy and 23 of them were able to undergo cytoreduction and HIPEC. A breakdown of the chemotherapy group by histology and the agents used were not reported. Preoperative chemotherapy seemed to correlate with reduced both overall survival and progression-free survival (PFS). The investigators noted, however, that a selection bias could have occurred and the patients treated with chemotherapy could be the ones with aggressive disease.

Whether the particularly aggressive histologies may benefit more from preoperative or postoperative chemotherapy remains an open question. The signet ring cell carcinoma variance is typically a poorly differentiated tumor with a worse survival compared with mucinous adenocarcinoma.[23] Chua and colleagues[24] reported on 33 patients with signet ring cell carcinoma of colorectal (15 cases) or appendiceal (18 cases) origin. In the appendiceal group, 11 patients received systemic chemotherapy with FOLFOX (5-FU, oxaliplatin, and leucovorin) with or without bevacizumab before CRS. The median survival was 27 months in the combined chemotherapy with CRS/HIPEC group and 15 months for the chemotherapy-only patients. In a recent retrospective study of a larger series (142 patients) of appendiceal adenocarcinoma, either poorly differentiated (114 cases) or with signet ring histology (28 cases), Lieu and colleagues[25] evaluated the role of systemic chemotherapy with modern agents; 78 patients with metastatic disease received upfront systemic chemotherapy. The overall radiographic response rate was 44% and an additional 42% of the patients treated had stable disease. The median PFS was 6.9 months and the median overall survival (OS) 1.7 years. The majority of the patients received oxaliplatin combined with 5-FU or capecitabine and 17% of patients received irinotecan; 26 patients also received bevacizumab. There was no statistically significant difference between the regimens in response rate, PFS, or OS. Forty-five patients received second-line chemotherapy but only 13% responded. The PFS in that cohort was only 2.3 months. In multivariate analysis, a response to chemotherapy was associated with improved PFS but not OS. Only complete cytoreduction improved OS.

When the investigators from the University of Texas MD Anderson Cancer Center evaluated the role of systemic chemotherapy in unresectable appendiceal neoplasms with less aggressive histology, a potential benefit was more clear.[26] Fifty-four patients received at least 2 cycles of chemotherapy. The overall response rate, including stable disease, was 56%. Sixteen patients underwent CRS postchemotherapy. This was a cohort of patients with better prognosis. Only 30% of tumors had signet ring cell histology and 45% were well differentiated. The median PFS was 7.6 months and the OS was 56 months. The agents used were mainly 5-FU and capecitabine combined with platinum but also irinotecan, bevacizumab, and cetuximab. One-third of the patients received 5-FU or capecitabine alone. Cetuximab and other epidermal growth factor receptor inhibitors are used similarly to colorectal cancer although their association with the KRAS and BRAF mutations has not been properly investigated or defined in appendiceal tumors. Therefore, even in the absence of prospective data, it seems that systemic chemotherapy with modern agents may have a role in histologically aggressive as well as the primarily unresectable appendiceal tumors.

Sugarbaker and colleagues[27] conducted a prospective study evaluating the role of neoadjuvant chemotherapy with FOLFOX in PMCA. Between 2005 and 2009 they treated 34 consecutive patients. Although 65% of the patients on chemotherapy had stable disease by CT evaluation, intraoperative findings demonstrated disease progression in 50% of the patients, and 29% of patients had a combined partial and complete response by histopathology. That indicates the limitations of imaging studies in the preoperative setting. In a retrospective analysis of 77 patients with PMCA who underwent cytoreduction in the authors' institution,[28] preoperative chemotherapy correlated with worse OS and relapse-free survival (RFS). Most patients received an oxaliplatin-based or irinotecan-based regimen; the subgroup of patients who received additional bevacizumab seemed to have better outcomes, but the difference was not statistically significant. There was a concern that preoperative chemotherapy might delay the surgery and, therefore, hinder the attempt for complete and timely cytoreduction.

The role of chemotherapy in the adjuvant setting after complete CRS and HIPEC is even less clear. There is a lack of prospective analysis and a majority of data are from small patient cohorts and case reports.[29] Many patients with tumors of aggressive histology are treated empirically similar to adjuvant therapy for colorectal cancer, despite that the most common pattern of recurrence after complete cytoreduction is locoregional disease and subsequent surgical resections may improve survival. Traditionally, most patients with suboptimal CRS and good performance status receive postoperative systemic chemotherapy for palliation or with the goal to facilitate a second cytoreduction if there is a significant response.

There is a need to determine if there is any contribution of systemic chemotherapy in the management of appendiceal tumors, a need to identify subtypes with a more aggressive biologic behavior that may benefit from chemotherapy, and a need to prospectively explore various chemotherapy agents instead of just applying the same regimens as for colorectal cancer. This effort requires prospective phase II and III trials, which are difficult to conduct because of the rarity of the disease. The significance of various molecular targets, as in colorectal adenocarcinoma, lung, and breast cancer, should be investigated.

Although the histology (ie, poorly differentiated PMCA or signet ring cells) has prognostic value, the complex behavior of these tumors may be better understood by molecular profiling. Leptin; the mucin core proteins, MUC2 and MUC5ACl; and the mammalian target of rapamycin (mTOR) are more frequently expressed in mucinous adenocarcinomas compared with adenomas.[30] The mTOR-immunopositive group of patients had decreased disease-free survival (DFS), an outcome that could be potentially modified by the use of the mTOR inhibitors class of agents. These findings were supported by an earlier observation of high expression but variable distribution of MUC2 in DPAM and PMCA. The MUC2 expression correlated with high density of enteric bacteria and, specifically, *H pylori*.[31] A previously published study by Yajima and colleagues[32] reported higher levels of p53 protein expression in mucinous carcinomas compared with mucinous adenomas, although there was no difference in expression between adenomas and carcinomas in the nonmucinous tumors. Logan-Collins and colleagues[33] explored the vascular endothelial growth factor (VEGF) expression in mucinous adenocarcinomas of the appendix after prior cytoreduction. There was increased expression in 94% of their specimens. Higher VEGF expression was associated with worse OS. This retrospective analysis indicates there may be a role for angiogenesis in the growth of peritoneal lesions. It needs to be validated by prospective clinical data. Yoon and colleagues[42] showed than 9 proteins were more frequently altered in the adenocarcinoma versus adenoma group: cyclin D1, β-catenin, Ki-67, nuclear factor κB, VEGF, E-cadherin, p53, MUC2, and MUC5AC. Furthermore, the number of altered protein markers, p53 overexpressionnuclear factor κB positivity, and β-catenin loss correlated with adverse clinical outcomes.

The notion that appendiceal cancer is biologically similar and, therefore, should be treated with chemotherapy identical to colon was challenged in a recent study by Levine and colleagues.[36] A prospectively maintained tissue bank of peritoneal metastases from appendiceal and colorectal cancers after CRS and HIPEC and 3 years of follow-up was used. The majority of appendiceal cancers were low histologic grade. Global gene expression analysis and unsupervised hierarchical clustering were performed. Three main clusters were produced: two clusters consisted of predominantly appendiceal samples and a third consisting of colorectal samples. The results of survival analysis were intriguing: the colorectal samples had the worst prognosis, with no survival at 5 years. Despite their low histologic grade, however, the appendiceal cancer clusters had statistically different survival curves compared with each other and they were labeled low risk and high risk. The MUC2, MUC5AC, and trefoil factors 1 and 2 genes correlated with worse prognosis. Additional genes, such as SRC and TGF-beta, were shown differentially regulated in the high-risk group. The study demonstrated a distinct molecular profile and, therefore, different biology between colorectal and appendiceal cancer. The results may suggest that targeted agents, such as Src inhibitors (the investigators discuss dasatinib) or vaccine therapy, could be considered for clinical trials.

In summary, despite more than 5 decades of using systemic chemotherapy in appendiceal cancer, understanding of its role is still limited. It seems that chemotherapy may be helpful in advanced, high-grade disease, particularly when complete cytoreduction is not feasible. This information, however, is mainly derived from retrospective single- institution data and general medical oncology practice is based on the erroneous notion that appendiceal and colorectal cancers are similar and they can therefore, be treated with identical chemotherapy regimens.

MORTALITY AND MORBIDITY WITH PERITONECTOMY AND HIPEC

The postoperative morbidity rates reported in the literature range from 14% to 70%.[43–49] Patients with complications are identified clinically with fatigue, increasing inflammatory parameters, dehydration, and occasionally pancytopenia that may aggravate the situation. Complications that occur may depend on[50–54]

- Metachronous peritoneal carcinomatosis ($P = .009$)
- PCI >13 ($P = .012$)
- Five or more affected regions ($P = .04$)
- Incomplete initial cytoreduction ($P = .035$)
- Blood transfusion requirements due to intraoperative blood loss ($P = .28$)
- Three or more anastomosis ($P = .018$)

Table 2
Compilation of recent series from multiple institutions across the world of peritoneal carcinomatosis of appendiceal origin treated with CRS and HIPEC

Author/Center	Year	N	Histology	Drugs	Temp (°)	CC-0	DFS	OS	Mortality
Stewart et al[55] (Wake Forest)	2006	110	DPAM: (50%) Intermediate: (16%) PMCA: 27% High-grade nonmucinous: 7%	MMC	42	R0 (n = 31) R1 (n = 17)		1 y: 79.9% 3 y: 59% 5 y: 53.4%	4% 30-d Mortality
Sardi et al[37] (Mercy-Baltimore)	2009	56	DPAM: 39.2% PMCA: 60.7%	MMC	42			DPAM (3 y): 80% PMCA (3 y): 52%	0% (Postoperative)
Vaira et al[56] (Italy)	2009	60	Adenocarcinoma appendix: 71.6% DPAM: 28.3%	MMC + Cisplatin	41.5	—	5 y: 80% 10 y: 70%	5 y: 94% 10 y: 84.6%	0% (Postoperative)
Sideris et al[57] (Montreal)	2009	37	PMCA (29%) DPAM: grade 0: 21% grade 1: 50%	MMC (HIPEC) 5-FU (EPIC)	42–43	64%	—	5 y: 59% (HIPEC) 5 y: 58% (EPIC)	0% (Postoperative)
Järvinen et al[58] (Finland)	2010	33	Pseudomyxoma peritonei appendix	—	—	—	—	5 y: 67% 10 y: 31%	2.7% (30-d Mortality)
Elias et al[59] (France)	2010	41	Adenocarcinoma appendix	MMC (HIPEC) MMC + 5-FU (EPIC)	40–43	71.5%	89 Mo	3 y: 63.2% 5 y: 63.2%	4.8% (Postoperative)
Ko et al[60] (Korea)	2010	55	Adenocarcinoma appendix	—	—	—	3 y: 66.4% 5 y: 53.3%	3 y: 72.2% 5 y: 64%	—
Youssef et al[61] (UK)	2011	456	Pseudomyxoma peritonei appendix	MMC	42	66%	9.2 y (mean)	5 y: 69% 10 y: 74%	1.65% In-hospital mortality
Chua et al[34] (Australia)	2011	46	Mucinous and nonmucinous adenocarcinoma appendix	MMC	42	72%	20.5 Mo	3 y: 59% 5 y: 45% 7 y: 34%	4%
Austin et al[62] (UPMC-Pittsburgh)	2012	282	PMCA (75%) DPAM (25.2%)	MMC	42	49.3	—	3 y: 67.4 5 y: 52.7	1.1% (60-d Mortality)
El Halabi et al[35] (Mercy-Baltimore)	2012	77	PMCA	MMC	42	PCI >20 65% PCI <20 96%		1 y: 88% 3 y: 56% 5 y: 40%	0%

Reported mortality rates are in the range of 0% to 20% in the world literature and 0% to 8% at active peritoneal carcinomatosis centers. A major impact in reducing morbidity and mortality is the learning curve of CRS with HIPEC, suggesting that surgeons should first visit established peritoneal surface malignancy centers before performing these operative procedures.[32] The morbidity and mortality rates of CRS and HIPEC are similar to other major gastrointestinal surgeries but these can be further reduced in high-volume peritoneal surface malignancy centers.

Table 2[34,35,37,55–62] shows a compilation of recent series from multiple institutions across the world of peritoneal carcinomatosis of appendiceal origin treated with CRS and HIPEC. As shown, the mortality rates from CRS/HIPEC ranges in these series from 0% to 4.8%.

QUALITY OF LIFE AFTER CRS AND HIPEC

Despite the reported initial impairment QOL, several studies show an improvement of QOL after CRS and HIPEC in long-term survivors.[63–67] Schmidt and colleagues[63] evaluated QOL after CRS and HIPEC in 67 patients with peritoneal carcinomatosis using the EORTC QLQ-C30 questionnaire. The mean score for global health status of long-term survivors was significantly decreased compared with the control population (62.6 vs 73.3) showing particularly an impairment of role and social functioning.

McQuellon and colleagues[64] reported that patients initially have a decrease of physical, functional, and well-being scores, but this does increase relative to baseline levels during follow-up at 3, 6, and 12 months. One year after surgery, 74% of the patients resumed greater than 50% of their normal activities. They also concluded that significant number of patients show depressive symptoms at the time of surgery (32%) as well as 1 year after surgery (24%).[67]

Tuttle and colleagues[66] showed a return of QOL measurements to baseline 4 months after surgery in a prospective analysis of 35 patients. Eight and 12 months after CRS and HIPEC, QOL was significantly improved. In conclusion, the existing studies show that CRS and HIPEC can be performed with acceptable postoperative QOL and even may improve QOL in a selected group of long-term survivors.

SUMMARY

Appendiceal tumors historically were considered rare tumors but their incidence is rising. Appendiceal mucinous neoplasms represent a homogeneous group of neoplasms and, if confined to the appendiceal mucosa, are cured by appendectomy, whereas any proliferation of neoplastic epithelium beyond the mucosa or rupture of the appendix places patients at risk for peritoneal dissemination. There is significant interobserver variability when classifying these tumors based on Ronnett's criteria.[12] In addition, there is clinical variability in the behavior of tumors within this classification system; a small percentage of patients with DPAM demonstrate a more aggressive clinical picture, whereas a variable spectrum of biologic behavior may be seen in patients with PMCA. Historically, these tumors were treated with nonaggressive, serial debulking procedures, mainly for symptom management, with selective use of intraperitoneal chemotherapy. Tumor recurrence was high and cure was uncommon. Sugarbaker[18] introduced the concept of radical CRS to remove all macroscopic tumor deposits, followed by perioperative intraperitoneal chemotherapy to treat residual microscopic disease. The peritoneal-based nature of this appendicular malignancy makes it an ideal candidate for aggressive locoregional therapies. Decisions regarding clinical management require clear communication among treating physicians, so adoption of a uniform reporting system for appendiceal mucinous neoplasms with peritoneal metastases by the World Health Organization and American Joint Committee on Cancer represents a major advancement in the field.

Improved patient survival has been demonstrated, with the use of CRS and HIPEC with reduced tumor recurrence and less need for potentially morbid reoperative interventions. Current evidence demonstrates that peritoneal carcinomatosis from mucinous appendiceal neoplams has a median survival of 51 to 156 months, a 10 year overall survival upto 70%, while maintaining overall morbidity of 20 - 50% and mortality of 1-10%.[62] Meaningful long-term survival can be achieved in patients with PMCA even with extensive peritoneal disease. Extensive multivisceral resections can be performed even in the setting of recurrent disease, with low major morbidity at experienced centers. Once controlled for complete cytoreduction, a PCI greater than 20 that suggests extensive disease should not be an exclusion criterion for surgery even in high-grade disease. Instead, complete cytoreduction of extensive disease is a more important factor, and all efforts should be made at surgery to achieve it.[35] This requires longer operative time and advanced surgical expertise in treating such disease. Delaying CRS/HIPEC may complicate the surgical approach and lower the possibility of complete cytoreduction.[35] The number of lymph nodes to be harvested in appendiceal cancer has not been standardized. Multi-institutional efforts should be made to classify further patients with positive lymph node into subcategories based on the ratio or number of positive lymph nodes.

Despite more than 5 decades of using systemic chemotherapy in appendiceal cancer, understanding of its role is limited. There is an urgent need to design and conduct phase II prospective trials that use and further explore available preclinical data and attempt to integrate cytotoxics with targeted agents. Those trials may need to be collaborative and multicenter because of the rarity of the disease. In the meantime, because a majority of patients are treated empirically, there is a risk of unnecessary toxicity and the benefit to survival outcomes is uncertain. Questions will arise about the effectiveness of short duration precytoreduction chemotherapy for patients with PMCA and lymph node involvement.

Due to the complexity in decision making, these patients are better managed through a multidisciplinary approach, preferably by a team with expertise in peritoneal surface malignancy. In conclusion, appropriate patient selection, complete cytoreduction, and low morbidity are modifiable factors in this disseminated malignancy, and aggressive management by experienced surgeons can lead to long-term survival.

REFERENCES

1. Connor SJ, Hanna GB, Frizelle FA. Appendiceal tumors: retrospective clinicopathologic analysis of appendiceal tumors from 7,970 appendectomies. Dis Colon Rectum 1998;41(1):75.
2. McCusker ME, Coté TR, Clegg LX, et al. Primary malignant neoplasm's of the appendix: a population-based study from the surveillance, epidemiology and end-results program, 1973-1998. Cancer 2002;94(12):3307.
3. Elting AW. Primary carcinoma of the vermiform appendix, with a report of three cases. Ann Surg 1903;37(4):549–74.
4. AJCC cancer staging manual. 7th edition. American Joint Committee on Cancer, 2010, Springer.
5. Prystowsky JB, Pugh CM, Nagle AP. Current problems in surgery: appendicitis. Curr Probl Surg 2005;42:688–742.

6. Gustafsson B, Siddique L, Chan A, et al. Uncommon cancers of the small intestine, appendix and colon: an analysis of SEER 1973-2004, and current diagnosis and therapy. Int J Oncol 2008;33:1121–31.
7. Misdraji J. Appendiceal mucinous neoplasms: controversial issues. Arch Pathol Lab Med 2010;134(6):864–70.
8. Higa E, Rosai J, Pizzimbono CA, et al. Mucosal hyperplasia, mucinous cystadenoma, and mucinous cystadenocarcinoma of the appendix. A re-evaluation of appendiceal "mucocele". Cancer 1973;32(6):1525–41.
9. Carr NJ, McCarthy WF, Sobin LH. Epithelial noncarcinoid tumors and tumor-like lesions of the appendix. A clinicopathologic study of 184 patients with a multivariate analysis of prognostic factors. Cancer 1995;75(3):757–68.
10. Misdraji J, Yantiss RK, Graeme-Cook FM, et al. Appendiceal mucinous neoplasms: a clinicopathologic analysis of 107 cases. Am J Surg Pathol 2003;27(8):1089–103.
11. Pai RK, Longacre TA. Appendiceal mucinous tumors and pseudomyxoma peritonei: histologic features, diagnostic problems, and proposed classification. Adv Anat Pathol 2005;12(6):291–311.
12. Ronnett BM, Zahn CM, Kurman RJ. Disseminated peritoneal adenomucinosis and peritoneal mucinous carcinomatosis. A clinicopathologic analysis of 109 cases with emphasis on distinguishing pathologic features, site of origin, prognosis, and relationship to "pseudomyxoma peritonei". Am J Surg Pathol 1995;19(12):1390–408.
13. Deschamps L, Couvelard A. Endocrine tumors of the appendix: a pathologic review. Arch Pathol Lab Med 2010;134(6):871–5.
14. Rindi G, Klöppel G, Couvelard A, et al. TNM staging of midgut and hindgut (neuro) endocrine tumors: a consensus proposal including a grading system. Virchows Arch 2007;451(4):757–62.
15. Subbuswamy SG, Gibbs NM, Ross CF, et al. Goblet cell carcinoid of the appendix. Cancer 1974;34(2):338–44.
16. Roy P, Chetty R. Goblet cell carcinoid tumors of the appendix: an overview. World J Gastrointest Oncol 2010;2(6):251–8.
17. Tang LH. Epithelial neoplasms of the appendix. Arch Pathol Lab Med 2010;134(11):1612–20.
18. Sugarbaker PH. Epithelial appendiceal neoplasms. Cancer J 2009;15(3):225–35.
19. Halabi HE, Gushchin V, Francis J, et al. Prognostic significance of lymph node metastases in patients with high-grade appendiceal cancer. Ann Surg Oncol 2012;19(1):122–5.
20. Ross A, Sardi A, Nieroda C, et al. Clinical utility of elevated tumor markers in patients with disseminated appendiceal malignancies treated by cytoreductive surgery and HIPEC. Eur J Surg Oncol 2010;36(8):772–6.
21. Sugarbaker PH. Technical handbook for the integration of cytoreductive surgery and perioperative intraperitoneal chemotherapy into the surgical management of gastrointestinal and gynecologic malignancy. 4th edition. Grand Rapids (MI): Ludann company; 2005.
22. Gonzalez –Moreno S, Gonzalez Bayon LA, Ortega Perez G. Hyperthermic intraperitoneal chemotherapy: rational and technique. World J Gastrointest Oncol 2010;2(2):68–75.
23. Kang H, O'Connell JB, Maggard MA, et al. A 10-year outcomes evaluation of mucinous and signet-ring cell carcinoma of the colon and rectum. Dis Colon Rectum 2005;48:1161–8.
24. Chua TC, Pelz JO, Kerscher A, et al. Critical analysis of 33 patients with peritoneal carcinomatosis secondary to colorectal and appendiceal signet ring cell carcinoma. Ann Surg Oncol 2009;16:2765–70.

25. Lieu CH, Lambert LA, Wolff RA, et al. Systemic chemotherapy and surgical cytoreduction in poorly differentiated and signet ring cell adenocarcinomas of the appendix. Ann Oncol 2012;23:652–8.

26. Shapiro JF, Chase JL, Wolff RA, et al. Modern systemic chemotherapy in surgically unresectable neoplasm's of appendiceal origin. Cancer 2010;116: 316–22.

27. Sugarbaker PH, Bijelic C, Chang D, et al. Neoadjuvant FOLFOX chemotherapy in 34 consecutive patients with mucinous peritoneal carcinomatosis of appendiceal origin. J Surg Oncol 2010;102(6):576–81.

28. El Halabi HM, Ledakis P, Gushchin V, et al. The role of cytoreductive surgery in patients with carcinomatosis from high-grade appendix cancer in the era of modern systemic chemotherapy. J Clin Oncol 2011;29(Suppl):4080.

29. Chen CF, Huang CJ, Kang WY, et al. Experience with adjuvant chemotherapy for pseudomyxoma peritonei secondary to mucinous adenocarcinoma of the appendix with oxaliplatin/fluorouracil/leucovorin (FOLFOX4). World J Surg Oncol 2008;11(6):118.

30. Chang MS, Byeon SJ, Yoon SO, et al. Leptin, MUC2 and mTOR in appendiceal mucinous neoplasms. Pathobiology 2012;79(1):45–53.

31. Semino-Mora C, McAvoy T, Nieroda C, et al. Pseudomyxoma peritonei: is disease progression related to microbial agents? A study of bacteria, MUC2 and MUC5AC expression in disseminated peritoneal adenomucinosis and peritoneal mucinous carcinomatosis. Ann Surg Oncol 2008;15(5):1414–23.

32. Yajima N, Wada R, Yamagishi S, et al. Immunohistochemical expressions of cytokeratins, mucin core proteins, p53, and neuroendocrine cell markers in epithelial neoplasm of appendix. Hum Pathol 2005;36(11):1217–25.

33. Logan-Collins JM, Lowy AM, Robinson-Smith TM, et al. VEGF expression predicts survival in patients with peritoneal surface metastases from mucinous adenocarcinoma of the appendix and colon. Ann Surg Oncol 2007;15(3):738–44.

34. Chua TC, Al-Alem I, Saxena A, et al. Surgical cytoreduction and survival in appendiceal cancer peritoneal carcinomatosis: an evaluation of 46 consecutive patients. Ann Surg Oncol 2011;18:1540–6.

35. El Halabi H, Gushchin V, Francis J, et al. The role of cytoreductive surgery and heated intraperitoneal chemotherapy in patients with high-grade appendiceal carcinoma and extensive peritoneal carcinomatosis. Ann Surg Oncol 2012;19: 110–4.

36. Levine EA, Blazer DG 3rd, Kim MK. Gene expression profiling of peritoneal metastases from appendiceal and colon cancer demonstrates unique biologic signatures and predicts patient outcomes. J Am Coll Surg 2012;214(4):599–606.

37. Omohwo C, Nieroda CA, Gushchin V, et al. Complete cytoreduction offers long term survival in patients with peritoneal carcinomatosis from appendiceal tumors of unfavourable histology. J Am Coll Surg 2009;209(3):308–12.

38. Gonzalez-Moreno S, Brun E, Sugarbaker PH. Lymph node metastases in epithelial malignancies of the appendix with peritoneal dissemination does not reduce survival in patients treated by cytoreductive surgery and perioperative intraoperative chemotherapy. Ann Surg Oncol 2005;12(1):72–80.

39. Smith JW, Kemeny N, Caldwell C, et al. Pseudomyxoma peritonei of appendiceal origin. The Memorial Sloan-Kettering Cancer Center experience. Cancer 1992;70: 396–401.

40. Gough DB, Donohue JH, Schutt AJ, et al. Pseudomyxoma peritonei. Long-term patient survival with an aggressive regional approach. Ann Surg 1994; 219:112–9.

41. Baratti D, Kusamura S, Nonaka D, et al. Pseudomyxoma peritonei: clinical pathological and biological prognostic factors in patients treated with cytoreductive surgery and hyperthermic intraperitoneal chemotherapy (HIPEC). Ann Surg Oncol 2008;15(2):526–34.

42. Yoon SO, Kim B, Lee HS, et al. Differential protein immunoexpression profiles in appendiceal mucinous neoplasms: a special reference to classification and predictive factors. Mod Pathol 2009;22:1102–12.

43. Rohani P, Scotti SD, Shen P. Use of FDG-PET imaging for patients with disseminated cancer of the appendix. Am Surg 2010;76(12):1338–44.

44. Verwaal VJ, van Tinteren H, van Ruth S, et al. Predicting the survival of patients with peritoneal carcinomatosis of colorectal origin treated by aggressive cytoreduction and hyperthermic intraperitoneal chemotherapy. Br J Surg 2004;91: 739–46.

45. Stephens AD, Alderman R, Chang D, et al. Morbidity and mortality analysis of 200 treatments with cytoreductive surgery and hyperthermic intraoperative intraperitoneal chemotherapy using coliseum technique. Ann Surg Oncol 1999;6:790–6.

46. Saxena A, Yan TD, Morris DL, et al. A critical evaluation of risk factors for complications after cytoreductive surgery and perioperative intraperitoneal chemotherapy for colorectal peritoneal carcinomatosis. World J Surg 2010;34:70–8.

47. Saxena A, Chua TC, Yan TD, et al. Postoperative pancreatic fistula after cytoreductive surgery and perioperative intraperitoneal chemotherapy: incidence, risk factors, management and clinical squeal. Ann Surg Oncol 2010;17(5):1302–10.

48. Kerscher AG, Mallalieu J, Pitroff A, et al. Morbidityand mortality of 109 consecutive cytoreductive procedures with hyperthermic intraperitoneal chemotherapy (HIPEC) performed at a community hospital. World J Surg 2010;34:62–9.

49. Glehen O, Osinsky D, Cotte E. Intraperitoneal chemohyperthermia using a closed abdominal procedure and cytoreductive surgery for the treatment of peritoneal carcinomatosis: morbidity and mortality analysis of 216 consecutive procedures. Ann Surg Oncol 2003;10(8):863–9.

50. Esquivel J, Vidal-Jove J, Steves MA, et al. Morbidity and mortality of cytoreductive surgery and intraperitoneal chemotherapy. Surgery 1993;113(6):631–6.

51. Kusamura S, Younan R, Baratti D, et al. Cytoreductive surgery followed by intraperitoneal hyperthermic perfusion: analysis of morbidity and mortality in209 peritoneal surface malignancies treated with closed abdomen technique. Cancer 2006;106(5):1144–53.

52. Verwaal VJ, van Tinteren H, Ruth SV, et al. Toxicityof cytoreductive surgery and hyperthermic intra-peritoneal chemotherapy. J Surg Oncol 2004;85(2):61–7.

53. Franko J, Gusani NJ, Holtzman MP, et al. Multivisceral resection does not affect morbidity and survival after cytoreductive surgery and chemoperfusion for carcinomatosis from colorectal cancer. Ann Surg Oncol 2008;15(11):3065–72.

54. Moradi BN, Esquivel J. Learning curve in cytoreductive surgery and hyperthermic intraperitoneal chemotherapy. J Surg Oncol 2009;100:293–6.

55. Stewart JH IV, Shen P, Russel GB, et al. Appendiceal neoplasms with peritoneal dissemination: outcomes after cytoreductive surgery and intraperitoneal hyperthermic chemotherapy. Ann Surg Oncol 2006;13(5):624–34.

56. Vaira M, Cioppa T, De Marco G, et al. Management of pseudomyxoma peritonei by cytoreduction+HIPEC (hyperthermic intraperitoneal chemotherapy): results analysis of a twelve-year experience. In Vivo 2009;23(4):639–44.

57. Sideris L, Mitchell A, Drolet P. Surgical cytoreduction and intraperitoneal chemotherapy for peritoneal carcinomatosis arising from the appendix. Can J Surg 2009;52(2):135–41.

58. Järvinen P, Järvinen HJ, Lepistö A, et al. Survival of patients with pseudomyxoma peritonei treated by serial debulking. Colorectal Dis 2010;12(9):868–72.
59. Elias D, Glehen O, Pocard M, et al. A comparative study of complete cytoreductive surgery plus intraperitoneal chemotherapy to treat peritoneal dissemination from colon, rectum, small bowel, and nonpseudomyxoma appendix. Ann Surg 2010;251(5):896–901.
60. Ko YH, Park SH, Jung CK, et al. Clinical characteristics and prognostic factors for primary appendiceal carcinoma. Asia Pac J Clin Oncol 2010;6(1):19–27.
61. Youssef H, Newman C, Chandrakumaran K, et al. Operative findings, early complications, and long-term survival in 456 patients with pseudomyxoma peritonei syndrome of appendiceal origin. Dis Colon Rectum 2011;54(3):293–9.
62. Austin F, Mavanur A, Sathaiah M, et al. Aggressive management of peritoneal carcinomatosis from mucinous appendiceal neoplasms. Ann Surg Oncol 2012; 19(5):1386–93.
63. Schmidt U, Dahlke MH, Klempnauer J, et al. Perioperative morbidity and quality of life in long-term survivors following cytoreductive surgery and hyperthermic intraperitoneal chemotherapy. Eur J Surg Oncol 2005;31:53–8.
64. McQuellon RP, Loggie BW, Fleming RA, et al. Quality of life after intraperitoneal hyperthermic chemotherapy (IPHC) for peritoneal carcinomatosis. Eur J Surg Oncol 2001;27:65–73.
65. McQuellon RP, Loggie BW, Lehman AB, et al. Long-term survivorship and quality of life after cytoreductive surgery plus intraperitoneal hyperthermic chemotherapy for peritoneal carcinomatosis. Ann Surg Oncol 2003;10:155–62.
66. Tuttle TM, Zhang Y, Greeno E, et al. Toxicity and quality of life after cytoreductive surgery plus hyperthermic intraperitoneal chemotherapy. Ann Surg Oncol 2006; 13:1627–32.
67. McQuellon RP, Danhauer SC, Russell GB, et al. Monitoring health outcomes following cytoreductive surgery plus intraperitoneal hyperthermic chemotherapy for peritoneal carcinomatosis. Ann Surg Oncol 2007;14:1105–13.

Urethral Cancer

Petros D. Grivas, MD, PhD[a], Matthew Davenport, MD[b],
James E. Montie, MD[c], L. Priya Kunju, MD[d], Felix Feng, MD, PhD[e],
Alon Z. Weizer, MD, MS[c],*

KEYWORDS

- Urethra • Cancer • Tumor • Therapy

KEY POINTS

- Outcomes of urethral cancer are heavily influenced by location, with distal (anterior) cancers presenting earlier and at lower stage with better chance of cure.
- Current epidemiologic data suggest that urothelial carcinoma (formerly called transitional cell carcinoma) is the most common diagnosis, and that men are affected more commonly than women. Recurrent lower urinary tract symptoms or persistent urethral stricture should warrant further urologic work-up including thorough physical examination, imaging of the lower urinary tract, and cystoscopy.
- Magnetic resonance imaging provides the best anatomic detail to define the local extent of urethral cancer in both men and women.
- Localized anterior tumors in both men and women may be managed primarily with endoscopic resection, segmental resection of the urethra, or partial penectomy in men. Radiation may represent an alternative in women or in cases in which surgical resection would negatively affect functional outcomes.
- Posterior tumors are best managed with multimodal therapy. Primary chemotherapy and/or radiation for locally advanced tumors based on histology should be considered, followed by endoscopic and radiologic assessment of response. In complete response, radiation (+/− radiosensitizer) could be considered for local control. For incomplete response, surgery with or without postoperative radiation (+/− radiosensitizer) should be considered. Systemic chemotherapy should be considered for metastatic disease.
- Rare tumor registries are needed to better optimize care for patients with rare cancers. Regionalization of care for rare cancers may improve outcomes.

Disclosures: None.
[a] Division of Hematology/Oncology, Department of Internal Medicine, University of Michigan, 1500 East Medical Center Drive, Ann Arbor, MI 48109, USA; [b] Department of Radiology, University of Michigan, 1500 East Medical Center Drive, Ann Arbor, MI 48109, USA; [c] Department of Urology, University of Michigan, 1500 East Medical Center Drive, Ann Arbor, MI 48109, USA; [d] Department of Pathology, University of Michigan, 1500 East Medical Center Drive, Ann Arbor, MI 48109, USA; [e] Department of Radiation Oncology, University of Michigan, 1500 East Medical Center Drive, Ann Arbor, MI 48109, USA
* Corresponding author. 7312 CCC SPC 5946, 1500 East Medical Center Drive, Ann Arbor, MI 48109-5946.
E-mail address: aweizer@umich.edu

INTRODUCTION

The differences in the anatomy and histology of the male and female urethra create challenges for the clinician in diagnosing and treating patients with urethral cancer. Gender, cause, location of the disease within the urethra, histology, and extent of the disease when it is diagnosed can strongly influence what treatment options are available to the patient, as well as the ultimate prognosis.[1]

The difficulty in treating primary urethral cancer is multifactorial. Although the rarity of the disease has prevented prospective studies, the problem is more severe in that most data on treatment are derived from case studies and small case series. As such, it has been necessary to extrapolate treatment from different cancers and general oncologic principles to guide therapy. In addition, the morbidity of the disease and impact of treatment options on urinary and sexual function heavily influence treatment decisions and disease prognosis. There has been no research into the impact of the disease or treatment on quality of life. Perhaps the greatest limitation is that urethral carcinoma is not a single entity. The anatomy of the urethra makes treatment options different in men and women. Within gender, differences in where the tumor arises in the urethra influence histology, treatment options, and prognosis. Therefore, it is difficult to develop adequate experience considering the subtleties of these different entities to make progress in optimizing outcomes for patients with this disease.

This article first describes the anatomy of urethral cancer, which is critical in understanding the natural history of this disease. It also describes the epidemiology, possible risk factors, diagnosis, and staging of urethral cancer. Because of the rarity of this disease and lack of evidence guiding treatment, treatment is discussed using a case-based format with best practices and alternatives for each scenario. Our management of urethral cancer and review recent studies are also described. In addition, possible ways to improve treatment outcomes for this rare and challenging disease are discussed.

ANATOMY/HISTOLOGY

There are major differences between the female and male urethras.[2] Anatomic differences give insight into the cause of the disease in some patients. These differences influence the underlying histology of urethral cancers by gender and also the patterns of disease spread. Understanding the anatomy and histology of the urethra also affects the selection of treatment with surgery (and type), radiation (and type), and chemotherapy (and regimen), including the use of multimodal strategies, which is often crucial in the successful management of the disease.

Female Urethra

The urethra extends from the bladder neck to the urethral meatus and measures from 3 to 5 cm (**Fig. 1**). The urethra is surrounded by the anterior vagina posteriorly, the bladder superiorly, and the pubic symphysis anteriorly where the distal one-third of the urethra is fixed. Paired Skene glands insert on the urethra on either side. The proximal urethra closest to the bladder neck comprises predominantly transitional epithelium similar to the bladder and upper urinary tract. However, the female trigone has a greater tendency to develop squamous metaplasia as a normal variant, and thus the proximal urethra may have a percentage of cells with squamous features. The distal urethra has more squamous and glandular features predominated by nonkeratinized stratified squamous epithelium. The urethra is surrounded by a layer of smooth muscle. A layer of striated muscle surrounds the distal two-thirds or anterior urethra and is involved in conscious urinary control. Urethral mucosal coaptation as well as

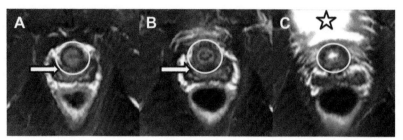

Fig. 1. Normal female urethral anatomy on T2-weighted magnetic resonance imaging (MRI) (with fat saturation). (*A*) Distal female urethra (*circle*); note the proximity to the anterior vaginal wall (*arrow*). (*B*) Proximal urethra (*circle*); note the proximity to the anterior vaginal wall (*arrow*). (*C*) Proximal urethra (*circle*) entering bladder (*star*). Note the target-like zonal anatomy of the female urethra (dark outer ring, striated muscle; intermediate middle layer, smooth muscle and submucosa; inner ring, mucosa and stratified epithelium). (*From* Hricak H, Secaf E, Buckley DW, et al. Female urethra: MR imaging. Radiology. 1991;178(2):527–35; with permission.)

the bladder neck also contribute to urinary continence. These factors are important when considering partial resection of the urethra for localized tumors.

The blood supply to the urethra is from the internal pudendal artery and venous drainage is via the pelvic plexus. Lymphatic drainage for the distal (anterior) urethra is to the inguinal lymph nodes with the proximal urethra draining to the pelvic lymph nodes. This difference in drainage influences patterns of locoregional tumor spread.

Male Urethra

The male urethra extends from the bladder neck to the penile meatus and is divided into an anterior and posterior urethra (**Fig. 2**). The posterior urethra extends distally from the bladder neck, and includes the portion of the urethra traversing the prostate (prostatic urethra) as well as the portion extending across the urogenital diaphragm (membranous urethra). The prostatic urethra is composed of transitional cell epithelium, whereas the membranous urethra is composed of stratified columnar cells. The anterior urethra includes the bulbar urethra and the penile urethra. The bulbar urethra is between the membranous urethra and the penile urethra, traverses most

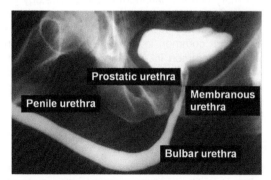

Fig. 2. Normal male urethra depicted on retrograde urethrogram. The penile urethra and bulbar urethra comprise the anterior (distal) urethra, whereas the membranous urethra and prostatic urethra comprise the posterior (proximal) urethra.

of the length of the penis, and is composed of columnar epithelium and pseudostratified cells. The most distal portion of the urethra (penile urethra) traverses the glans and is composed predominantly of stratified squamous epithelium.

The prostatic urethra is surrounded by the transition zone of the prostate. Paired ejaculatory ducts drain into the prostatic urethra at the verumontanum, which is in the middle of the prostatic urethra. This is the primary entry point of prostatic secretions, seminal vesicle secretions, and sperm into the urethra. Cowper glands are paired glands that drain into the membranous urethra. The glands of Littre are found on the dorsal surface of the pendulous urethra.

The arterial supply to the urethra comes from the paired bulbourethral arteries, which are branches of the internal pudendal artery. Venous drainage is into the deep dorsal vein of the penis and ultimately into the pelvic venous plexus. Lymphatic drainage from the urethra in the male is similar to that in the female, with the anterior urethra draining predominantly to the inguinal lymph nodes, and the posterior urethra draining to the hypogastric, internal iliac, and remaining pelvic lymph nodes.

EPIDEMIOLOGY

The historical assumption has been that urethral cancers are more common in women than in men. However, most of the literature has consisted of single-center case reports and case series, so there is an inherent bias in the literature toward reporting population(s) typically seen at tertiary care centers. To address this bias, Swartz and colleagues[3] used the United States National Cancer Institute Surveillance, Epidemiology and End Results (SEER) database from 1973 to 2002 to identify patients with primary urethral carcinoma. This data source comprised 9 reporting centers from across the United States. They concluded that the commonly held belief was incorrect: 67% of all urethral cancers reported to the database (N = 1615 total cases) occurred in men. They also challenged the previously held assumption that squamous cell carcinoma was the most common histologic subtype. Their results showed that 55% of cases were urothelial carcinomas, 22% were squamous cell carcinomas, and 16% were adenocarcinomas. The remaining 5.3% of cases comprised rare (eg, melanoma [1.4%]) or unclassified entities (1.7%).

Another more recent epidemiologic study from the National Cancer Registry of the Netherlands confirmed that, even in women, urothelial carcinoma is the predominant cell type (45%), with adenocarcinoma being the second most common (29%), followed by squamous cell carcinoma (19%).[4]

The incidence of primary urethral carcinoma during the study period in the study by Swartz and colleagues[3] was 4.3 cases per million in men and 1.5 cases per million in women, with a higher incidence seen in African American men (5 cases/million). Adenocarcinoma was more common in African American women and squamous cell carcinoma was more common in African Americans than in American white people. The incidence of primary urethral carcinoma increased for all populations and histologic subtypes with advancing age (peak age 75–84 years) but the overall incidence of all forms of primary urethral cancer decreased during the study period, suggesting that this is becoming an even rarer cancer.[3]

CLINICAL PRESENTATION

Primary urethral cancer can represent a diagnostic dilemma to the treating physician, leading to delays in diagnosis. Almost all men present with symptoms, and the presentation of a younger man (40s) with obstructive urinary symptoms should raise suspicion in the treating physician.[1] Men typically present with symptoms of obstructive voiding symptoms, hematuria, and a palpable urethral mass. Although the cause is unknown, chronic inflammation is thought to be a primary driver in the development of urethral cancer. Up to 50% of men with urethra cancer have a history of urethral stricture disease and almost 25% report a history of sexually transmitted infections.[5] Human papilloma virus 16 has been reportedly linked to the development of squamous cell carcinoma of the urethra.[6]

In patients with a known preexisting diagnosis (eg, stricture, infection, urethritis), the diagnosis of urethral cancer can often be delayed because men continue to be treated based on the assumption that their symptoms are caused by the preexisting disease. In this setting, rapid recurrence of symptoms following treatment or worsening symptoms despite intervention should lead the clinician to investigate for the possibility of primary urethral carcinoma.

In men without a history of inflammation, the diagnosis is often delayed because the patient is treated for other more common causes such as benign prostatic hyperplasia (BPH) or urinary tract infection.[7] Again, further investigation is warranted if a urinary tract infection recurs quickly or symptoms do not fully resolve. The initial diagnosis of BPH creates a greater challenge because, despite medical therapy, men often do not have improvement of their symptoms for 4 to 6 weeks; during this time, a masquerading urethral cancer can undergo disease progression. A thorough physical examination is necessary when evaluating this patient population. This examination should include a complete genital and rectal examination, as well as inspection and palpation of the perineum. Because the disease initially spreads by direct extension, palpation of the entire urethra as well as visual inspection of the urethral meatus is critical.

Roughly 98% of women with urethral cancer present with symptoms. Similar to men, women can present with urinary obstructive or irritating symptoms, hematuria, or a palpable mass. Many women are initially treated for a urinary tract infection because this represents the overwhelming cause of lower urinary tract complaints in women. Similar to urothelial cancer of the bladder in women, urethral cancer is often diagnosed late because of repeated treatment of urinary tract infections.[8] There is a critical need to obtain a urine culture before treating women with lower urinary tract symptoms and hematuria. Absence of a positive urine culture or failure to resolve symptoms despite appropriate antibiotic coverage in women should prompt referral to urologist. Although stricture disease is less common in women, chronic inflammation or irritation in the form of infection, urethral polyps, caruncles, or urethral diverticula (**Fig. 3**) can give clues to the presence of urethral carcinoma.[9]

Thorough pelvic examination of women with persistent symptoms is important. A palpable mass can indicate a urethral cancer (**Fig. 4**), diverticulum (see **Fig. 3**), or

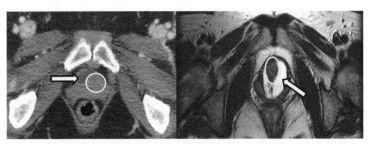

Fig. 3. Urethral diverticula (*arrows*) displacing the urethra (*ovals*) in 2 different patients, shown with axial contrast-enhanced computed tomography scan of the pelvis (*left*) and axial T2-weighted pelvic MRI (*right*).

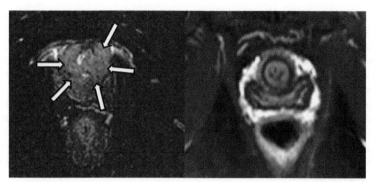

Fig. 4. Carcinoma of the female urethra (*arrows*) on T2-weighted MRI with fat saturation (*left*). A normal urethra is presented for comparison (*right*). The urethral cancer shows abnormal soft tissue thickening, with obliteration of the normal targetlike zonal anatomy (dark outer ring, striated muscle; intermediate middle layer, smooth muscle and submucosa; inner ring, mucosa and stratified epithelium). (*Data from* Hricak H, Secaf E, Buckley DW, et al. Female urethra: MR imaging. Radiology. 1991;178(2):527–35.)

polyp. In addition, extension of urethral cancer to the vulva and anterior vaginal wall is common, and can be readily identified by a speculum examination.

DIAGNOSTIC STUDIES

The diagnosis of urethral cancer requires a high level of suspicion for a primary urethral problem. Similar to urinary bladder cancer, diagnosis requires history and physical examination, laboratory evaluation, direct visualization, tissue diagnosis, and imaging to assess the local and systemic extent of the disease.

History should include a complete review of systems to elicit potential causes for the symptoms, prior urologic history and procedures, and history of prior radiation therapy for pelvic malignancies. Inquiry about the character, intensity, timing, frequency, and duration of urinary symptoms can be helpful. Constitutional symptoms related to malignancy, such as fatigue, weakness, fever, anorexia, night sweats, or cachexia, should be queried. History of medical comorbidities, family history of cancer, as well as immunosuppression is important. In addition, the history of other malignancies such as melanoma may raise suspicion for possible metastasis to the lower urinary tract. The use of quality-of-life instruments such as the American Urological Association symptom score and the Incontinence Symptom Index may add additional insight into the details of the urinary complaints and the extent to which they affect a patient's life.

As stated earlier, a more extensive physical examination should be performed when common symptoms present in an unusual patient population or when there is persistence of symptoms despite appropriate treatment. In addition to a complete physical examination, a male genital examination should include direct visualization of the urethral meatus, palpation of the urethra and scrotal contents, inspection of the perineum, and a digital rectal examination. Bladder palpation can help identify urinary retention in patients with obstructing masses. Palpation of inguinal lymph nodes can identify lymphatic spread in up to one-third of patients.[10]

Appropriate physical examination in women includes a bimanual examination, which includes assessment of the cervix, bladder, and urethra, and a speculum examination, which includes direct visualization of the urethral meatus and anterior vaginal wall. A protruding mass can occasionally be inspected. Women with urethral diverticula may have pain related to a stone, tumor, or infection within an obstructed diverticulum.[11]

Laboratory studies are occasionally helpful, but should include a comprehensive metabolic panel including serum electrolytes, glucose, creatinine, urea, and liver function panel. A complete blood count as well as coagulation panel should be ordered in anticipation of potential endoscopy with biopsy. Urine microscopy and analysis can identify microscopic or gross hematuria that might lead to cystoscopy. Urine culture should be obtained in women, because urinary tract infection is still the most common diagnosis in women of all age groups with irritating voiding symptoms.[12] The absence of a urinary tract infection in men or women with irritating voiding symptoms should lead to the consideration of cystourethroscopy using a flexible cystoscope. Urine cytology should be performed in all patients with gross or confirmed microscopic hematuria. Although the sensitivity of urine cytology for urethral carcinoma is low,[5] if positive, it can reinforce additional evaluation with imaging as well as direct visualization with cystoscopy. Serum prostate-specific antigen (PSA) should be considered, especially if prostate cancer or prostatitis is in the differential diagnosis.

The next most frequent step is direct visualization of the urethra with a flexible cystoscope. For patients reporting poor emptying, an ultrasound scan to assess the postvoid residual may help identify urinary retention. Urinalysis can allow identification and treatment of a superimposed urinary tract infection before performing cystoscopy.

Before taking a patient to the operating room to confirm the diagnosis with tissue sampling, imaging should be performed. Most patients diagnosed during a hematuria evaluation have already undergone computed tomography (CT) urogram. This study is not adequate for assessment of the urethra (primarily because of poor soft tissue contrast resolution), but it is useful in detecting lymph node enlargement and visceral metastasis.

Magnetic resonance imaging (MRI) is typically the imaging modality of choice in the evaluation of patients with urethral cancer because, unlike CT, it provides exquisite soft tissue contrast.[13,14] However, because this is a rare disease and the imaging protocols are nonstandard, image interpretation requires special expertise. Detailed descriptions of appropriate imaging protocols are beyond the scope of this article, but have been described in other reports.[15–19]

In both men and women, MRI can assess the local disease extent, including extension into the corpora spongiosum or cavernosum in men, and involvement of the vagina in women. In addition, invasion of pelvic bones and adjacent organs (prostate and rectum) can be identified. In women who are suspected of having a urethral diverticulum, MRI can confirm the diagnosis, assess the location of the diverticulum, and help determine whether it contains neoplastic tissue.[11]

Additional imaging studies should be directed to evaluate the presence of metastases. Depending on the degree of suspicion, chest radiograph or CT can be used to detect potential lung nodules. CT is more sensitive for lung nodules than chest radiography, but it carries a higher cost and greater radiation exposure. A radionuclide bone scan is indicated in patients with an increased serum alkaline phosphatase or serum calcium, or in patients with unusual bone pain or tenderness on palpation. Other imaging should be based on the patient's history, suspicion that the urethral mass represents a metastasis instead of a primary malignancy, and/or underlying tumor histology. Although there is no strong evidence to support this for primary urethral cancer, CT of the brain should be considered in patients with small cell histology or neurologic symptoms/signs.[20] CT positron emission tomography (PET) is generally not indicated for patients with primary urethral cancer, but may be useful if there is concern for metastases.[14]

Cystourethroscopy is the most sensitive test for detecting cancer of the lower urinary tract.[21] In patients with a presentation of gross or microscopic hematuria, a hematuria evaluation should include a urine cytology, CT urogram (assuming no contraindication), and visual inspection with cystoscopy. In patients with an obvious lesion in the lower urinary tract on CT urogram, visualization with flexible cystoscopy in the office can be skipped in favor of a rigid cystoscopy under anesthesia, which allows better visualization and the ability to confirm the diagnosis with biopsy. However, in the absence of an obvious mass, flexible cystoscopy in the office provides a sensitive means of identifying tumor within the lower urinary tract. Identification of mucosal irregularity, erythema, or friability warrants further investigation with a cystoscopy in the operating room under general anesthesia.

Under a general or regional (spinal) anesthetic, patients are placed in the dorsal lithotomy position and prepped and draped in the usual sterile fashion. Antibiotics are given to cover typical urogenital flora. Typically, a 22-French rigid cystoscope is introduced into the urethra and direct visualization of the mucosa is performed as the scope is directed toward the bladder. Flexible biopsy forceps can be introduced to biopsy concerning lesions. Hemostasis is achieved with Bugbee electrocautery. For early discrete tumors, a resectoscope with an electrified cutting loop can be introduced per urethra to completely resect the tumor. Care must be taken if the tumor appears close to the striated external sphincter in both men and women because aggressive resection can result in urinary incontinence. In the distal urethra of men, endoscopic resection can be challenging because of the limited working space in the urethra. In women, the shorter urethra creates greater risk of incontinence if aggressive resection is performed. Because many urethral cancers create and/or arise in the setting of urethral stricture(s), it is often not possible to directly visualize the entire urethra. In the setting of known urethral cancer, it is not advisable to dilate the urethra, because this may result in further pain, bleeding, and disruption of the tumor. In patients with associated urinary retention, tissue diagnosis should be combined with placement of a suprapubic catheter (if possible) to alleviate urinary tract obstruction. Optimal renal function is important for the delivery of systemic chemotherapy (when indicated) and urinary diversion is important in patients who are considered for organ preservation with radiation therapy.

A critical portion of the cystoscopy procedure is a physical examination under anesthesia. Patients with locally extensive or advanced disease are often difficult to examine in the office setting because of pain. Anesthesia allows careful inspection and palpation of the external genitalia and urethra to localize disease, which may be crucial in women with cancer arising in a urethral diverticulum because the tumor may not be visualized during endoscopy. In this circumstance, palpation with percutaneous biopsy may be the best way to obtain a tissue diagnosis.

A bimanual examination in women should include palpation of the anterior vaginal wall and pubic arch to assess tumor involvement. In men, a rectal examination can be used to assess involvement of the prostate as well as potential extension to involve the membranous urethra and pubic arch.

Palpation under anesthesia can also allow better assessment of inguinal lymphadenopathy. Enlarged nodes can sometimes be biopsied in the operating room under ultrasound guidance, particularly if there is concern that the urethral lesion may represent metastatic disease from another primary tumor.

PATHOLOGY AND STAGING

Results of the tissue diagnosis have implications for both treatment and prognosis. Similar to other cancers, grade and pathologic stage are obtained from the biopsy specimen and/or resection of the lesion. Combined with the examination under anesthesia and imaging results, the clinical stage can be assessed. Staging for primary urethral cancer is listed in **Table 1**.[22] As discussed later, staging is the primary factor influencing the type and extent of treatment.

The histology of urethral cancer depends on the location. In general, proximal (prostatic urethra in men, proximal third in women) tumors are commonly conventional urothelial carcinomas, whereas distal carcinomas (membranous, bulbar, or penile urethra in men, distal two-thirds in women) are commonly squamous cell carcinomas. Also, the morphologic distinction between high-grade urothelial carcinoma and nonkeratinizing squamous cell carcinoma can be challenging. Adenocarcinoma may arise at any site along the urethra and is commonly associated with diverticula and prostatic adenocarcinoma. In women, adenocarcinoma may arise in periurethral glands and involve the mucosa secondarily. Squamous cell carcinoma was historically thought to be the most common type of primary urethral cancer, and was reported to account for 80% of all urethral cancers.[23,24] However, as described earlier, it is likely that urothelial carcinoma is the most frequent type of urethral cancer histology in both men and women.[3,4] Other rare types of primary urethral cancer have been reported in the literature and include lymphoma, melanoma, paraganglioma, sarcoma, small cell, and undifferentiated tumors.[1] Because of the true rarity of these histologic types, there is a small literature on the management of these tumors. **Fig. 5** shows typical urethral cancer histology and its characteristic features.

Table 1
Tumor-node-metastasis staging of urethral cancer

Primary Tumor (T)	
Tx	Primary tumor cannot be assessed
T0	No evidence of primary tumor
Ta	Noninvasive papillary, polypoid, or verrucous carcinoma
Tis	Carcinoma in situ
T1	Tumor invades subepithelial connective tissue
T2	Tumor invades corpus spongiosum, prostate, or periurethral muscle
T3	Tumor invades corpus cavernosum, beyond prostatic capsule, anterior vagina, or bladder neck
T4	Tumor invades other adjacent organs (eg, bladder)
Regional Lymph Nodes (N)	
Nx	Regional lymph nodes cannot be assessed
N0	No regional lymph node metastasis
N1	Metastases in a single lymph node, ≤ 2 cm in greatest dimension
N2	Metastases in a single node >2 cm but ≤ 5 cm in greatest dimension, or in multiple nodes (≤ 5 cm)
N3	Metastases in lymph node >5 cm in greatest dimension
Distant Metastases (M)	
Mx	Distant metastases cannot be assessed
M0	No distant metastases
M1	Distant metastases

From Edge SB, Byrd DR, Compton CC, et al. American Joint Committee on Cancer staging manual. 7th edition. New York: Springer; 2010. p. 507; with permission.

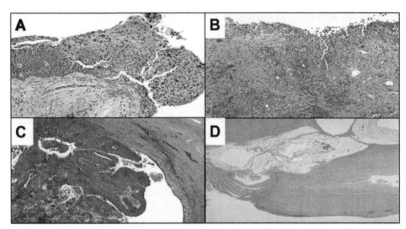

Fig. 5. Histology of urethral carcinoma. (*A*) Squamous cell carcinoma in situ of the penile urethra. (*B*) Invasive high-grade urothelial carcinoma involving prostatic urethra. Note the carcinoma in situ involving the prostatic urethral mucosa. (*C*) Papillary urothelial carcinoma involving penile urethra (history of cystectomy with pT3 urothelial carcinoma in bladder). (*D*) Mucin-secreting adenocarcinoma involving penile urethra (arising from proximal penile urethra).

TREATMENT OF PRIMARY URETHRAL CANCER

There are several issues that must be considered when discussing treatment options for patients with primary urethral cancer. Perhaps the most important consideration is the potential for cure. In general, for both men and women, anterior (distal) urethral cancers have the greatest opportunity for cure because of their greater accessibility and their earlier presentation. Posterior tumors are less likely to be cured because the disease is often more advanced at the time of presentation.[25] In conjunction with cure, the physician and patient must consider the impact of intervention on urinary and sexual function, as well as body image. Although penile urethral lesions can often be cured by aggressive surgical intervention in men (partial urethrectomy with penectomy), the negative consequences are often difficult for patients to tolerate. Similar to penile cancer, for which there is now more effort to preserve function without compromising cancer control,[26] these factors need to be part of the discussion in surgical decision making for primary urethral cancer. The various general treatment options are discussed later, followed by case discussion and an algorithm for how patients with urethral cancer can be rationally treated based on gender, location, grade/stage, histology, performance status, and medical comorbidities.

Treatment Modalities

Surgery for urethral cancer
The goal of surgical intervention should be the excision of the cancer with an adequately negative margin. If a negative margin cannot be achieved, then neoadjuvant chemotherapy and/or radiation should be considered before surgical intervention. In addition, if chemotherapy combined with radiation would offer better functional outcomes with the same potential for eradication, then patients should be counseled about the potential risks and benefits of the different alternatives. Because many patients have urethral stricture disease as an underlying cause, reconstruction may be required at a later time for patients undergoing radiation for preservation.

Description of surgical techniques is beyond the scope of this article and can be found in other references.[1]

Endoscopic resection through a resectoscope is an option for some men and women with primary urethral cancer. This technique tends to work for patients with localized low-grade disease (clinical stage <T2), in whom the location allows adequate visualization and reduces the risk of iatrogenic incontinence.[27] However, this approach carries the highest risk of recurrence and the potential for the development of urethral stricture disease. The ideal lesion for this approach is small, low grade, and noninvasive. In women, this approach may be more feasible given the short length of the urethra and the better capability to visualize the tumor during resection.

Segmental resection with reconstruction is another reasonable alternative for localized disease in which the urinary and sexual function may not be compromised. For very distal urethral tumors in men, the urethra can be surgically removed with a clean margin, and the healthy urethra can be mobilized and advanced to create a new urethral meatus. However, this may result in unintentional spraying of the urinary stream. If it is not possible to advance the urethra because of the length of the resected segment, then several options exist for reconstruction. One option is to leave the man with a hypospadic urethral meatus, which allows him to sit to void as long as the opening is along the penile shaft. Another alternative is to perform urethral reconstruction at a later date by replacing the urethral mucosa with buccal mucosa. Delayed reconstruction should be considered after a period of 3 to 6 months to make sure there is no recurrence in the proximal urethra. Another alternative is to leave the patient with a perineal urethrostomy requiring the patient to sit to void.[28] The same may be accomplished in women. However, because of the shorter urethral length in women, there is a higher potential for compromising urinary control and this approach should be limited to very distal urethral tumors.

Isolated tumors in the penile urethra may be amenable to segmental resection with primary reanastomosis. However, this should be reserved for patients with very isolated tumors in which no more than 2 to 3 cm of urethra need to be resected to achieve a negative margin, because a primary anastomosis could result in penile shortening and curvature of erection.

Partial/total penectomy with perineal urethrostomy

In cases in which there is involvement of the corpora cavernosum, more extensive surgery is typically required. For distal urethral tumors, preference should be given to partial rather than total penectomy. Similar to penile cancer, the goal of partial penectomy is preservation of enough length to be able to stand to void. Because the literature is limited, there are no conclusive data assessing the length of negative margin needed to reduce the probability of recurrence. In cases in which an adequate penile length cannot be achieved, total penectomy should be considered. Another possibility is to remove the involved urethral and penile tissue, while preserving penile length. In this case, it may still be necessary to perform a perineal urethrostomy, but preservation of penile tissue may result in functional and psychological benefit. For patients with anterior penile lesions requiring total penectomy and perineal urethrostomy, it may be helpful to involve a plastic surgeon and psychiatric evaluation for consideration of delayed reconstruction, and to help with coping around the time of the surgery and after care. For anterior tumors that involve corpora cavernosum without significant urethral stricture disease, radiation may represent a reasonable alternative with or without concomitant radiosensitizing chemotherapy (eg, 5-fluorouracil, cisplatin, carboplatin, mitomycin C).[24]

In general, segmental resection is not reasonable in women except for very distal tumors; consideration of chemoradiation is probably more appropriate.[23]

Total urethrectomy with urinary diversion, or cystectomy and urinary diversion

Some low-grade posterior urethral tumors in men may be amenable to endoscopic resection, but this is rarely an option. Most cases of posterior urethral cancer in both women and men present with locally advanced disease. As such, total urethrectomy (including penectomy in men) with bladder neck closure and some form of urinary diversion to the skin from the bladder may be an alternative. This technique should only be considered as a primary treatment modality if it appears that the tumor can be completed resected with a clean margin. However, use of multimodal therapy may have a better chance at local control in this scenario compared with surgery alone. Primary chemotherapy, based on the underlying the histology, with or without radiation, followed by reassessment with cystoscopy and imaging after such therapy may allow a patient to avoid surgery in the setting of good local response. In this case, consolidation with radiation therapy may result in good local control, although continued endoscopic surveillance is required to detect possible recurrence. In cases in which cancer control is not adequate, surgery is likely indicated with or without adjuvant chemotherapy and/or radiation.

Options for diversion include closure of the bladder neck with either a continent catheterizable stoma to the native bladder or an incontinent diversion (ileovesicostomy) using a segment of small bowel connected to the bladder, with the distal end brought out through a stoma. In these cases, it is necessary to reduce the capacity of the bladder so that the system will drain well. Failure to close adequately the bladder neck can result in urine leak that may require surgical reintervention.

For advanced disease that has failed other therapies (chemotherapy, radiation), if disease is localized or for palliative reasons it is often necessary to perform an emasculation in men or a total urethrectomy with resection of anterior vaginal wall in women. Both genders require cystectomy combined with urinary diversion. The most common form of diversion is an ileal conduit that is incontinent to the skin. An alternative in patients with the potential for cure is to perform a right colon pouch using both terminal ileum and right colon to create a continent catheterizable system. The patient must have a colonoscopy before this surgery to exclude the possibility of colon disorder.

For many patients in this setting, wide local excision of the perineum/scrotum with inguinal lymphadenectomy may be part of this surgery if lymph nodes are enlarged. This surgery requires a plastic surgeon as part of the surgery team to cover the surgical area with myocutaneous flaps.

In general, prophylactic lymphadenectomy is not routinely indicated because, unlike penile cancer, there is no proven survival benefit in patients with urethral cancer. However, in patients with palpable inguinal nodes, lymphadenectomy should be considered to reduce the local morbidity created by erosion of tumor into the femoral vessels. There are no data to support radiation therapy for either prophylaxis or treatment of enlarged inguinal lymph nodes.

Radiation therapy for urethral cancer

Radiation therapy for urethral cancer seems to offer comparable results with surgery in select settings.[29] In the setting of anterior urethral disease, external beam radiation therapy and/or brachytherapy may be an alternative to segmental urethral resection or partial penectomy. For women, radiation is often preferred rather than surgery for most forms of urethral cancer other than superficial distal tumors because of the morbidity involved with surgery (eg, sexual dysfunction, urinary incontinence).

Radiotherapy alone may be adequate for distal tumors less than or equal to stage T2, whereas the addition of a radiosensitizer may be beneficial for more advanced lesions. For very locally advanced tumors, it is likely that neoadjuvant chemotherapy (with or without radiation) followed by assessment of disease response may inform decision making regarding the potential use of radiation or surgery.

For proximal urethral carcinoma in women, radiation is usually the modality of choice. Proximal tumors often present with more advanced disease, and the concurrent addition of chemotherapy has shown benefit.[30] Primary chemoradiation in proximal advanced tumors has also been used in men with promising results, especially with squamous cell histology, and can be considered as the initial multimodality approach.[31–35] Surgical intervention can follow in that case, and especially if there is an incomplete response.[31] Radiation is also suggested after surgery for advanced disease in men if there are positive surgical margins, evidence of lymphovascular invasion, and/or in those thought to be at high risk for local recurrence. Moreover, radiation alone can be used for symptom palliation in patients with locally advanced symptomatic lesions who are not surgical or chemotherapy candidates. Further details on radiation can be found in a prior *Clinics* article by Koontz and Lee[29]

Complications associated with radiation include urethral stricture, radiation cystitis/urethritis, bowel irritation, fibrosis, infection, bleeding, and, rarely, fistula formation or secondary cancers; the overall risk of complication is approximately 20%. Complications may require surgical intervention to correct stricture or fistula, or to resect with urinary diversion if repair is not possible. This risk should be considered by physicians and patients who consider organ preservation for the treatment of distal lesions that could be managed effectively and with lesser risk by either segmental urethral resection or partial penectomy.[29]

Chemotherapy for urethral cancer

Data regarding the role of systemic chemotherapy in urethral cancer are limited and often derived from single-center retrospective case series. Because of the rarity of the disease, high-level evidence derived from prospective, randomized trials is lacking. It can be argued that chemotherapy has a role in locally advanced disease, either alone or combined with radiation therapy; this multimodality approach has been associated with promising clinical or pathologic responses.[31,32] The selection of chemotherapy depends on tumor histology. Squamous cell carcinomas have been traditionally treated with cisplatin/5-fluorouracil,[31] or mitomycin C/5-fluorouracil chemotherapy.[32–35] Either regimen can be combined with radiation therapy in the primary treatment setting. In patients with bulky disease, in which radiation field is extended and local therapy can occur at a later point, primary systemic chemotherapy with platinum/5-fluorouracil can be used, whereas the addition of paclitaxel could be suggested in patients with good performance status and organ function, based on data extrapolation from squamous cell carcinoma of different origin (eg, head/neck). In urothelial carcinoma, bladder cancer regimens can be used; methotrexate/vinblastine/adriamycin/cisplatin (MVAC) and methotrexate/vinblastine/cisplatin (CMV) are the 2 regimens that have shown survival benefit in the neoadjuvant setting in bladder cancer.[36,37] Gemcitabine/cisplatin regimen was shown to be equivalent to MVAC in advanced disease and has become the regimen of choice for metastatic urothelial cancer.[38] There is controversy regarding the optimal chemotherapy regimen for urethral adenocarcinoma, considering the rarity of this histologic type; however, data could probably be extrapolated from adenocarcinoma of different origin. Small cell carcinoma is usually treated with the combination of platinum/etoposide, whereas melanoma or lymphoma management is usually based on treatment recommendations for these distinct histologic types.

Treatment Recommendations

In general, the recommendations presented later are based on the personal opinion of the authors. Our overall goal is to achieve optimal cancer control while reducing morbidity and mortality. Because most tumors arising in the urethra are probably of urothelial origin, based on the registry data discussed earlier, our management is largely derived from data on urothelial bladder cancer.[39] It has been suggested that the pattern of spread may vary among histologic types, with squamous cell carcinoma exhibiting more direct contiguous local tissue invasion, whereas adenocarcinoma may spread more in the lymphatics.[1] In addition, recent data from divergent histologies of bladder cancer suggest that they respond as well to conventional cisplatin-based therapy as does conventional urothelial carcinoma, questioning the need to extrapolate from data regarding same histologic types of different origin.[40,41]

For low-risk disease (low-grade, Ta/T1 or very focal T2 disease) in men, we in general advocate segmental resection either through endoscopic resection, distal urethral resection, or partial penectomy. For low-risk disease in women, if a tumor can be managed with endoscopic resection, that is the preferred modality. For all other distal low-risk tumors in women, primary radiation should be considered unless the tumor is so distal that surgical resection would not compromise urinary continence. For men with more advanced distal urethral disease, partial penectomy is the preferred approach; however, chemotherapy followed by radiation could be considered if there is a good response to chemotherapy.

For posterior low-risk tumors in men, endoscopic resection could be considered for noninvasive disease as long as it will not affect sphincter function. However, for more advanced disease, we advocate either primary chemoradiation or primary chemotherapy followed by reassessment after 3 cycles. If there is a good response, radiation can be considered, but if not, then aggressive surgical intervention followed by radiation (if indicated) is our preferred approach. In women with proximal urethral disease, chemotherapy combined with radiation is indicated. Surgery should be reserved in this setting for women who have failed radiation therapy or for women with bulky disease for which radiation is considered insufficient. In these cases, a neoadjuvant chemotherapy approach followed by reassessment in a fashion similar to treatment in men is appropriate. Routine lymph node dissection is not indicated except for enlarged nodes on imaging (eg, CT/MRI/ultrasonography) or palpable inguinal lymphadenopathy.

Outcome/Prognosis

The recommendations given earlier represent an idealized version of our management of urethral cancer. In the clinical setting, patients seldom present in an ideal manner and therefore therapeutic decision making is often individualized. In addition, because multimodal care is frequently crucial, there may be different individual clinician experiences with this disease that influence care. In the future, a prospective global registry of all cases of urethral cancer could allow assessment of outcomes based on initial management to better define patterns of care. Understanding this entity has ramifications for penile cancer (a less rare disease) as well as management of the urethra following cystectomy for bladder cancer (a more common problem).

Two recent studies offer insight into outcomes of contemporary management of urethral cancer in both men and women.[42,43] In addition, both of these studies shed light on factors influencing outcomes for this rare disease.

Rabbani[43] used the SEER registry to identify 2065 men diagnosed with primary urethral cancer from 1988 to 2006. Patients were excluded from analysis if they had a diagnosis of bladder cancer in the registry. The last 5 years of analysis represented a disproportionate percentage of patients in the cohort (46%). Rabbani[43] confirmed the finding of Swartz and colleagues[3] that urothelial carcinoma was the most common histology of urethral cancer (78%). The author also found that two-thirds of the patients presented with less than or equal to T1 disease. Most patients were managed with simple surgical excision (61%). Only 10% of patients received radical resection and approximately 10% of patients received some form of radiation therapy.

Median follow-up for the cohort was 2.5 years. Median age at diagnosis was 73 years. Radical surgery and radiation were more commonly used for advanced-stage disease. Overall survival at 5 and 10 years was 46% and 29%, respectively. In a multivariate Cox proportional hazards model, advanced age, higher grade, higher stage, positive lymph nodes and/or metastases, urothelial histology, and no surgical intervention were associated with increased likelihood of mortality. Patients with adenocarcinoma tended to do better, possibly reflecting the greater likelihood that these were distal urethral tumors. Five-year and 10-year cancer-specific survival was 68% and 60%, respectively. The same factors were predictive in the disease-specific survival setting. In a subset analysis of 453 patients with nonmetastatic T2 to T4 urethral cancer, Rabbani[43] found a significant benefit for cancer-specific survival with surgery compared with radiation ($P = .018$). A major limitation of this study is that there was no information on tumor location or use of chemotherapy in this administrative dataset. Although there was an attempt to exclude patients with bladder cancer, there is a possibility of misclassification. However, for nonmetastatic disease in men, it seems that surgical intervention offers the best chance for disease control, representing the only modifiable predictive factor studied in this cohort.[43]

In a separate study evaluating primary urethral cancer in women, Champ and colleagues[42] identified 722 women from the SEER registry queried from 1983 to 2008. Median age was 69 years with 25% of women being classified as African American. Unlike Swartz and colleagues,[3] and more consistent with historical data, Champ and colleagues[42] showed an even distribution between urothelial, squamous, and adenocarcinoma. Unlike what Rabbani[43] had reported, women seemed more likely to present with invasive disease (50% ≥T2). Although 69% of women had some form of surgical resection, roughly 42% of women also received radiation. This rate is much higher than that seen in men with urethral cancer. In addition, roughly 23% of women received radiation either before or after surgical intervention.

Five-year and 10-year overall survival was 43% and 32%, respectively, similar to what Rabbani[43] reported in men with urethral cancer. However, 5-year and 10-year cancer-specific survival was only 53% and 46%, respectively, which is lower than what has been reported in men. This result may reflect the higher percentage of invasive disease in women on presentation. In a multivariate analysis confined to 359 women with nonmetastatic primary urethral cancer, race (African American), advanced-stage, node-positive disease at the time of surgery, nonsquamous histology, and advanced age were associated with worse cancer-specific survival. Surgery was associated with improved cancer-specific survival. The addition of radiation or radiation alone was not associated with improved cancer-specific survival, even when the investigators addressed changes in radiation practice between external beam and brachytherapy over the study period. This finding is contrary to commonly held practice patterns for urethral cancer in women, although selection bias could heavily influence the investigators' results given the lack of granularity in the administrative dataset and the lack of data on the use of chemotherapy. The current use of chemotherapy as a radiosensitizer is likely to offer a benefit compared with monotherapy, especially for more advanced disease that usually requires a combination of surgery, radiation, and chemotherapy to achieve disease control. The investigators also found that African American women were more likely to present with more advanced disease, which suggests that surgical resection and better awareness are needed to influence disease outcomes for women with urethral cancer.[42]

Case Presentations

The following are a series of anecdotal case presentations designed to highlight important aspects of urethral cancer management in men and women.

Case 1

A 66-year-old man with no medical comorbidities and excellent performance status noted a firm, painless lump on the tip of his penis associated with difficulty urinating and intermittent hematuria. Physical examination showed a 2-cm lump on the distal penis without any skin/mucosal abnormalities and without palpable inguinal lymph nodes. Otherwise, physical examination (including digital rectal examination) was normal. MRI pelvis/genitalia confirmed the mass within the urethra but did not reveal any enlarged lymph nodes; CT chest/abdomen with contrast was normal. Laboratory evaluation with a comprehensive metabolic panel and complete blood count was normal.

1. What is the most appropriate diagnostic approach to establish diagnosis?

This tumor arises from the urethra and not from the penile epithelium. Urethroscopy with tumor biopsy is necessary to establish the diagnosis. Cytology does not seem to be a reliable diagnostic method. If the rectum were to have been involved by physical examination or MRI, flexible sigmoidoscopy would be recommended before treatment planning.

2. What is the most common histologic type of urethral carcinoma?

In almost all reports, the most common (50%–70%) histologic type is squamous cell carcinoma.[5,44,45] However, SEER registry data showed a higher (55%) rate of urothelial carcinoma.[3] Adenocarcinoma is the third most common histologic type; more rare types include small cell carcinoma, lymphoma, and melanoma.

3. Biopsy revealed moderately differentiated squamous cell carcinoma of the urethra invading in the submucosa (cT1). What is the most appropriate treatment option?

Distal urethral carcinoma is amenable to surgical resection, with good results in several series.[5,46] Low-stage tumors in the distal urethra have a better prognosis compared with high-stage tumors in the proximal urethra; the cure rate for low-stage distal tumors can be as high as 70% to 90%.[47] Tumor location was also prognostic in a series from Memorial Sloan Kettering Cancer Center, in which patients with distal tumors did better compared with those with proximal tumors.[5] The presence of earlier symptoms can account for this difference, resulting in a lower initial stage of distal lesions. A series of 27 men from MD Anderson Cancer Center revealed 100% survival at the time of last follow-up for low-grade fossa navicularis lesions. Radiation therapy alone was not adequate in this cohort; however, it is suggested that this can be offered in patients who do not wish to, or cannot, undergo surgery. Distal urethrectomy with or without partial penectomy is recommended for low-stage distal tumors.[48] For tumors isolated to the very distal urethra, partial penectomy may not be necessary.

For tumors in men involving the meatus or fossa navicularis, we have found that distal urethrectomy with a negative margin followed by urethral advancement can result in good oncologic and cosmetic results, although spraying of urine can be a problem. For noninvasive tumors with a favorable grade, more extensive urethral resection can be performed with immediate or delayed urethral reconstruction using buccal mucosa. As opposed to penile carcinoma, benefit from prophylactic inguinal lymph node dissection has not been shown in urethral carcinoma, although it is indicated for patients with palpable inguinal adenopathy.

Case 2

A 59-year-old man with a history of urethral stricture for 15 years presented with worsening difficulty urinating. He was experiencing fatigue, fevers, and night sweats. Cystourethroscopy with urethral biopsy showed invasive, moderate to poorly differentiated squamous cell carcinoma. MRI of the pelvis showed an irregularly enhancing mass within the penis invading the corpus spongiosum and corpora cavernosa, with direct invasion of the penile bulb (**Fig. 6**). There was involvement of the penile urethra, bulbar urethra, and membranous urethra, with possible extension into the prostatic urethra. Pelvic MRI and CT abdomen/pelvis showed bilateral inguinal adenopathy, with the largest inguinal lymph node measuring 4.0 × 2.4 cm. There were small bilateral external iliac lymph nodes. Chest radiograph was negative and the patient's performance status was excellent. Laboratory evaluation included a comprehensive metabolic panel and complete blood count which were normal.

1. What is the stage of his urethral carcinoma?

Tumor involves the corpora cavernosum (T3) and there are enlarged nodes (>2 cm): Clinical stage cT3N2.

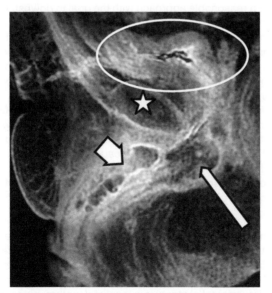

Fig. 6. Sagittal, T1-weighted, contrast-enhanced magnetic resonance image (with fat saturation) showing urethral cancer invading the corpora spongiosum and cavernosum (*arrowhead*), and penile bulb (*arrow*). Note the normal symphysis pubis (*star*) and thick-walled urinary bladder (*oval*).

2. What is the most appropriate treatment option?

This is a high-stage tumor; multimodality therapy with chemotherapy, radiation, and surgery could be used. The optimal combination or sequence of these modalities is controversial and solid evidence derived by randomized clinical trials is lacking because of the rarity and heterogeneity of the disease. A retrospective review of 21 patients (10 women, 11 men, mean age 59 years) with primary urethral carcinoma treated at Wayne State and Karmanos Cancer Institute reported that the best outcome for patients with locally advanced tumors was achieved with multimodality therapy.[31] Nine patients were treated with primary chemotherapy consisting of cisplatin/5-fluorouracil combined concurrently with radiation using 45 Gy to pelvis plus 25 to 30 Gy to the primary lesion, with or without surgery; 5 patients were disease free with a median follow-up for the cohort of 42 months. Only 1 out of 8 patients treated with chemoradiation followed by surgical resection had residual tumor in the surgical specimen, suggesting that urethral carcinoma can be responsive to chemoradiation. In a series of 18 men with invasive tumors (17 squamous cell, 1 adenocarcinoma), 2 cycles of neoadjuvant chemotherapy with mitomycin C 10 mg/m^2 on days 1 and 29/5-fluorouracil 1000 mg/m^2 on days 1 to 4 and days 29 to 32 combined with external beam radiation (45–55 Gy in 25 fractions over 5 weeks) resulted in 83% (15/18) complete response rate.[32] Five of the 15 responders had recurrence, whereas complex urethral reconstruction was needed in 3 out of 10 patients with long disease-free survival. All 3 nonresponders had persistent disease after salvage surgery and they died of disease, which challenges the role of surgery in that salvage setting. Five-year disease-free and overall survival were 83% and 60%, respectively, suggesting that chemoradiation is a reasonable option in invasive squamous cell tumors of male urethra.

In this case, because of bulky disease, it was thought that any attempted radiation field would be large and associated with significant toxicity. Therefore, it was decided that induction chemotherapy without radiotherapy using cisplatin, 5-fluorouracil, and paclitaxel would be a reasonable approach with the goal to downstage the tumor. The choice of this regimen was based on data derived from squamous cell carcinoma of head and neck; however, there are no robust data to support this triplet regimen as induction therapy in urethral cancer. The patient had only stable disease after 2 cycles and had moderate treatment-related toxicity. Because there was no response to this aggressive systemic regimen, a local modality was pursued. The patient underwent radical penectomy, pelvic lymph node dissection, ileovesicostomy, and resection of a perineal mass. Final pathology confirmed the presence of squamous cell carcinoma invading the corpora cavernosum and adjacent adipose tissue, with adjacent flat carcinoma in situ; there was a focally positive soft tissue margin and 1 out of 5 nodes were involved with extranodal extension. Because of the positive margin that can increase the risk of locoregional recurrence, he underwent adjuvant radiation therapy with weekly infusions of cisplatin as a radiosensitizer. He is currently disease free 6 months after completion of radiation.

Case 3

A 54-year-old woman with a long history of recurrent urinary tract infections presented with difficulty urinating accompanied by burning dysuria. She was treated with antibiotics without resolution of her symptoms. Urine cytology showed atypical cells, and urinalysis showed persistent microscopic hematuria. Cystourethroscopy revealed the presence of a circumferential stricture in the distal urethra; biopsy confirmed squamous cell carcinoma involving the submucosa. MRI pelvis showed tumor restricted to the urethra with no extension into the periurethral musculature. There were no enlarged lymph nodes. CT chest/abdomen showed no enlarged lymph nodes or distant metastasis. She runs 3.2 km every day and has not had surgery or radiation therapy previously.

1. What is the clinical stage of this tumor?

This is a low-stage (cT1N0) distal urethral carcinoma.

2. What is the recommended treatment option?

Considering the early stage and distal location, local modalities can be considered. A high incidence of local recurrence was noted historically for all forms of single modality therapy (46%–64%), suggesting the need for clinical trials with combination preoperative irradiation followed by definitive surgical procedures.[49] In 1 series, all histologic types seemed to respond equally to radiation. Another report suggested radiation therapy as the treatment of choice for women with primary carcinoma of the urethra, with surgical resection being reserved mainly for recurrent or resistant disease.[50] However, surgery was suggested as the treatment of choice for distal urethral lesions. In another report of 20 women with carcinoma of the entire urethra, combined radiation and surgery was the suggested treatment. The reported 3-year and 5-year survival rates were 33% and 21%, respectively.[51] In another series, a 21% recurrence rate with tumors less than or equal to T2 stage treated with partial urethrectomy was reported.[52] A series of 5 patients from Japan used surgical resection in 2 patients, radiation therapy in 2 patients, and surgery with adjuvant chemotherapy in another case; 3 patients were disease free, whereas 2 patients were alive with residual/recurrent disease from 5 to 87 months after diagnosis.[53] A report from Boston discussed that low-stage female urethral carcinoma can be curable by radiation therapy alone, with a 60% to 80% 5-year survival. Preservation of bladder function and bladder control can be expected with good radiation practice.[54] The investigators suggested that, except for stage Tis or small T1 lesions of the distal urethra that can be treated with limited surgical resection, radiation therapy should be considered as an alternative to more extensive surgery for low-stage bulky disease.

A Canadian retrospective experience with 34 women with primary urethral cancer was reported (15 squamous cell carcinomas, 13 urothelial carcinomas, 6 adenocarcinomas). Primary tumor was greater than 4 cm in 8 patients, involved the proximal urethra in 19 patients, and extended to adjacent structures in 22 patients. Inguinal or iliac lymphadenopathy was present in 9 patients. Radiotherapy was given only to the primary tumor in 15 patients, and to the primary tumor and regional lymph nodes in 19 patients. Brachytherapy with or without external beam radiation was given in 20 patients; 21 patients experienced a relapse. The 7-year actuarial overall and cause-specific survivals were 41% and 45%, respectively. Brachytherapy reduced the risk of local recurrence, but this was mainly in patients with bulky disease. Large tumor size was the only independent adverse predictor of recurrence and cancer death.[55]

Results from a series of 44 women with urethral cancer were also reported. Stage was T1 in 8, T2 in 5, T3 in 22, and T4 in 9 patients. Seven patients were treated with surgery alone, 25 patients were treated with radiation alone, and 12 patients were treated with both modalities. The 5-year overall and cause-specific survival was 42% and 40%, respectively; at the time of last follow-up, 11 women were alive. Recurrence occurred in 27 women, 23 of whom died. Recurrence was local in 8, local and distant in 15, and distant in 4 patients. The severe complication rate was 29% (2 out of 7) for women treated with surgery, 24% (6 out of 25) for women treated with radiotherapy, and 8% (1 out of 12) for women treated with both modalities. Tumor size and histology were independent prognostic factors for survival and local tumor control. Only 1 out of 10 women with a tumor greater than 4 cm was alive at 5 years;

no women with adenocarcinoma were alive at 5 years.[56] Data from MD Anderson Cancer Center suggested that primary carcinoma of the female urethra can be curable with radiation, although the complication rate was significant. In this report, an overall survival rate of 41% was reported in 84 patients, with a 74% survival rate in patients with only partial urethral involvement.[57] In a series of 42 patients from Iowa, combined external beam radiation therapy and brachytherapy produced fewer local failures (14%) compared with all radiation-treated patients or patients treated with surgery (60%).[58] However, 5-year survival rates were similar between those treated with surgery and those treated with radiation. The typical radiation dose used in most series is 55 to 70 Gy, with a 20% to 40% complication rate (eg, stricture, necrosis, fistula, abscess, cellulitis, cystitis).[59]

The heterogeneity of the published data renders interpretation of the literature difficult. The National Cancer Institute (NCI) recommends radiation therapy with or without surgical resection (anterior exenteration with urinary diversion) or surgery alone (open excision or anterior exenteration) for the management of distal urethral tumors in women. The choice of surgery depends on the stage, location, physician's experience, and patient's preference. It is discussed that a 2-cm tumor-free margin is preferable with surgical resection.[60]

In case 3, the patient met with Urology and Radiation Oncology, and chose to undergo urethrectomy and continent urinary diversion. A T1-stage squamous cell carcinoma was confirmed; however, there was a focally positive proximal margin. Adjuvant radiation therapy was implemented to reduce the risk of locoregional recurrence.

Case 4

A 63-year-old woman with a history of diabetes mellitus, hypertension, and chronic kidney disease presents with difficulty urinating and a sense of fullness in her urethra. Cystourethroscopy revealed urethral papillary tumors involving her entire urethra. Biopsy revealed small cell carcinoma. MRI pelvis confirms diffuse urethral involvement and enlarged bilateral inguinal nodes (largest 2.3 × 1.6 cm). CT chest/abdomen showed a 2-cm mass in the right hepatic lobe; CT-guided biopsy confirmed the presence of small cell carcinoma.

1. What is the next treatment step?

The origin of extrapulmonary neuroendocrine carcinoma remains elusive; it has been suggested that it may arise from differentiation of a multipotent stem cell.[61] It is an extremely rare type of urethral cancer with only a few cases reported.[62–65] Four out of 5 reported cases were treated primarily with surgical resection. Cisplatin-based chemotherapy was used adjuvantly in 1 of these cases, and as primary treatment in the fifth reported case. The data regarding the management of this neoplasm are sparse, and often extrapolated from small cell lung cancer (SCLC). In SCLC, concurrent chemotherapy and radiation therapy has proved to provide overall survival benefit when the disease is limited to a single radiation field (limited-stage SCLC). However, extrapolation of data from cancers derived from other organs bearing the same histology should always be interpreted with caution. This patient had extensive disease, therefore systemic chemotherapy was the appropriate next step; a regimen with platinum/etoposide is typically used. She underwent 4 cycles of renally dosed carboplatin/etoposide and is scheduled for restaging scans.

SUMMARY AND FUTURE DIRECTIONS

Urethral cancer is a rare disease with limited data in the literature to guide treatment decisions. The most common histologic types are urothelial carcinoma, squamous cell carcinoma, and adenocarcinoma. Older age, history of bladder cancer, prior radiation therapy, and chronic inflammation of urethra are considered potential risk factors. The different anatomy of urethra between men and women, as well as tumor location, stage/grade, and histologic type, all contribute to the diagnostic and management complexity of this rare and heterogeneous entity. Early stage anterior (distal) lesions can be approached via local therapies, such as surgical resection or radiation. However, proximal lesions are often more advanced and require multimodal therapy using chemotherapy, radiation, and surgery in various combinations and sequences with the goal of optimizing patient outcome and minimizing morbidity. Prognosis can vary, whereas selection bias can influence the results of retrospective case series. Prospective tumor registries with real-time documentation of the intervention and monitoring can help increase the experience with this rare malignancy. Case discussion in multidisciplinary tumor boards as well as referral to cancer centers with experience in genitourinary oncology is strongly recommended. International expert collaborations are needed to share experiences and design clinical trials that can answer essential questions and provide evidence-based guidelines. Education of both patients and providers is important to increase awareness and encourage enrollment in clinical trials when these become available. At the postgenomic era, deep genetic sequencing of urethral tumors could better characterize their heterogeneous biology, contributing to the identification of potential therapeutic targets and/or biomarkers of prognostic and/or predictive value. Translational research is important, with the development of preclinical models that can be used to understand underlying disease mechanisms.

REFERENCES

1. Sharp DS, Angermeier KW. Surgery of penis and urethral carcinoma. In: Wein AJ, editor. Wein: Campbell-Walsh urology. 10th edition. Philadelphia: Elsevier Saunders; 2011. p. 934–55.
2. Gormley EA. Anatomy of the urethra. In: Graham SD, Keane TE, editors. Glenn's urologic surgery. Philadelphia: Lippincott Williams & Wilkins; 2010. p. 211–4.
3. Swartz MA, Porter MP, Lin DW, et al. Incidence of primary urethral carcinoma in the United States. Urology 2006;68(6):1164–8.
4. Derksen JW, Visser O, de la Riviere GB, et al. Primary urethral carcinoma in females: an epidemiologic study on demographical factors, histological types, tumour stage and survival. World J Urol 2012.
5. Dalbagni G, Zhang ZF, Lacombe L, et al. Male urethral carcinoma: analysis of treatment outcome. Urology 1999;53(6):1126–32.
6. Wiener JS, Effert PJ, Humphrey PA, et al. Prevalence of human papillomavirus types 16 and 18 in squamous-cell carcinoma of the penis: a retrospective analysis of primary and metastatic lesions by differential polymerase chain reaction. Int J Cancer 1992;50(5):694–701.
7. Wei JT, Calhoun E, Jacobsen SJ. Benign prostatic hyperplasia. In: Litwin MS, Saigal CS, editors. Urologic diseases in America. US Department of Health and Human Services, Public Health Service, National Institutes of Health, National Institute of Diabetes and Digestive and Kidney Diseases. Washington, DC: US Government Printing Office; 2007. p. 45–69.
8. Johnson EK, Daignault S, Zhang Y, et al. Patterns of hematuria referral to urologists: does a gender disparity exist? Urology 2008;72(3):498–502 [discussion: -3].
9. Dalbagni G, Zhang ZF, Lacombe L, et al. Female urethral carcinoma: an analysis of treatment outcome and a plea for a standardized management strategy. Br J Urol 1998;82(6):835–41.

10. Vapnek JM, Hricak H, Carroll PR. Recent advances in imaging studies for staging of penile and urethral carcinoma. Urol Clin North Am 1992;19(2): 257–66.

11. Foley CL, Greenwell TJ, Gardiner RA. Urethral diverticula in females. BJU Int 2011;108(Suppl 2):20–3.

12. Dielubanza EJ, Schaeffer AJ. Urinary tract infections in women. Med Clin North Am 2011;95(1):27–41.

13. Kawashima A, Sandler CM, Wasserman NF, et al. Imaging of urethral disease: a pictorial review. Radiographics 2004;24(Suppl 1):S195–216.

14. Stewart SB, Leder RA, Inman BA. Imaging tumors of the penis and urethra. Urol Clin North Am 2010;37(3):353–67.

15. Ryu J, Kim B. MR imaging of the male and female urethra. Radiographics 2001; 21(5):1169–85.

16. Hahn WY, Israel GM, Lee VS. MRI of female urethral and periurethral disorders. AJR Am J Roentgenol 2004;182(3):677–82.

17. Pretorius ES, Siegelman ES, Ramchandani P, et al. MR imaging of the penis. Radiographics 2001;21(Spec No):S283–98 [discussion: S98–9].

18. Kayes O, Minhas S, Allen C, et al. The role of magnetic resonance imaging in the local staging of penile cancer. Eur Urol 2007;51(5):1313–8 [discussion: 8–9].

19. Kirkham AP, Illing RO, Minhas S, et al. MR imaging of nonmalignant penile lesions. Radiographics 2008;28(3):837–53.

20. Kalemkerian GP. Staging and imaging of small cell lung cancer. Cancer Imaging 2011;11:253–8.

21. Cohan RH, Caoili EM, Cowan NC, et al. MDCT urography: exploring a new paradigm for imaging of bladder cancer. AJR Am J Roentgenol 2009;192(6): 1501–8.

22. Edge SB, Byrd DR, Compton CC, et al. American Joint Committee on Cancer Staging Manual. 7th edition. New York: Springer; 2010. p. 507.

23. Madeb R, Golijanin DJ, Messing E, et al. Urethral cancer in women. Amsterdam: Wolters Kluwer; 2012 [updated April 16, 2012; cited 2012 July 1, 2012].

24. Madeb R, Golijanin DJ, Messing E, et al. Urethral cancer in men. Amsterdam: Wolters Kluwer; 2012 [updated April 16, 2012; cited 2012 July 1, 2012].

25. Karnes RJ, Breau RH, Lightner DJ. Surgery for urethral cancer. Urol Clin North Am 2010;37(3):445–57.

26. Philippou P, Shabbir M, Malone P, et al. Conservative surgery for squamous cell carcinoma of the penis: resection margins and long-term oncological control. J Urol 2012;188(3):803–8.

27. Konnak JW. Conservative management of low grade neoplasms of the male urethra: a preliminary report. J Urol 1980;123(2):175–7.

28. Salgado CJ, Monstrey S, Hoebeke P, et al. Reconstruction of the penis after surgery. Urol Clin North Am 2010;37(3):379–401.

29. Koontz BF, Lee WR. Carcinoma of the urethra: radiation oncology. Urol Clin North Am 2010;37(3):459–66.

30. Hara I, Hikosaka S, Eto H, et al. Successful treatment for squamous cell carcinoma of the female urethra with combined radio- and chemotherapy. Int J Urol 2004;11(8):678–82.

31. Gheiler EL, Tefilli MV, Tiguert R, et al. Management of primary urethral cancer. Urology 1998;52(3):487–93.

32. Cohen MS, Triaca V, Billmeyer B, et al. Coordinated chemoradiation therapy with genital preservation for the treatment of primary invasive carcinoma of the male urethra. J Urol 2008;179(2):536–41 [discussion: 41].

33. Licht MR, Klein EA, Bukowski R, et al. Combination radiation and chemotherapy for the treatment of squamous cell carcinoma of the male and female urethra. J Urol 1995;153(6):1918–20.

34. Lutz ST, Huang DT. Combined chemoradiotherapy for locally advanced squamous cell carcinoma of the bulbomembranous urethra: a case report. J Urol 1995;153(5):1616–8.

35. Tran LN, Krieg RM, Szabo RJ. Combination chemotherapy and radiotherapy for a locally advanced squamous cell carcinoma of the urethra: a case report. J Urol 1995;153(2):422–3.

36. Grossman HB, Natale RB, Tangen CM, et al. Neoadjuvant chemotherapy plus cystectomy compared with cystectomy alone for locally advanced bladder cancer. N Engl J Med 2003;349(9):859–66.

37. Griffiths G, Hall R, Sylvester R, et al. International phase III trial assessing neoadjuvant cisplatin, methotrexate, and vinblastine chemotherapy for muscle-invasive bladder cancer: long-term results of the BA06 30894 trial. J Clin Oncol 2011; 29(16):2171–7.

38. von der Maase H, Sengelov L, Roberts JT, et al. Long-term survival results of a randomized trial comparing gemcitabine plus cisplatin, with methotrexate, vinblastine, doxorubicin, plus cisplatin in patients with bladder cancer. J Clin Oncol 2005;23(21):4602–8.

39. Advanced Bladder Cancer Meta-analysis Collaboration. Neoadjuvant chemotherapy in invasive bladder cancer: a systematic review and meta-analysis. Lancet 2003;361:1927–34.

40. Canvasser NE, Weizer AZ, Tallman CT, et al. Variant histology in bladder cancer: survival outcomes in a large single-institution cystectomy series. J Urol 2012; 187(4). E706–E.

41. Scosyrev E, Messing EM. Do mixed histological features affect survival benefit from neoadjuvant platinum-based combination chemotherapy in patients with locally advanced bladder cancer? BJU Int 2011;108(5):700.

42. Champ CE, Hegarty SE, Shen X, et al. Prognostic factors and outcomes after definitive treatment of female urethral cancer: a population-based analysis. Urology 2012;80(2):374–82.

43. Rabbani F. Prognostic factors in male urethral cancer. Cancer 2010;117(11):2426–34.

44. Dinney CP, Johnson DE, Swanson DA, et al. Therapy and prognosis for male anterior urethral carcinoma: an update. Urology 1994;43(4):506–14.

45. Gillitzer R, Hampel C, Wiesner C, et al. Single-institution experience with primary tumours of the male urethra. BJU Int 2008;101(8):964–8.

46. Zeidman EJ, Desmond P, Thompson IM. Surgical treatment of carcinoma of the male urethra. Urol Clin North Am 1992;19(2):359–72.

47. Anderson KA, McAninch JW. Primary squamous cell carcinoma of anterior male urethra. Urology 1984;23(2):134–40.

48. Bracken RB, Henry R, Ordonez N. Primary carcinoma of the male urethra. South Med J 1980;73(8):1003–5.

49. Bracken RB, Johnson DE, Miller LS, et al. Primary carcinoma of the female urethra. J Urol 1976;116(2):188–92.

50. Turner AG, Hendry WF. Primary carcinoma of the female urethra. Br J Urol 1980; 52(6):549–54.

51. Kamat MR, Kulkarni JN, Dhumale RG. Primary carcinoma of female urethra: review of 20 cases. J Surg Oncol 1981;16(2):105–9.

52. Dimarco DS, Dimarco CS, Zincke H, et al. Surgical treatment for local control of female urethral carcinoma. Urol Oncol 2004;22(5):404–9.

53. Touyama H, Mukouyama H, Miyazato T, et al. Primary carcinoma of the female urethra: report of five cases. Hinyokika Kiyo 1997;43(4):303–5 [in Japanese].

54. Sailer SL, Shipley WU, Wang CC. Carcinoma of the female urethra: a review of results with radiation therapy. J Urol 1988;140(1):1–5.

55. Milosevic MF, Warde PR, Banerjee D, et al. Urethral carcinoma in women: results of treatment with primary radiotherapy. Radiother Oncol 2000;56(1):29–35.

56. Grigsby PW. Carcinoma of the urethra in women. Int J Radiat Oncol Biol Phys 1998;41(3):535–41.

57. Garden AS, Zagars GK, Delclos L. Primary carcinoma of the female urethra. Results of radiation therapy. Cancer 1993;71(10):3102–8.

58. Foens CS, Hussey DH, Staples JJ, et al. A comparison of the roles of surgery and radiation therapy in the management of carcinoma of the female urethra. Int J Radiat Oncol Biol Phys 1991;21(4):961–8.

59. Forman JD, Lichter AS. The role of radiation therapy in the management of carcinoma of the male and female urethra. Urol Clin North Am 1992;19(2):383–9.

60. Reis LO, Ferreira F, Almeida M, et al. Urethral carcinoma: critical view on contemporary consecutive series. Med Oncol 2011;28(4):1405–10.

61. Kobori O, Oota K. Neuroendocrine cells in serially passaged rat stomach cancers induced by MNNG. Int J Cancer 1979;23(4):536–41.

62. Altintas S, Blockx N, Huizing MT, et al. Small-cell carcinoma of the penile urethra: a case report and a short review of the literature. Ann Oncol 2007;18(4):801–4.

63. Vadmal MS, Steckel J, Teichberg S, et al. Primary neuroendocrine carcinoma of the penile urethra. J Urol 1997;157(3):956–7.

64. Parekh DJ, Jung C, Roberts R, et al. Primary neuroendocrine carcinoma of the urethra. Urology 2002;60(6):1111.

65. Rudloff U, Amukele SA, Moldwin R, et al. Small cell carcinoma arising from the proximal urethra. Int J Urol 2004;11(8):674–7.

Current Treatment of Anal Squamous Cell Carcinoma

Rob Glynne-Jones, FRCP, FRCR[a],*, Andrew Renehan, PhD, FRCS[b,c]

KEYWORDS

- Squamous cell carcinoma of the anus • Human papilloma virus
- Chemoradiotherapy • Salvage surgery

KEY POINTS

- With our current sophisticated radiological staging procedures and ability to spare critical normal tissues with intensity-modulated radiotherapy, a "one-size-fits-all" approach for anal cancer is probably inappropriate.
- Radiotherapy dose escalation and intensification of the concurrent chemotherapy might improve local control, but is just as likely to adversely affect colostomy-free survival.
- Integration of biologic therapy with conventional chemotherapies looks hopeful.
- Patients with anal cancer should be treated from diagnosis by a specialised multidisciplinary team.

EPIDEMIOLOGY AND PATHOGENESIS
Incidences and Trends

Anal cancer is an uncommon malignancy with an incidence ranging between 1.0 to 2.5 per 100,000 population in many western countries. In 2011, an estimated 5820 new cases (2140 men and 3680 women) were registered in the United States[1]; in the United Kingdom, in 2007, there were 790 new cases (292 men and 498 women).[2] The incidence of anal cancer has been increasing over the past 3 decades in Denmark,[3] Sweden[4] and Scotland,[5] most markedly in women. The exception is the United States, where the increases have been greater in men compared with women.[6,7]

Conflict of interest statements: Rob Glynne-Jones has received honoraria for lectures and advisory boards and has been supported in attending international meetings by Merck, Pfizer, Sanofi-Aventis, and Roche. He has also received unrestricted grants for research from Merck-Serono, Sanofi-Aventis, and Roche. Andrew Renehan has received honoraria for lectures and advisory boards from Sanofi Pasteur MPS.

[a] Radiotherapy Department, Centre for Cancer Treatment, Mount Vernon Hospital, Northwood, Middlesex HA6 2RN, UK; [b] Department of Surgery, Christie NHS Foundation Trust, Wilmslow Road, Manchester, M20 4BX, UK; [c] Institute of Cancer Sciences, University of Manchester, Christie Campus, Manchester, M20 4BX, UK
* Corresponding author.
E-mail address: rob.glynnejones@nhs.net

Hematol Oncol Clin N Am 26 (2012) 1315–1350
http://dx.doi.org/10.1016/j.hoc.2012.08.011
0889-8588/12/$ – see front matter © 2012 Elsevier Inc. All rights reserved.

Risk Factors and Etiology

Squamous cell carcinoma (SCC) accounts for more than 90% of anal cancer and is commonly associated with human papilloma virus (HPV) infection.[8] Risk factors include a history of receptive anal intercourse, a history of other HPV-related cancers, human immunodeficiency virus (HIV) infection, immunosuppression after solid organ transplantation,[9,10] social deprivation,[5] and cigarette smoking.[11–14] There is no clear association with dietary habits and chronic inflammatory diseases, and the presence of hemorrhoids does not appear to predispose to anal cancer development.[15,16]

Among men who have sex with men (MSM) in the United States, the incidence of anal cancer is approximately 35 per 100,000. In men who are HIV seropositive, the incidence increases further to 75 to 135 per 100,000. The incidence is also increased among seropositive women (30 per 100,000).[17]

The evidence supporting the role of HPV in the etiology of anal cancer comes from several different lines. A meta-analysis investigated HPV prevalence in anal intraepithelial neoplasia (AIN) grades 1 to 3 and carcinoma from 93 studies conducted in 4 continents and using polymerase chain reaction assays.[18] HPV was identified in 84.5% of cases, paralleling the prevalence seen in cervical and vulval carcinoma in women.[19] In common with cervix cancer, HPV 16 and 18 are the 2 commonest genotypes detected. Prospective data also links HPV seropositivity and risk of subsequent anal and perianal skin cancer.[20] HIV-positive and HIV-negative homosexual men are more likely than the general population to be infected with HPV, often with more than 1 subtype,[21] and are more likely to demonstrate HPV-associated AIN.

Anal Intraepithelial Neoplasia

In a similar manner to cervical carcinogenesis, it is believed that anal cancer arises in most cases through a precursor lesion: AIN. In turn, AIN is graded from 1 to 3 in severity. The prevalence of AIN in the population is generally low and the progression to invasive carcinoma is also low.[22] The prevalence of AIN in HIV-negative homosexual men is high (greater than 36%),[23] however, and almost universal among HIV-positive MSM. In these patients, progression to invasive carcinoma is more likely and is influenced by HIV seropositivity, low CD4 count, and the HPV gentotype.[24,25]

The natural history from AIN to invasive carcinoma in HIV-positive individuals is also influenced by HIV treatment; namely, highly active antiretroviral therapy. HIV-positive individuals now live longer and have longer exposure to the effects of HPV. Anal SCC is now the commonest malignancy in HIV-positive individuals in the United States.[26]

HPV Vaccination

Prophylactic HPV vaccination against HPV-16 and HPV-18 has been shown to be highly effective in preventing cervical dysplasia and thus cervical cancer.[27] Recently, the quadrivalent HPV vaccine (against HPV types 6, 11, 16, and 18) has also been shown to be highly effective in preventing HPV-16 and HPV-18 associated anal dysplasia,[28] and thus, in theory, may prevent a large proportion of cases of anal SCC in the future.

The role of HPV may have therapeutic implications, as patients with HPV-positive tumors in some anatomic sites appear to be more radiosensitive.[29,30] This finding may be partly explained because HPV is associated with the proteins E6 and E7, which affect tumor-suppressor proteins p53 and Rb in normal cells,[31] and have apoptotic cellular effects to prevent abnormal cell division.

PRESENTATION AND DIAGNOSIS
Presentation and the Role of the MDT

For UK and European treatment series,[32–35] mean ages at presentation are between 60 and 70 years; for US series,[36–38] mean ages are typically a decade earlier, an observation to take into account when comparing outcomes.

Common presenting symptoms are anal pain, bleeding, anal discharge, pruritis ani, and ulceration. Once the anal sphincters are involved, patients complain of discharge and soiling before frank fecal incontinence and tenesmus. In locally advanced disease, perianal infection and fistula formation may occur. Cases may present with enlarged inguinal lymph nodes in the absence of anal symptoms. Clinically palpable (inguinal) lymph nodes occur in 16% to 25% of cases,[33,35,36,38,39] depending on the clinical setting. Distant metastases at presentation are generally reported as less than 5% in treatment series[33,35,38]; the proportion for all-comer series is unclear.

Increasingly, new cases may present through a variety of other routes: incidental excision of anal tag or hemorrhoidectomy, through AIN surveillance clinics (particularly for high-risk patients), through transplant clinics, and as carcinoma arising within existing perianal Crohn disease (although most of these are mucinous adenocarcinomas rather than SCC).[40]

Within the United Kingdom, each of the 32 cancer networks is required to establish a specialized anal cancer multidisciplinary team (MDT), which meets regularly. The MDT includes a team of colorectal surgeons, clinical oncologists, radiologists, gynecologists, and pathologists, supported by a dedicated MDT coordinator, advanced nurse specialist, and data manager. All patients with a new diagnosis of anal SCC are reviewed in the MDT before initial treatment. In general, no more than 2 consultant surgical core members within the network should perform all salvage surgical operations for anal cancer.[41]

Anatomy and Lymphatic Drainage

For this article, we use the definitions of the anal canal and anal margin used by the National Comprehensive Cancer Network (NCCN).[42] For the anal canal, the superior functional border, separating it from the rectum, has been defined as the palpable upper border of the anal sphincter and puborectalis muscles of the anorectal ring. It is approximately 3 to 5 cm in length, and its inferior border starts at the anal verge, the lowermost edge of the of the sphincter muscles, corresponding to the introitus of the anal orifice. The anal margin starts at the anal verge and includes the perianal skin over a 5-cm to 6-cm radius from the squamous mucocutaneous junction.

The most proximal portion of the anal canal drains to perirectal nodes and nodes along the superior rectal vessels to the inferior mesenteric system, and thence to the para-aortic nodes. There is also drainage to the internal iliac and obturator nodes.[43] The canal above the dentate line drains to internal pudendal nodes, and to the internal iliac system. Venous drainage of the upper half of the canal is mainly by the superior rectal vein to inferior mesenteric vein, whereas drainage of the lower half is by the inferior rectal vein, to the internal pudendal vein and internal iliac vein. Hence, metastases may occur either to liver via the portal system, or lung via the systemic circulation, partly depending on tumor position. The canal below the dentate line drains to the medial group of superficial inguinal nodes with some communication with femoral nodes and to external iliac nodes. Involved nodes are often palpable, but historical pathology studies, using a "clearing" technique, demonstrated that almost half of all involved lymph nodes were smaller than 5 mm in diameter.[44] The inguinal, femoral, and iliac lymph nodes are the most frequent sites for nodal metastases.[45]

Histopathology

Assessment of the integrity of the biopsy specimen should be documented. The size of the tumor in terms of the greatest dimension if possible, and after local excision, the resection margins (specified in mm), both deep and at the periphery, are required to decide if further treatment is advisable. Hence, all the relevant resection margins should ideally be inked.

This article does not discuss the diagnosis of non-SCC anal malignancies. Traditionally, SCC has been subdivided into basaloid or cloacogenic types, but these are now recognized as an SCC variant that lacks terminal differentiation; specific prognostic significance is questionable,[46] and does not indicate differences in management (**Fig. 1**).[47] Verrucous carcinomas are another variant and are sometimes described as giant condylomas or Buschke-Lowenstein tumors, which are often larger but may have a better prognosis than SCC. Grading is subject to considerable interobserver variability, however, and there is considerable heterogeneity in larger tumors. Hence, although high-grade tumors are generally accepted to have a worse prognosis, this has not been confirmed in multivariate analysis from historical surgical series.[48]

Molecular Pathology and Prognostic Factors

Over the past 2 decades, chemoradiation has become the standard treatment (detailed later) and offers an excellent response rate and prognosis for most patients, but there is still considerable heterogeneity as regards their outcomes. Hence, biologic factors/biomarkers that affect outcomes would be useful to provide prognostic information and, in turn, inform individualized therapies.

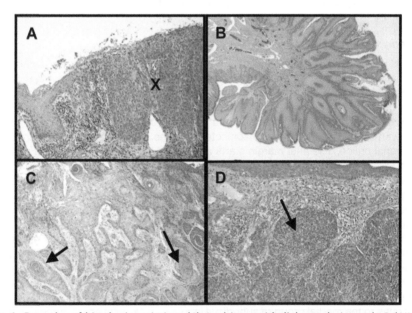

Fig. 1. Examples of histologic variation. (*A*) Anal intraepithelial neoplasia grade 3 (AIN 3: marked as "x") adjacent to normal squamous epithelium. (*B*) HPV-related condyloma mimicking an SCC. (*C*) Keratinizing SCC (*keratin pearls indicated by arrow*). (*D*) Basaloid differentiation (*indicated by arrow*) of squamous cell carcinoma (hematoxylin and eosin stain; original magnification ×20, all images). (*Courtesy of* Bipasha Chakrabarty.)

A recent systematic review examined 29 different biomarkers belonging to 9 different functional classes: tumor suppressors, epidermal growth factor receptor (EGFR), apoptosis regulation, proliferation index, angiogenesis, tumor-specific markers (eg, squamous cell carcinoma antigen and carcinoembryonic antigen), Hedgehog signaling, and telomerase.[49] Thirteen biomarkers were associated with outcome in at least one study, but the tumor-suppressor genes p53 and p21 were the only biomarkers shown to have prognostic value in more than one study. Notably, overexpression of p53 is common in anal carcinomas.[50] Alterations in p53 protein function may result from either mutations in its gene or sequestration by other cellular proteins, such as the E6 viral oncoprotein of the HPV virus.[51] In an analysis of 240 patients randomized in the United Kingdom Coordinating Committee on Cancer Research Anal Cancer Trial I (UKCCCR ACT I), the presence of mutated p53 predicted a poorer cause-specific survival.[52] Anal carcinomas appear to have a high proliferative index[53,54]; however, only 2 studies have shown its prognostic significance.

In the interpretation of these data, it is important to take residual confounding into account. Thus, for example, some biomarkers may be associated with more advanced disease and may be prognostic Because of coincidence with advanced stage. Prognostic studies are best addressed where treatment is standardized in a narrow stage range.[55]

STAGING AND INITIAL ASSESSMENT
TNM Staging

Early trials used the International Union Contra Cancer staging system in which T stage is based on anatomic extent and the proportion of the circumference of the anal canal involved by tumor. Since 2000, studies have used the unified American Joint Committee on Cancer/International Union against Cancer (AJCC/UICC) staging system incorporating primary tumor size (T), lymph node status (N), and distant metastases (M). The seventh edition of the AJCC/UICC classification for anal cancer is shown in **Table 1**.[56]

Clinical and Standard Radiological Assessment

Accurate initial clinical staging is clinically important for several reasons[40]:

1. Determination of distant metastases: generally deems the case noncurative;
2. Prognosis and treatment response: in general terms, risk of local disease relapse increases with increasing T size;
3. Gross tumor volume: for planning radiotherapy (RT) delivery;
4. Determination of inguinal node involvement: as inguinal node positivity materially changes the planned RT schedule;
5. Defining follow-up;
6. Defining early anal margin tumors suitable for local excision; and
7. Defining stage for future trial entry.

Clinical examination and digital rectal examination (DRE) remain valuable methods for assessing tumor loco-regional extent. Direct proctoscopy is often difficult in more advanced lesions because of pain. Examination under anesthetic allows more detailed palpation of the anorectal and pelvic structures and may be required for biopsy. Vaginal examination is essential in female patients to assess extension into the postvaginal wall or even breaching of the vaginal mucosa. Clinical assessment of inguino-femoral lymph nodes is helpful to identify palpable nodes, but more accurate assessment of whether there is disease involvement relies of radiological assessment and other techniques.

Table 1
Seventh Edition of the American Joint Committee on Cancer/International Union against Cancer TNM staging for anal canal cancer

Primary Tumor (T)	
Tx	Primary tumor cannot be assessed
Tis	Carcinoma in situ [Bowens disease, high-grade intraepithelial lesion (HSIL), anal intraepithelial neoplasia (AIN) II-III]
T1	Tumor smaller than 2 cm in greatest dimension
T2	Tumor between 2 cm and 5 cm in greatest dimension
T3	Tumor larger than 5 cm in greatest dimension
T4	Tumor invading adjacent organs [vagina, urethra, bladder, sacrum]

Regional lymph nodes (N)	
NX	Regional nodes cannot be assessed
N0	No regional lymph node metastasis
N1	Metastasis in perirectal nodes
N2	Metastasis in unilateral internal iliac and/or inguinal nodes
N3	Metastasis in perirectal and/or bilateral internal iliac or inguinal nodes

Distant Metastasis (M)	
M0	No distant metastasis
M1	Distant metastasis

Anatomic stage/Prognostic groups			
0	Tis	N0	M0
I	T1	N0	M0
II	T2	N0	M0
	T3	N0	M0
IIIA	T1	N1	M0
	T2	N1	M0
	T3	N1	M0
	T4	N0	M0
IIIB	T4	N1	M0
	Any T	N2	M0
IV	Any T	N3	M0
	Any T	Any N	M1

From Edge SB, Byrd DR, Compton CC, et al. AJCC Cancer staging manual. 7th edition. New York: Springer; 2009; with permission.

Although clinical examination is an important initial component of staging assessment, radiological modalities offer additional information and are essential parts of the anal cancer MDT assessment (**Fig. 2**). Given that definitive chemoradiation is the standard of care, however, there are few data to confirm the performance characteristics of radiological staging, as there can be no histopathological correlation (ie, a lack of a referent standard). Transrectal ultrasound (TRUS) allows a 360° view of the anal canal, and can accurately assess the depth of tumor infiltration and involvement of the sphincter mechanism and fistula tracts. TRUS, however, offers a limited field of view and is poor at assessing lymph node involvement in the mesorectum and pelvis. Magnetic resonance imaging (MRI) provides excellent clarity regarding the primary tumor for RT planning, and offers more accurate information on nodal involvement, particularly in the mesorectum and inguinal regions, than clinical staging with computed tomography (CT).[57] MRI is favored for assessing loco-regional disease extent,[58] as this provides good contrast resolution and multi-planar anatomic detail. The intermediate to high signal intensity tumor is well de-lineated on T2 and short tau inversion recovery (STIR)-weighted sequences, and primary tumor extent into surrounding structures.[59] TRUS may be superior to MRI for detecting small, superficial tumors; MRI is more effective for N staging. To move to more conformal RT (using intensity-modulated RT [IMRT] or volumetric-modulated arc therapy, detailed later in this article) and run future phase III trials, we need clear definitions of nodal involvement by MRI criteria and subclin-ical areas, which potentially harbor microscopic disease.

Role of Fluorodeoxyglucose Positron Emission Tomography

Current NCCN treatment guidelines include fluorodeoxyglucose positron emission tomography integrated with CT (FDG-PET/CT) as part of the pretreatment diagnostic workup.[60] FDG-PET/CT can evaluate primary tumor size, lymph node status, and image distant metastases, and can detect uptake in normal-sized but involved nodes with a high positive predictive value, but offers limited accuracy for lymph nodes smaller than 8 mm. As this is a size limit for CT and MRI, a false-negative result is likely to remain false negative in all 3 modalities. PET appears to be highly specific for nodal spread in other pelvic malignancies, such as vulva and cervix.[61] PET/CT can also be used for radiation therapy treatment planning by defining sites of metabolically active tumor. Yet, precise anatomic detail is still poor.

An Italian group examined PET/CT to define stage and assist target volume delinea-tion, and found a change in clinical stage in 18.5% of the 27 patients, leading to a change in treatment intent in 3.7%.[62] The largest UK published series to date found PET/CT changed clinical stage in 23% of patients. The sensitivity of PET was also found to be superior for detection of regional nodal metastases; 89% versus 62% and overall PET changed management in 16% of cases.[63] Others[64] have found that PET/CT complements standard clinical staging information in 10% to 24% of cases, but has little value posttreatment. A recent study from Mount Vernon found that PET/CT diagnosed distant metastatic disease undetected by CT scan in 5%, and altered staging in 42% of patients overall.[65] Currently in the United Kingdom, PET/CT is not part of routine staging and is mainly used to justify radical surgical salvage.

PET/CT should be increasingly used in standard staging protocols. With the advent of advanced planning techniques, such as IMRT, altered RT treatment volumes based on PET/CT imaging may lead to potentially lower toxicity, improved dose accuracy, and a paradigm shift away from therapeutic techniques dependent on the assumption of malignant involvement to those in which we can be more confident of optimal target delineation.

Assessment of Inguino-femoral Nodes

The importance of the accurate prediction of inguino-femoral lymph node involvement is set against the broadly 2 approaches to initial treatment. In the United Kingdom and some European countries, centers follow a 2-phase RT regimen: the phase I dose (typically 30.6 Gy) is a prophylactic treatment of the inguino-femoral and pelvic side-wall lymphatic fields; the phase II dose (to 50.4 Gy) in used in patients with clinically evident nodal disease. The alternative approach is the elective treatment of the inguino-femoral nodes either by RT or surgical nodal dissection.

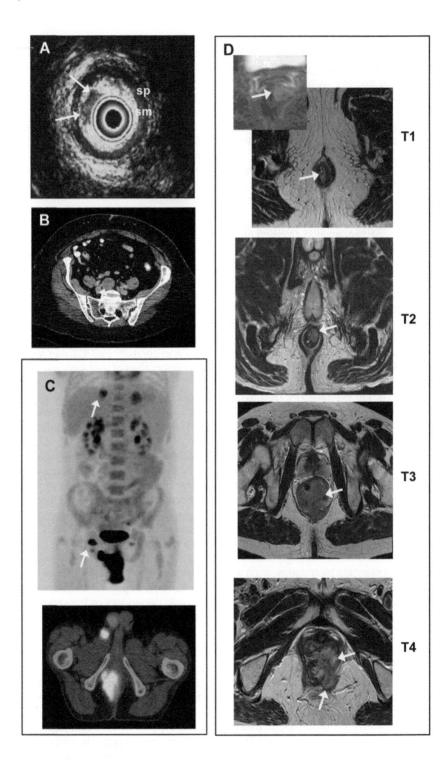

For early-stage disease (T size ≤3 cm), the risk of inguinal nodal involvement is less than 5%.[66] In contrast, the risk of involvement for clinically staged T3 or T4 may approach 20%.[67] Clinical examination and CT supplemented by fine-needle aspiration cytology (FNAC) has traditionally been the standard of care,[67] but is probably insufficiently accurate. Lymph node metastases in the groin are difficult to assess partly because fewer than 50% of involved lymph nodes will measure less than 5 mm in diameter,[44] and hence, many involved lymph nodes will simply not be palpable or imaged on CT. Reactive nodes in the groins are often enlarged and palpable and may easily be confused with pathologically involved lymph nodes. FNAC of groin nodes with the use of ultrasound may be slightly more accurate,[68] but there are sampling limitations, and negative results do not always give confidence that this is a truly negative result. Excision biopsy, if followed by RT, is likely to lead to added morbidity, such as lymphedema.

More recently, inguinal-femoral node staging by FDG-PET/CT has been advocated, because positive lymph nodes may be more easily identified than with other imaging modalities.[61,64]

Sentinel lymph node biopsy (SLNB) has been validated in lymph node staging of small breast tumors to spare the need for major axillary dissection. In anal cancer, the rationale is to spare formal inguinal irradiation, but SLNB has yet to fulfill its initial hopes in this setting. There is undoubtedly an important training issue for the surgeon undertaking SLNB, as in one study, 24% of patients had a postoperative complications in the groin.[69] Future trials in this question have to be set against the established observation that the risk of metachronous inguinal node metastasis in patients treated with prophylactic groin radiation is low (4%).[37] SLNB may be useful in the setting of loco-regional recurrence after chemoradiation to decide whether radical inguinal dissection is required at the time of salvage radical anorectal surgery.

INITIAL TREATMENT
The Evidence for Chemoradiation

Initial studies of Nigro and colleagues[70,71] demonstrated high rates of local control (LC) with the use of low doses (approximately 30 Gy) of irradiation with concurrent mitomycin and 5-fluoruracil (MMC/5-FU). Cummings and colleagues[72] reported a series of 190 patients treated with RT alone or chemoradiation (CRT) using 7 sequential regimens and concluded retrospectively improved LC with CRT with the addition of MMC to 5-FU. The definitive evidence for the advantage of CRT is based on 2 phase III trials that compared RT with RT and concurrent MMC/5-FU: the UKCCCR ACT I trial[35] and the European Organization for Research and Treatment of Cancer (EORTC)

Fig. 2. Radiological staging is an essential part of the anal cancer MDT assessment. (*A*) Many centers around the world use transrectal ultrasound, which is useful for the staging of early lesions, as in this figure. This is a T1 tumor (*arrowed*). sp, sphincter; sm, submucosa. (*B*) CT imaging of the chest, abdomen, and pelvis are required for staging. This may reveal extrapelvic disease. In this figure, the arrow indicates an enlarged involved para-aortic lymph node. (*C*) Increasingly, PET-CT is helpful in the staging of anal cancer. This figure demonstrates the "hot" primary tumor, a right-inguinal involved lymph node, and a left lobe liver metastasis. (*D*) In the United Kingdom, MR scanning is the key imaging modality for pretreatment staging. Even for small lesions, experienced radiologists can stage T1 lesions (insert: STIR weighted). This modality is particularly useful to define T4 lesions invading adjacent structures. ([*B–D*] *Courtesy of* Rohit Kochher.)

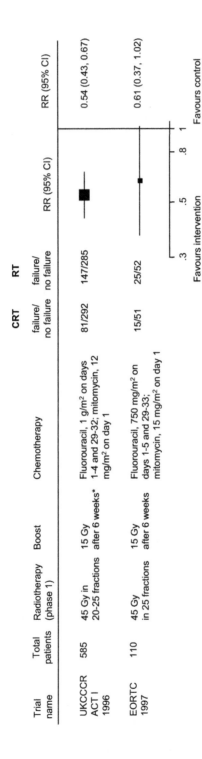

The table content of the figure:

Trial name	Total patients	Radiotherapy (phase 1)	Boost	Chemotherapy	CRT failure/no failure	RT failure/no failure	RR (95% CI)	RR (95% CI)
UKCCCR ACT I 1996	585	45 Gy in 20-25 fractions	15 Gy after 6 weeks*	Fluorouracil, 1 g/m² on days 1-4 and 29-32; mitomycin, 12 mg/m² on day 1	81/292	147/285		0.54 (0.43, 0.67)
EORTC 1997	110	45 Gy in 25 fractions	15 Gy after 6 weeks	Fluorouracil, 750 mg/m² on days 1-5 and 29-33; mitomycin, 15 mg/m² on day 1	15/51	25/52		0.61 (0.37, 1.02)

Favours intervention   Favours control

Fig. 3. Evidence that chemoradiation improves LC compared with RT alone. The results from the trials are similar but the studies varied in the proportion of early (T1 and T2) tumors between 16% in the EORTC 22861 study, and 41% in ACT I. The T-staging classification also varies, because early trials used the 1978 International Union Contra Cancer (UICC), or the 1985 UICC classification based on anatomic extent, and the proportion of the circumference involved by tumor. Hence, the outcomes from these studies have not been combined to give an overall summary estimate "diamond." CI, confidence interval; RR, relative risk.

trial.[32] Both trials showed very comparable results that CRT improves disease-free survival (DFS) compared with RT alone (**Fig. 3**). By the late 1990s, primary CRT with concurrent MMC/5-FU became standard treatment. This continues today, although a small minority of investigators continue to use external beam RT alone followed by a small volume boost either with photons or electrons (particularly for small T1 tumors).

Interstitial implantation of radioactive sources as a sole modality or as a boost after external beam RT[73,74] has been used in parts of Europe. Scandinavian retrospective series[75] have described the use of high doses in the region of 60 Gy external beam RT with results that compare favorably with the randomized trials. High rates of LC have been observed in a series from Institute Gustave Roussy of 91% for T1 and T2 tumors,[76] and in a study from San Francisco in patients who were node negative with T1 and T2 tumors had a high 5-year survival rate of 92%.[77] In contrast to this experience in specialist centers, multicenter anal cancer trials[35] demonstrate that even T1 and T2 lesions appear to obtain the benefit from the addition of chemotherapy. Together with sequential phase II studies,[72,78–82] these randomized trials have helped to refine techniques of RT and the efficacy of relatively low total radiation doses. However, the optimal schedules, radiation dose, technique, duration of gap, and chemotherapy choice have been repeatedly questioned and remain in some cases the subject of ongoing clinical trials.

Optimizing Chemotherapy Schedules

The Radiation Therapy Oncology Group (RTOG)-8704 trial demonstrated the advantage of adding 2 courses of MMC at a dose of 10 mg/m^2.[83] With a median dose of 48 Gy and a boost of 9 Gy to histologically confirmed residual disease, the RTOG-8704 confirmed the superiority of MMC/5-FU over 5-FU alone when combined with RT.

The US Intergroup RTOG 98-11 phase III trial[36] randomly assigned 682 patients with anal canal tumors (35% with T3/T4 tumors, and 26% with clinically involved lymph nodes) to either neoadjuvant 5-FU and cisplatin for 2 cycles before concurrent chemoradiation with 5-FU and cisplatin (n = 341), or the standard arm of concurrent chemoradiation with MMC/5-FU (n = 341). The primary end point was 5-year DFS. The neoadjuvant cisplatin-based chemotherapy arm failed to improve DFS, locoregional control, distant relapse, or overall survival (OS). In fact, trends favored the control arm of mitomycin. Recent presentation of the trial data suggest the outcome for cisplatin could be significantly inferior.[84] By contrast, the requirement for a colostomy was significantly higher in the cisplatin arm compared with the mitomycin arm (19% vs 10%; $P = .02$). Hematological toxicity was worse with mitomycin. Similar compliance to both chemotherapy and RT in each arm suggests that the differences did not relate to excess toxicity. Both neoadjuvant and concurrent cisplatin was used in the same experimental arm of the trial, however, making analysis of the individual role of each strategy difficult. In total, 10% of patients developed long-term toxicity after CRT, with 5% requiring a colostomy for treatment-related problems.

The Action Clinique Coordonees en Cancerologie Digestive (ACCORD)-03 phase III trial[85] tested 2 cycles of neoadjuvant chemotherapy (NACT) with 5-FU and cisplatin and also radiation dose escalation in a factorial 2 × 2 trial design in 307 patients with SCC cancers larger than 40 mm and/or with pelvic or inguinal involved nodes. The primary end point was colostomy-free survival (CFS). Secondary end points included LC, OS, and cancer-specific survival. The trial compared 45 Gy in 25 daily fractions plus a 15-Gy boost after 3 weeks gap with a higher boost dose of 20 to 25 Gy (ie, 65–70 Gy total dose), but found no benefit in CFS at doses higher than 59 Gy. Toxicity-related dose reductions during CRT were required in 19% of the concomitant cycles.

Selected doses of chemotherapy were lower than those prescribed for patients with primary head and neck or esophagus cancer. Newer techniques of irradiation, such as IMRT, should reduce this toxicity by better sparing organs at risk, thereby preventing chemotherapy dose reductions.

Preliminary results of the ACT II multicenter, randomized trial, which recruited 940 patients, have been presented.[86] Patients received 5-FU (1000 mg/m^2/d on days 1–4, 29–32) and RT (50.4 Gy in 28 daily fractions), and were randomized to receive MMC (12 mg/m^2, day 1; n = 471) or cisplatin (60 mg/m^2 on day 1, 29; n = 469). A second randomization directed 2 courses of consolidation therapy (n = 448) 5 and 8 weeks after CRT (5-FU/cisplatin, ie, weeks 11, 14), or no consolidation (n = 446). Response was assessed clinically at 11 and 18 weeks, and by CT at 24 weeks. Preliminary results showed almost identical complete response rates (95%) in both arms, with 3-year recurrence-free survival rates of 75% in T1/T2 tumors overall, and 68% for more advanced T3/T4 tumors.[86] Hence, neither strategy, ie, CRT with cisplatin versus CRT with MMC, nor chemotherapy consolidation with cisplatin was more effective for achieving complete clinical response (cCR), reducing tumor relapse or cancer-specific deaths than the standard of MMC/CRT. Acute hematological toxicity was more pronounced for MMC, but nonhematological toxicity similar.

In summary, The RTOG-9811, ACCORD-03, and ACT II phase III trials in anal cancer showed no benefit for cisplatin-based induction and maintenance chemotherapy, or radiation dose escalation above 59 Gy. Neither the RTOG-9208 trial nor the ACCORD-03 trial support the view that radiation dose escalation within a CRT schedule increases LC in anal cancer. The present authors feel that 5-FU and MMC (12 mg/m^2, day 1) is the recommended standard. A recent update of the RTOG98-11 presented suggests that, with more mature follow-up, there is a significant advantage in 5-year DFS for 5-FU/MMC over induction cisplatin and CRT with 5-FU/cisplatin (**Tables 2** and **3**).

Optimizing RT Dose Schedule

The determination of optimal dose fractionation is limited by a lack of data regarding the pattern of failure. No randomized study has described the site(s) of local failure (within, marginal to, or outside of the RT field). Therefore, it remains uncertain whether most loco-regional failure is attributable to inadequate clinical target volumes, insufficient radiation dose, or intrinsic radioresistance.

Brachytherapy may potentially increase dose to the primary tumor in T3/T4 tumors[87] but requires skill and expertise to avoid radionecrosis owing to an unsatisfactory dose distribution. A low dose-rate iridium interstitial implant was originally advocated as a boost following RT alone[74] after an interval of 6 weeks, but this technique does not achieve current standards of conformal treatment. This delaying strategy influenced the design of the 2 early European phase III studies,[32,35] in which a brachytherapy boost delivered 25 Gy following CRT after an interval of 6 weeks. Enthusiasm that brachytherapy achieves better outcomes in terms of LC probably reflects patient selection; patients with smaller tumors or good responders to CRT are preferentially selected for brachytherapy boost.

Other Chemotherapy Considerations

Other considerations are as follows (**Table 4**):

1. All the phase III trials to date used a continuous 4-day or 5-day infusion of 5-FU in the first and fifth weeks of RT. None have used a prolonged venous infusion or an oral fluoropyrimidine during the RT phase, as in rectal cancer. Because the dose and intensity of the chemotherapy administered concurrently with radiation are

Table 2
Characteristics of the randomized trials of different chemoradiation regimens in anal cancer

Trial Name (Years)	No. of Patients	Design	RT Dose	Testing 1	Testing 2	Planned Gap	Primary End Point
RTOG 87-04/ECOG (1988–1991)	291	5-FU/RT vs 5-FU/MMC/RT	Phase I 45 Gy–56 Gy median 48 Gy then biopsy of residual disease; 9 Gy boost if +	Addition of MMC 10 mg/m² d 1 and 29 to 5-FU-based CRT		4–6 wk after 45–50.4 Gy if biopsy +	Disease-free survival
RTOG 98-11 (1998–2005)	644	NACT cisplatin/5-FU then 5-FU/cisplatin/RT (ie, 4 courses) vs 5FU/MMC/RT	Phase I 45 Gy/25# in 5.0–6.5 wk T3/T4, N+ or residual T2 boost to 54–59 Gy	NACT with 5-FU 1000 mg/m² d 1–4, 29–32 and cisplatin 75 mg/m² then CRT 5-FU/cisplatin vs MMC 10 mg/m² d 1 and 29 and 5-FU 1000 mg/m² d 1–4, 29–32 CRT		Max 10-d gap for skin intolerance, but median OTT = 49 d	Disease-free survival
ACT II (UKCCCR) (2001–2008)	940	2 × 2 factorial 5-FU/ MMC vs 5-FU cisplatin CRT and consolidation 5-FU/cisplatin vs control	Phase I 30/6 Gy/17# in 3.5 wk then Phase II 19.8 Gy/11# conformal Total 50.4 Gy/28#/38 d no gap	Cisplatin 60 mg/m² d 1 and 29 vs 12 mg/m² MMC day 1 with 5-FU 1000 mg/m² d 1–4, 29–32 CRT	Consolidate 2 courses 5-FU 1000 mg/m² and Cisplatin 60 mg/m²	No gap; OTT 38 d	Relapse- free survival
ACCORD-03 (1999–2005)	307	2 × 2 factorial NACT (5-FU/cisplatin- 2 cycles) vs no NACT Standard vs high-dose boost for responders	Phase I 45 Gy/25#/33 d 3 wk gap then 15-Gy boost standard arms 20 Gy–25 Gy boost (high-dose arms) for responders 40% received brachytherapy boost	NACT with 5-FU 800 mg/m² d 1–4, 29–32 and cisplatin 80 g/m² on days 1 and 29 then CRT 5-FU/cisplatin on days as above with RT	Dose escalation of RT boost 15-Gy boost standard arms 20 Gy–25 Gy boost (high-dose arms) for responders	3 wk after 45 Gy CRT completed	Colostomy-free survival Secondary end points included local control, overall survival, and cancer-specific survival.

Abbreviations: 5-FU, 5-Fluorouracil; ACCORD, Action Clinique Coordonees en Cancerologie Digestive; Cisplatin, Cisplatinum; CRT, chemoradiation; ECOG, Eastern Cooperative Oncology Group; Gy, Gray; HDRT, high-dose radiotherapy; MMC, Mitomycin C; NACT, neoadjuvant chemotherapy; NS, not significant; OTT, overall treatment time; RT, radiotherapy; RTOG, Radiation Therapy Oncology Group; UKCCCR ACT, United Kingdom Coordinating Committee on Cancer Research Anal Cancer Trial.

Table 3
Outcomes of the randomized trials of different chemoradiation regimens in anal cancer

Studies (Authors)	No. of Patients	Median Follow-up	Complete Response	Local Failure Rate	DFS/RFS	Colostomy Rate/ Colostomy-Free Survival	Overall Survival
RTOG 87-04 (Flam et al,[83] 1996)	291	3 y	Path CR (biopsy) 86% 5-FU 92.2% (MMC) at 4–6 wk post	16% at 4 y	DFS 51% 5-FU vs 73% with 5-FU/MMC at 4 y	Colostomy rate: 22% with 5-FU vs 9% with 5-FU, MMC; P = .002 Colostomy-free survival: 59% with 5-FU vs 71% with 5-FU/MMC, at 4 y; P = .014	71% with 5-FU vs 78.1% with 5-FU/MMC; P = .31
RTOG 98-11 (Ajani et al,[36] 2008)	644	2.5 y	No data on clinical response provided	25% with 5-FU, MMC vs 33% with 5-FU, cisplatin	DFS 60% with 5-FU, MMC vs 54% 5-FU, cisplatin at 5 y; NS P = .17	Colostomy rate: 10% with 5-FU, MMC vs 19% with 5-FU, cisplatin; P = .02 at 5 y	75% with 5-FU, MMC vs 70% with 5-FU, cisplatin; P = .1 at 5 y
UKCCCR ACT II (James et al,[86] 2009)	940	36 mo	94.5% 5-FU/MMC/RT vs 95% 5-FU/Cis/RT at 18 wk, ie, 12 wk post boost	11% with MMC; 13% with cisplatin	RFS 75% in both arms at 3 y	Colostomy rate same in both arms (5% with maintenance vs 4% without)	85% with maintenance at 3 y; 84% without; not significant
ACCORD-03 (Peiffert et al,[85] 2012)	307	50 mo	Overall 79% complete clinical response at 2 mo post boost	Arm A 28% Arm B 12% Arm C 16% Arm D 22% overall 19% at 5 y	Tumor-free survival Arm A 64% Arm B 78% Arm C 67% Arm D 62%	5 y colostomy-free survival Arm A 70% Arm B 82% Arm C 77% Arm D 73%	5 y specific survival Arm A 77% Arm B 89% Arm C 81% Arm D 76%

Abbreviations: 5-FU, 5-Fluorouracil; ACCORD, Action Clinique Coordonees en Cancerologie Digestive; Cis, Cisplatinum; CRT, chemoradiation; DFS, disease-free survival; HDRT, high-dose radiotherapy; MMC, Mitomycin C; NACT, neoadjuvant chemotherapy; NS, not significant; RFS, relapse-free survival; RT, radiotherapy; RTOG, Radiation Therapy Oncology Group; UKCCCR ACT, United Kingdom Coordinating Committee on Cancer Research Anal Cancer Trial.

Table 4
Reported phase I and II trials of different treatments in anal cancer

Trial Names (Authors)	No. of Patients	Design	RT Dose	Complete Response	Median F/U	3 y DFS	3 y CFS	OS
RTOG - 8314 (Sischy[156] 1989)	79	5-FU 1000 mg/m² d 2–5 and 30–33 MMC 10 mg/m²	40.8 Gy in 24 fractions over 4.5–5.0 wk	90% at 6–8 wk −ve biopsy	3 y	61%	No data	73% at 3 y
ECOG E7283 (Martenson et al,[81] 1995)	50	5FU 1000 mg/m² d 2–5, MMC 10 mg/m² d2 + RT + 5-FU 28 d later	40 Gy + 10–13 Gy boost	34/46 evaluable (74%) at 6–8 wk 1/11 with PR had −ve biopsy	No data	53% at 7 y	No data	58% at 7 y
ECOG E4292 (Martenson[157] 1996)	19	5-FU 1000 mg/m² d 1–4, Cisplatin 75 mg/m² d 1 + RT, + after 36 Gy	59.4 Gy/33 # 2 wk break at 36 Gy	15/19 (79%) at 8 wk post RT	No data maximum F/U 33/12	No data	No data	No data
Italian Study (Doci[158] 1996)	35	5-FU 750 mg/m² d 1–4, Cisplatin 100 mg/m² d 1 and on day 1 of RT and at 36 Gy if fit	36 Gy/20#/28 d then 18–24 Gy in 10# at 6 wk, ie, 2-wk gap	33/35 (94%) at 2 mo	37 mo	94% at 37 mo	86% at 37 mo	97% alive at 37 mo
RTOG - 92-08 (John et al,[80] 1996, Konski[159] 2008)	47	5-FU/MMC	2-k mandatory gap total 59.4 Gy	81% pCR at Biopsy 4–6 wk	12 y	5-y DFS estimated 53%	5 y 58% estimated	5-y OS est 67%
RTOG - 92-08 (Konski[159] 2008)	20	5-FU/MMC	No mandatory gap total 59.4 Gy	No data	8.8 y	5-y DFS estimated 80%	5 y 75% estimated	5-y OS est 85%
Portuguese study (Vaz[160] 1998)	36	2 cycles NACT 5-FU/cisplatin 2 cycles with RT	45 Gy/25#/33 d 1–2-mo gap 15–20-Gy boost	20/23 (87%)	20.6 mo	No data	No data	No data

(continued on next page)

Table 4
(continued)

Trial Names (Authors)	No. of Patients	Design	RT Dose	Complete Response	Median F/U	3 y DFS	3 y CFS	OS
French Study (Gerard[161] 1999)	26	Randomized phase II 5-FU 800 mg/m² d 1–4 + cisplatin 80 mg/m² vs cisplatin 30 mg/m² d 1–3	30 Gy/10 fractions/12 d + sacral fields 18 Gy/6#/21 d implant 15–25 Gy	23/26 overall 11/13 Group A vs 12/13 Group B	No data	No data	No data	91% at 4 y
ACT II pilot (Sebag-Montefiore[163] 2012) phase II	20	5-FU 1000 mg/m² d 1–4 MMC 10 mg/m² d 1 Cisplatin 60 mg/m² d 1 (all 3 drugs) and RT +3 maintenance 5FU/Cisplatin	45 Gy/25#/33 d 1–2-mo gap 15–20-Gy boost total 60–65 Gy	9/18 (50%) at 4–8 wk	4/12	No data	No data	No data
FNCLCC (Peiffert et al,[101] 2001)	80	2 cycles NACT 5-FU/cisplatin 2 cycles with RT	45 Gy/25#/33 d 1–2-mo gap 15–20-Gy boost	74/79 (93%)	29 mo	70% at 3 y	73% at 3 y	86% at 3 y
EORTC 22953 (Bosset et al,[150] 2003)	43	PVI 5-FU during whole treatment 2 doses of MMC 10 mg/m²	36 Gy/20#/28 d 16-d gap 23.4 Gy/13#/ 17-d boost	36/43 (84%) at 6 wk 39/43 (90.7%) at 8 wk (week 16)	30 mo	88% loco-regional at 3 y	81% at 3 y	3-y estimated rate 81%
TROG 99-02 (Matthews[162] 2005)	40	5-FU/MMC (5-FU 800 mg/m²/ d single dose MMC 10 mg/m² max 15 mg)	36 Gy/20#/28 d 2-wk gap 14.4 Gy/8# boost	No data	24 mo	25% primary relapse 24% groin relapse at 3 y	No data	No data

Study	N	Regimen	RT schedule	Response				
EORTC 22011 (Crehange[164] 2006) phase I	21	5-FU+MMC+RT vs cisplatin 25 mg/m² weekly +MMC 10 mg/m² + RT	36 Gy in 20# ~ over 28 d then 16-d gap then 23.4 Gy in 13#	19/21 (90.5%) at 8 wk	No data	No data	No data	No data
EXTRA phase II (Glynne-Jones et al,[151] 2008)	31	Capecitabine and MMC with RT	50.4 Gy/28#/38 d No gap	24/31 77% at 4 wk	14 mo	3/31 recurrences at 14/12	No data	No data
CALGB 9281 (Meropol et al,[100] 2008)	50	5-FU 1000 mg/m² d 1–4, Cisplatin100 mg/m² d 1, 29	Split course 30.6 Gy/17 #/then 3-wk gap then 14.4 Gy - total 45 Gy/25#	37/45 (82%)	4 y	61% at 4 y	50% at 4 y	68% at 4 y
PHASE I Brazilian study (Olivatto,[93] 2008)	10	5-FU days 1–4, Cisplatin d 1, 29 plus Cetuximab	45 Gy/25#/33 d 10-Gy boost	7/9 (78%)	No data	No data	No data	No data
M. D. Anderson Oxaliplatin phase I/II (Eng et al,[98] 2009)	20	Capecitabine 825 mg/m² bd M-F a Oxaliplatin 50 mg/m² weekly – modified to omit wk 3 and 6	T1 45 Gy25# T2 55 Gy/30# T3/T459 Gy/32#	90% in Group 1 and 100% in Group 2	19 mo	100%	100%	100%
EORTC 22011 (Matzinger et al,[94] 2009) Phase II leading to phase III	88	5-FU+MMC +RT vs cisplatin +MMC + RT	36 Gy in 20# ~ over 28 d then 16-d gap then 23.4 Gy in 13#	23/39 (59%) 5FU/MMC 27/37 (73%) MMC/Cisplatin at 8 wk	No data	No data	No data	No data
TOTAL	715							

Abbreviations: 5-FU, 5-Fluorouracil; ACT, Anal Cancer Trial; bd, twice daily; CALGB, Cancer and Leukemia Group B; CFS, colostomy-free survival; Cis, Cisplatinum; CRT, chemoradiation; DFS, disease-free survival; ECOG, Eastern Cooperative Oncology Group; EORTC, European Organization for Research and Treatment of Cancer; FNCLCC, National Federation of French Cancer Centres; F/U, follow-up; MMC, Mitomycin C; NACT, neoadjuvant chemotherapy; NS, not significant; OS, Overall survival; PR, partial response; pCR, pathologic complete response; PVI, prolonged venous infusion; RT, radiotherapy; RTOG, Radiation Therapy Oncology Group; TROG, Tasman Radiation Oncology Group.

almost invariably compromised by concerns for acute toxicity, it seems unlikely that such schedules would impact significantly on distant metastases.

2. The central role of MMC in anal cancer therapy is well accepted, yet the dose is still not standardized, and optimal doses are unknown. There is a suggestion that cumulative doses less than 28 mg/m^2 are safe,[88] but higher doses are associated with an increased risk of hemolytic uremic syndrome.[89]

3. The RTOG-8704 trial used an MMC dose of 10 mg/m^2 in weeks 1 and 5.[83] In contrast, the European trials[32,35] have used a single dose on day 1 of MMC at 12 mg/m^2 (capped at 20 mg total dose in the ACT II study). Although MMC has a rapid systemic elimination, there is little apparent excretion of MMC in urine or feces, suggesting rapid tissue uptake followed by a slow release of the drug from tumor and normal tissues. MMC may remain in hypoxic cells as a radiosensitizer for long periods. It has a recognized biphasic pattern of hematological toxicity. Hence, it is not clear whether a second dose of MMC on day 29 adds to the efficacy of CRT or not, although it clearly would add to toxicity.

4. In addition to the aforementioned phase III trials, 2 European phase II studies,[90,91] a large retrospective study,[92] and a Brazilian Phase I study[93] have all evaluated cisplatin dosing in concurrent chemotherapy and RT for anal cancer. However, cisplatin doses and schedules vary in all these studies between 60 and 80 mg/m^2 on days 1 and 29, without an obvious advantage to the higher dose. In contrast to clinical studies in cervical cancer, cisplatin has been explored in a weekly schedule in only a single, phase II study.[94]

5. The standard regimen recommended in head and neck cancers is high-dose (100 mg/m^2) cisplatin 3-weekly (for 3 cycles) concurrent with RT,[95,96] and it is felt important to deliver 3 full doses. This high-dose schedule is associated with significant acute and late toxicities, with a significant toxic death rate, and compliance is poor. In contrast, weekly cisplatin at a dose of 40 mg/m^2 is usually well tolerated with acceptable toxicity, in the treatment of nasopharyngeal carcinoma.[97] It seems unlikely that high-dose cisplatin (100 mg/m^2) would be deliverable with pelvic RT in anal cancer without excess toxicity, but the optimal dose of 60, 75, or 80 mg/m^2 remains undefined, although 75 mg/m^2 is clearly feasible in cervix cancer.

6. A phase II trial at the M. D. Anderson Cancer Center examined the combination of capecitabine and oxaliplatin with RT.[98] Preliminary results show encouraging response rates of 91% to 100% and CFS of 100%.

7. Carboplatin has also been integrated into chemoradiation schedules. A multicenter randomized study comparing 5-FU/carboplatin with 5-FU/MMC CRT was sponsored by the Societa Italiana Di Proctologia in the 1990s in Italy, but has never been published.

8. Historical reports from Sweden suggest bleomycin was less effective in combination with radiation than 5-FU and mitomycin or 5-FU and carboplatin in more advanced (T3/T4) anal cancer.[79]

9. The EORTC 22011-40014 randomized phase I/II study compared 5-FU and MMC in combination with radiation versus MMC and cisplatin concurrent with radiation.[94] The MMC/cisplatin arm used a cervical cancer schedule (25 mg/m^2 per week) with a total of 175/mg/m^2. Overall response rate at 16 weeks was 79.5% (31/39) with MMC/5-FU versus 91.9% (34/37) with MMC/cisplatin. With a median follow-up of 2 years, the 1-year progression-free survival was 76.3% in the control versus 94.2% in the MMC/cisplatin arm, and 1-year event-free survival was 74.4% versus 89.2% respectively. Despite these promising results, the schedule was not taken forward into the planned phase III design.

Neoadjuvant Chemotherapy

Previous investigators suggested a potential role for cisplatin in the neoadjuvant setting of advanced SCC of the skin,[99] and population studies from Sweden suggest that NACT has been widely used.[33] Three trials have prospectively examined the strategy of NACT before definitive CRT.

The Cancer and Leukemia Group B performed a small phase II study (CALGB-9281) in 45 patients with locally advanced anal cancer (T3 to T4, bulky N2 or N3) to investigate NACT with 2 cycles of cisplatin and 5-FU followed by MMC/5-FU chemoradiation[100]; 78% achieved a complete pathologic response rate in the mandated biopsy. After a 4-year follow-up, a 68% OS and a 61% DFS were achieved.

This study served as a pilot for the Intergroup RTOG-9811 trial, which compared cisplatin-based NACT before concurrent cisplatin-based chemoradiation[36] with the standard of MMC/5-FU concurrent CRT. NACT using cisplatin failed to improve OS, DFS, loco-regional control, and distant relapse when compared with the standard arm. With a median follow-up of 2.51 years, the 3-year and 5-year DFS rates were 67% and 61% respectively in the MMC arm versus 61% and 54% for the cisplatin arm. The 3-year and 5-year OS rates at 84% and 75% for the MMC arm compared with 76% and 70% respectively for the cisplatin arm were not significantly different ($P = .1$). The cumulative rate for a colostomy was significantly higher for the cisplatin arm compared with MMC (19% versus 10%; $P = .02$). The lack of any major difference in the compliance to both chemotherapy and RT in each arm suggest that none of the differences relate to toxicity or inadequate delivery of treatment.

However, the trial report[36] states "for patients with T3/T4 node-positive disease or *patients with T2 residual disease after 45 Gy* [our italics], the intent was to deliver an additional boost of 10–14 Gy in 2 fractions...." It would suggest that an excellent response to NACT could be followed by a limited dose of only 45 Gy. More than 60% of patients in both arms had T2 lesions. It is possible that most patients in the neoadjuvant arm received a systematically lower radiation dose, and this strategy may play as importance in radiation dose reduction in future trials.

Finally, the 4-arm INTERGROUP/ACCORD 03 study compared moderate-dose versus high-dose RT and NACT with 5-FU/cisplatin in a 2×2 factorial analysis. The primary end point was CFS. Secondary end points included LC, OS, and cancer-specific survival. A total of 307 patients were randomly assigned to 1 of 4 treatment arms. Interim analysis suggested this study would be underpowered.[101] Recently published updated results after a mean follow-up of 50 months, did not show any benefit of NACT compared with standard treatment,[85] and the optimal boost dose remains undefined.

Consolidation Chemotherapy Following Chemoradiation

In SCC of the cervix, small studies[102] and a meta-analysis[103] have shown consolidation chemotherapy after CRT to be well tolerated and effective in terms of outcomes. The addition of 3 cytotoxics to RT in a chemoradiation schedule proved too toxic in anal cancer,[86,104] although a maintenance chemotherapy strategy was adopted in ACT II on the basis of this pilot study.

The current ACT II trial randomly allocated 930 patients to 2 courses of consolidation 5-FU/cisplatin (5-FU 750 mg/m^2 for 4 days and cisplatin 60 mg/m^2 on day 1) following CRT versus control. Preliminary results do not encourage the present authors that there will be a statistically significant advantage to consolidation chemotherapy.[86]

Treatment of Small Cancers and Postoperative Adjuvant Treatment

Local excision of anal margin cancers is possible for very small lesions. These usually have to be smaller than 1 cm in diameter to allow a further 1-cm surgical clearance without damage to the anal sphincter muscles. Thus, these are the exception and should be discussed by the anal cancer–dedicated MDT before treatment. Anecdotal evidence from the authors' practices suggest that this is not infrequently attempted by surgeons less familiar with anal cancer pathology, with a resulting positive margin, and in the absence of visible tumor, it makes for less accurate delivery of the radiation field for the radiation oncologist.

Postoperative CRT should be considered in patients in whom completeness of excision cannot be guaranteed, when the resection margin is involved, or in the case of narrow margins. Some investigators argue that smaller fields can be treated, and the total dose can be lowered to 30 Gy for microscopic disease.[105,106]

Some patients may undergo initial abdominoperineal resection as definitive treatment of their anal cancer. This sometimes results from a small, poorly differentiated biopsy, which is not recognized as SCC histology, and is treated as a low rectal cancer. Postoperative chemoradiation should be considered when there is evidence of involvement of the circumferential resection margin ($\leq$1 mm), or numerous involved mesorectal lymph nodes. There are occasions when an "up-front" abdominoperineal resection is indicated (eg, if the patient has already received radical RT to the pelvis), but these cases are the exception.

SURVEILLANCE AND SALVAGE SURGERY
Assessment of Treatment Response

Despite refinements in CRT regimens for initial treatment of anal cancer, retrospective studies suggest 20% to 25% of cases develop local disease relapse at some point in the first 3 years.[107] Patients should be evaluated for recurrence every 3 to 6 months for 2 years, and 6 to 12 monthly until 5 years, with clinical examination including DRE and palpation of the inguinal lymph nodes. Patients tend to relapse loco-regionally rather than at distant sites.[108] Regular CT scans for metastatic surveillance outside trials remains controversial, although some have argued for regular pelvic MRI surveillance in the first 3 years. Intensive follow-up to detect potentially salvageable pelvic failure should be restricted to a maximum of 3 years in future trials, as only 7% of relapses occur beyond this time point.[108]

There is debate regarding when best to define lack of treatment response and persistent local disease. Some prospective studies examined clinical response at an early point of 4 weeks after completion of CRT, or biopsied the primary tumor at 4 to 6 weeks to assess pathologic response,[83] rather than waiting for longer periods to allow assessment of regression. The degree of tumor regression (>80%) after primary chemoradiation may predict CFS and DFS.[109] Most randomized studies assess clinically between 6 and 12 weeks following completion of CRT.

In practice, local ulceration may raise concern of ongoing disease, although definitive histology is required.[110] Positron emission tomography at 1 month might enhance assessment of clinical response.[64,111]

The differences in complete response rates between trials are in part explained by differences in how and when treatment response assessment was performed. In the most recent ACT II trial, cCR, ie, complete absence of tumor and clinically node negative, was assessed by DRE or imaging at 11 and 18 weeks with a mandated CT at 26 weeks after the start of CRT. Median follow-up was 5 years. Patients were excluded from analysis if assessment was either missing or not performed at one or more time points (n = 245). Hence, data from 695 patients could be analyzed for response. At week 11, 66% of patients achieved cCR with MMC and 56% with cisplatin, compared with 75% and 76% at 18 weeks, and 83% and 84% at 26 weeks, respectively (Glynne-Jones and colleagues,[86] 2012). By this argument, early surgical salvage may not have been appropriate for patients who did not achieve cCR at 11 weeks. On the other hand, some surgical groups have adopted an intensive approach to early detection of local treatment failure and relapse, arguing that in a proportion of patients there is a limited "window of opportunity" to resect local disease relapse, and a prolonged period of observation may allow disease progression beyond resectability. Thus, in the Manchester series of 254 patients treated with curative intent, of the 99 local relapses, 73 (74%) underwent salvage surgery.[34] The corresponding rate in the contemporaneous UKCCCR ACT I trial was 56%.[35]

Salvage Surgery

For most patients with local disease relapse from anal cancer, salvage surgery takes the form of a radical abdomino-perineal resection (APR). A small number of cases may be treated by local resection, but this is the exception. In a further small number of cases, it is necessary to consider a posterior or total pelvic exenteration. In using the term, *radical APR*, there is recognition that it is the norm that there is a need to extend this operation to encompass adjacent viscera (for example, the vagina in women) and irradiated soft tissue of the perianal area, perineum, and buttocks. It is important to emphasize that radical APR for local disease relapse from anal cancer is completely different from that for low rectal adenocarcinomas, in several aspects: the perineal skin resection during salvage anal cancer surgery is wider; the key oncological margin during salvage anal cancer surgery is the lateral margin at the level of the ischial tuberosity; the effects of radiation on perineal cutaneous tissue are greater; the en bloc resection of adjacent viscera or organs is common; and there is an almost universal need for plastic reconstruction of the perineal defect.

The characteristics and outcomes from series of patients undergoing salvage anal cancer surgery are reported elsewhere.[34,107] Two patterns emerge: (1) salvage radical surgery achieves a local pelvic disease control rate of approximately 60%; and (2) the 5-year postsalvage surgery survival rate is 40% to 60%.

Late Effects

Overall, 80% to 85% of patients with anal cancer treated initially by chemoradiation are cured. This excellent survivorship means that many will potentially experience severe G3/G4 late effects,[112] and up to 20% require a colostomy for these adverse late effects, particularly in the case of large primary tumors.[113] Other factors implicated in the expression of late morbidity are higher total doses,[114] large individual fraction size,[72] and longer duration of interstitial brachytherapy.[115] Brachytherapy dose may be relevant.[116] The late effects reflect aspects of the radiation rather than the type of chemotherapy. The symptoms are expensive in terms of on-going use of health care resources, as they provide a permanent burden on patients.

There is a wide spectrum of complications observed in anal cancer following RT from minor side effects to serious and life threatening complications. The symptoms of late anorectal damage tend to peak within the first 2 years, but radiation injury can present first after an interval of 5 to 10 years and may then follow an inexorably progressive course. Late complications of RT are infrequently reported and poorly recorded in phase III trials. A widespread agreement on a uniform classification for describing late morbidity of radiation was not in place until 1995.[117] Before this, the World Health Organization and Radiation Therapy Oncology Group/Eastern

Cooperative Oncology Group (RTOG/ECOG) systems, used in the EORTC, ACT I, and RTOG-8704 trials, were not specifically designed to capture radiation-induced morbidity.

The only late complication that the EORTC22921 could show to be different between the arms (RT versus CRT) was ulceration of the anal canal. In contrast, when fistula, skin ulceration stenosis, and fibrosis were combined, there was no difference on an actuarial basis.[32] The ACT I trial defined any toxicity occurring or persisting more than 6 months after completing initial RT as late morbidity. These were not scored or quantified,[118] but were descriptive in nature. There was no evidence of a treatment difference between RT and CRT for ulcers or radionecrosis, anorectal, genitourinary, or skin late morbidities. Details were not methodically collected after 2000, and hence could not be collated into a log rank analysis to examine the late effects over time. As a relevant, comprehensive, and clinically meaningful late end point, the overall incidence of anorectal ulceration and radionecrosis was chosen as a composite end point for late morbidity. Among good responders, no reports of late ulcers/radionecrosis at the primary site were provided for those patients who were not boosted, whereas the boosted reported 8% severe G3/G4 morbidity ($P = .03$). This late effect was more common in the subgroup, who received boost by implant (14%) compared with the EBRT boost subgroup (6%; $P = .003$), although posttreatment biopsies for suspicion of residual disease might have contributed in some to nonhealing and ulceration.

Similarly, the ACT II trial required regular descriptive reports of the presence or not of a range of late effects (bowel, urinary, and sexual) that were considered by the investigator as severe, and returned on a case report form, but were not formally graded. It is the personal opinion of one of the authors (R.G.J.) that the late effects experienced by survivors in the ACT II study is observably less than those patients in ACT I, particularly when compared with those who received an interstitial brachytherapy boost.

There are data on the requirement for colostomy to palliate severe late morbidity. No differences in late toxicity were observed between RT and chemoradiation in the EORTC and UKCCCR trials. Colostomy rates in randomized trials[32,35] and population studies[33] vary from 15% to 36%, and approximately 15% to 20% of colostomies are fashioned to deal with the results of treatment.[36,118]

In the EORTC trial, anal ulcers, fistulae, severe fibrosis, skin ulceration, and rectal stenosis were documented, but data at 5 years allowed comparison of only 5 patients in each arm, which is insufficient for valid comparisons. In the RTOG-8704 trial, only 2 patients in each arm required a stoma for treatment-related complications,[83] and there appeared to be no additional risk from the addition of MMC. In the RTOG-9811 trial, the rate of severe long-term toxic effects was similar in both arms, 11% versus 10%, but only 5% required a colostomy for treatment-related problems. Late effects appear to relate mostly to total radiation dose received in multivariate analysis rather than the type of chemotherapy.

Finally, radiation-induced pelvic and hip insufficiency fractures are increasingly being recognized and reported, and are also more common in women.[119,120]

Quality of Life

Few formal assessments of quality of life (QOL) have been reported within published randomized trials, and compliance to questionnaires is poor. Chemoradiation appears to improve QOL compared with RT alone.[121] In the ACCORD-03 study, assessment 2 months after completion of treatment did not show that NACT and high-dose RT, either alone or in combination, had a negative impact on QOL.[122] In fact, QOL appeared to improve over QOL at entry. Data on long-term QOL are sparse,[123] but appear satisfactory to patients despite objective impairment of sphincter function.[124,125]

TREATMENT OF METASTATIC DISEASE

Carcinoma of the anus has a low rate of distant metastasis.[126,127] In treatment series, hematogenous spread at presentation is noted in fewer than 5% of cases and predominantly involves lung or liver. CT of the thorax and abdomen is therefore preferred to a chest radiograph and liver ultrasound for the assessment of metastatic disease because of its higher sensitivity.[65,128]

Although single agent carboplatin has been examined,[129] the combination of 5-FU and cisplatin remains the most commonly used palliative regimen, as in a wide range of squamous cancers, which has been shown to affect OS.[130–137] Few reports included more than a handful of patients, however. Case reports suggest several cytotoxic agents are sometimes effective and responses can be sustained, but do not represent a cure. Single-center series show response rates of 20% to 60% in first line. A phase II study of 5-FU, carboplatin, and paclitaxel in metastatic SCCs from any primary source (7 patients with anal cancer) demonstrated a 50% cCR rate with a median duration of 26 months in those with anal cancer.[138]

Other trials have used either bleomycin-based regimens[139,140] or combinations of 5-FU and cisplatin[134] and shown partial remissions in about 60% of patients with limited benefit (**Table 5**). Historically, median survival has been short with a median survival, in a Norwegian retrospective series, of 12 months (range 3–54 months).[141] A recently published series used a regimen containing paclitaxel, ifosfamide, and cisplatin and reported excellent responses, some of which have been sustained over long periods.[142]

NEW DIRECTIONS
Intensity-Modulated Radiotherapy

Technical advances in radiation oncology, including functional and molecular imaging and IMRT delivery techniques are allowing greater treatment precision and dose escalation. IMRT allows the delivery and modulation of doses of RT to the tumor while sparing normal surrounding structures, such as perineal skin, the external genitalia, the bony confines of the pelvis (sacrum and pubis), the femoral head and neck, the bladder and small bowel, to a greater degree compared with conventional 2-dimensional or 3-dimensional planning. IMRT has found favor in tumor sites that show a marked dose-response curve (such as prostate cancer and head and neck cancer), and/or are in close proximity to many critical organs. This is particularly important if these critical organs are much more radiosensitive, or have a lower radiation tolerance than the tumor site itself. IMRT specifies a desired dose distribution with an optimal intensity. Tumor dose escalation is possible with reduced complication rates of clinical structures, and this has been shown to improve clinical outcomes in a number of sites. In anal cancer, a Canadian study[143] achieved a local DFS of 91% at 4 years with significant reductions in grade III toxicity. Yet, it would seem difficult to increase the dose to tumor while sparing the anal canal, as maximal dose predicts the risk of complications. Despite limited evidence, the maximum dose to the anal canal has been recommended as 55 Gy.[144]

A further US multicenter trial[145] achieved an 18-month local failure-free survival of 83.9% and a CFS of 83.7%. Grade 3 toxicity was 15.1%. As a result, IMRT dose escalation was possible with pelvic regions and inguinal nodes receiving 45 Gy. IMRT can also reduce the volume of pelvic bone marrow receiving 15 and 20 Gy (PBM-V15 and

Table 5
Prospective trials of treatments in advanced metastatic anal cancer

Trial Name (Authors)	No.	Design	Response Rate	Complete Response	Toxicity	Median Survival	Median Time to Progression/ Death
Wilking et al,[140] 1985	15	Vincristine, bleomycin, high-dose methotrexate	3/12 (25%) duration 1, 2, and 5 mo	None	5/15 G4		
ECOG E7282 (Jhawer et al,[139] 2006)	20	MMC, driamycin, cisplatin followed by Bleomycin-CCNU	12/20 (60%)	None	7/20 G3 and 2/20 G4 hematological toxicity	15 mo (range 6–20)	8 mo
Hainsworth et al,[138] 2001	(60) 4 with anal cancer	Paclitaxel, carboplatin and PVI of 5-FU	65% overall	2/4 50% in anal cancer	48% G3/4 leukopenia 17% G3/G4 diarrhea overall	No data	Median PFS 35 mo overall
TOTAL	39						

Abbreviations: 5-FU, 5-Fluorouracil; cisplatin, Cisplatinum; ECOG, Eastern Cooperative Oncology Group; MMC, Mitomycin C; PFS, progression-free survival; PVI, prolonged venous infusion.

PBM-V20), which is significantly associated with decreased white blood count and absolute neutrophil count nadir.[146] This sparing of normal tissues may allow improved compliance to treatment and lessen late morbidity, although there are likely to be more second malignancies observed.

Biologic Agents

Biologic therapy could be integrated into the chemoradiation component, or as a consolidation maneuver following chemoradiation, at a point when the cancer appears to express high levels of both vascular endothelial growth factor and epidermal growth factor to increase efficacy. There are no data of the efficacy of biologic agents combined with chemoradiation, although several trials are currently in progress (**Table 6**). A Brazilian study reported on 10 patients with cetuximab added to CRT.[93]

Anal cancers overexpress EGFR.[147,148] In addition, radiation itself induces EGFR activation, which contributes, at least in part, to the mechanism of accelerated proliferation, and can be expected to increase the capacity for tumor DNA damage repair. Overexpression of EGFR has been linked to radio-resistance[149,150]; hence, a promising avenue of treatment is to target the EGFR pathway.

Radiotherapy Technique and Treatment Fields

There are significant differences in approach within Europe. Treatment should aim to encompass the primary tumor and any palpable or imaged sites of nodal involvement within the high-dose volume. The inguinal nodes are usually included in the radiation fields in most cases, even in the absence of clearly demonstrable involvement. The incidence of nodal involvement increases with increasing primary tumor size up to at least 20% in patients with T3 disease. Some clinicians may treat clinically uninvolved inguinal nodes only in more advanced cases eg T3 to T4 primary disease, location of primary tumor within the canal, 1 cm or less from the anal orifice, or if there is involvement of pelvic lymph nodes (on CT or MRI criteria). The results of the ACT II trial and documentation of the sites of recurrence, should help to clarify the optimum field sizes.

Toxicity and Supportive Care During Radiotherapy

Recent trials in anal cancer report 10% to 20% rate of physician-reported, acute grade 3/4 diarrhea,[85,86] which may not define the true QOL effects of acute toxicity from the patient's perspective. CRT (particularly if Mitomycin C is used) is associated with high risks of G3 and G4 hematological toxicity.[36]

The EORTC trial had no toxic deaths.[32] In the UKCCCR ACT I trial,[35] there were 6 treatment-related deaths in the first 116 patients; after amending the protocol to provide antibiotics throughout treatment, there were no more septicemic deaths. In the RTOG study,[83] 20% of patients experienced G4/G5 toxicity with MMC/5-FU versus 7% of those on 5-FU alone. There were 4 (3%) treatment-related deaths in the MMC arm. In the recent ACT II trial, all patients were given prophylactic antibiotic cover during CRT.

Expected acute side effects include diarrhea, proctitis, urinary frequency and dysuria, loss of pubic hair and erythema, lymphedema, and moist desquamation of the skin in the groins and perineum. Skin effects rapidly disappear within 2 to 3 weeks after treatment is completed. Tolerance to treatment can be improved with anti-emetics, antidiarrheal agents, analgesia, skin care, advice regarding nutrition, and psychological support. Patients should be warned of the adverse effects of smoking, which may worsen acute toxicity during treatment and lead to a poorer outcome in

Table 6
Ongoing and unreported phase I and II trials of different treatments in anal cancer

Trial Name (Authors)	No.	Design	RT Dose	Complete Response	Median F/U	3 y DFS	3 y CFS	OS
RTOG-0529 phase II (Kachnic[165] 2010)	63	5-FU 1000 mg/m² d 1–4, and 29–33 2 doses of MMC 10 mg/m² d 1, 29 total dose = 20 mg/m²	IMRT dose acc to T stage 50.4 Gy/28# T2N0 54 Gy/30# for T3/T4N0	34/61 67% at 8 wk	No data	No data	No data	No data
ECOG E3205	62	NACT cisplatin/5-FU ×2 induction then 5-FU/cisplatin/cetuximab during RT in immunocompetent	54 Gy/30# for T3/T4N0	Study suspended 11/3/08	No data	No data	No data	No data
AMC045 NCT003244415	47	5-FU 1000 mg/m² d 1–4, cisplatin day 1, 29 cetuximab during RT in HIV+	54 Gy/30# for T3/T4N0		No data	No data	No data	No data
FNCLCC NCT00955140	77	Cisplatin and 5-FU with cetuximab	65 Gy		No data	No data	No data	No data
JCOG0903: SMART-AC Phase I/II	65	S1, MMC, and RT	???	Study ongoing	No data	No data	No data	No data
TOTAL	310							

Abbreviations: 5-FU, 5-Fluorouracil; CFS, colostomy-free survival; cisplatin, Cisplatinum; DFS, disease-free survival; ECOG, Eastern Cooperative Oncology Group; FNCLCC, National Federation of French Cancer Centres; F/U, follow-up; HIV, human immunodeficiency virus; IMRT, intensity-modulated radiotherapy; MMC, Mitomycin C; NACT, neoadjuvant chemotherapy; OS, overall survival; RT, radiotherapy; RTOG, Radiation Therapy Oncology Group; ???, unknown.

terms of DFS and CFS.[121] The use of vaginal dilators in sexually active women is recommended, although evidence of benefit is limited.

Patterns of Relapse

Patients can recur either at the primary tumor site, in the regional lymph nodes, or at distant sites, such as liver and lung.[126,127] Patients tend to relapse loco-regionally in the pelvis, rather than at distant sites, although loco-regional failure is commonly followed by distant failure. However, exact rates, for example, inguinal node failure without local failure are lacking and make for difficult comparisons between selective and prophylactic groin RT strategies.

In the UKCCCR ACT I trial,[35] only 21 (7%) of 285 patients treated with chemoradiation developed metastatic disease outside the pelvis in the absence of evidence of pelvic recurrence. Long-term follow-up of this study, with a median follow-up of 11.5 and 13.5 years in the RT and CRT groups respectively, shows 239 of 560 patients had a local relapse (153 RT; 86 CRT).[118] Only 4 of these patients had a distant relapse before their first recorded local relapse.

Is There a Role for Modifying the Schedules?

It is perhaps surprising that the strategy of continuous radiosensitization accepted in rectal cancer (ie, prolonged venous infusion or oral capecitabine) has infrequently been exploited in anal cancer.[94,151] Infusional 5-FU or the oral fluoropyrimidine capecitabine could have a useful role.[152] Preferential conversion to 5-FU by tumor potentially offers a therapeutic advantage over 5-FU. Other potential chemotherapy agents include gemcitabine, vinorelbine, paclitaxel, etoposide, topotecan, and biologic agents, all of which have been investigated in cervix cancer.

Overexpression of EGFR is common in SCC of the anus,[147] but KRAS and BRAF mutations appear rare,[153] so there may be a therapeutic role for EGFR inhibition using cetuximab as a single agent or in combination with irinotecan.[154] Data on the efficacy of biologic agents combined with chemoradiation are awaited.

SUMMARY

With our current sophisticated staging procedures and ability to spare critical normal tissues with IMRT, a "one-size-fits-all" approach for anal cancer is probably inappropriate. In the United Kingdom, many investigators believe that early T1 tumors are currently overtreated, whereas T3/T4 lesions have a 3-year DFS of 40% to 68%, and might benefit from more intensive treatment and a proactive approach to surgical salvage.[155] Radiotherapy dose escalation and intensification of the concurrent chemotherapy might improve LC, but is just as likely to adversely affect colostomy-free survival. So, we need trials to clarify these concepts. Integration of biologic therapy with conventional chemotherapies looks hopeful. Finally, it is in the interest of all patients to be offered participation in a clinical trial.

REFERENCES

1. Siegel R, Ward E, Brawley O, et al. Cancer statistics, 2011: the impact of eliminating socioeconomic and racial disparities on premature cancer deaths. CA Cancer J Clin 2011;61(4):212–36.
2. Office of National Statistics. Cancer registration statistics: four-digit codes. 2007. Available at: http://www.statistics.gov.uk/StatBase/Product.asp?vlnk=7720. Accessed May 30, 2010.

3. Frisch M, Melbye M, Moller H. Trends in incidence of anal cancer in Denmark. BMJ 1993;306(6875):419–22.

4. Goldman S, Glimelius B, Nilsson B, et al. Incidence of anal epidermoid carcinoma in Sweden 1970-1984. Acta Chir Scand 1989;155(3):191–7.

5. Brewster DH, Bhatti LA. Increasing incidence of squamous cell carcinoma of the anus in Scotland, 1975-2002. Br J Cancer 2006;95(1):87–90.

6. Johnson LG, Madeleine MM, Newcomer LM, et al. Anal cancer incidence and survival: the surveillance, epidemiology, and end results experience, 1973-2000. Cancer 2004;101(2):281–8.

7. Chiao EY, Krown SE, Stier EA, et al. A population-based analysis of temporal trends in the incidence of squamous anal canal cancer in relation to the HIV epidemic. J Acquir Immune Defic Syndr 2005;40(4):451–5.

8. Williams GR, Lu QL, Love SB, et al. Properties of HPV-positive and HPV-negative anal carcinomas. J Pathol 1996;180(4):378–82.

9. Penn I. Cancers of the anogenital region in renal transplant recipients. Analysis of 65 cases. Cancer 1986;58(3):611–6.

10. Sillman FH, Sentovich S, Shaffer D. Ano-genital neoplasia in renal transplant patients. Ann Transplant 1997;2(4):59–66.

11. Daling JR, Sherman KJ, Hislop TG, et al. Cigarette smoking and the risk of anogenital cancer. Am J Epidemiol 1992;135(2):180–9.

12. Holly EA, Whittemore AS, Aston DA, et al. Anal cancer incidence: genital warts, anal fissure or fistula, hemorrhoids, and smoking. J Natl Cancer Inst 1989; 81(22):1726–31.

13. Nordenvall C, Nilsson PJ, Ye W, et al. Smoking, snus use and risk of right- and left-sided colon, rectal and anal cancer: a 37-year follow-up study. Int J Cancer 2011;128(1):157–65.

14. Tseng HF, Morgenstern H, Mack TM, et al. Risk factors for anal cancer: results of a population-based case–control study. Cancer Causes Control 2003;14(9): 837–46.

15. Frisch M, Johansen C. Anal carcinoma in inflammatory bowel disease. Br J Cancer 2000;83(1):89–90.

16. Frisch M, Olsen JH, Melbye M. Malignancies that occur before and after anal cancer: clues to their etiology. Am J Epidemiol 1994;140(1):12–9.

17. Silverberg MJ, Lau B, Justice AC, et al. Risk of anal cancer in HIV-infected and HIV-uninfected individuals in North America. Clin Infect Dis 2012;54(7):1026–34.

18. De Vuyst H, Clifford GM, Nascimento MC, et al. Prevalence and type distribution of human papillomavirus in carcinoma and intraepithelial neoplasia of the vulva, vagina and anus: a meta-analysis. Int J Cancer 2009;124(7):1626–36.

19. Bosch FX, Manos MM, Munoz N, et al. Prevalence of human papillomavirus in cervical cancer: a worldwide perspective. International biological study on cervical cancer (IBSCC) Study Group. J Natl Cancer Inst 1995;87(11):796–802.

20. Bjorge T, Engeland A, Luostarinen T, et al. Human papillomavirus infection as a risk factor for anal and perianal skin cancer in a prospective study. Br J Cancer 2002;87(1):61–4.

21. Palefsky JM, Holly EA, Ralston ML, et al. Prevalence and risk factors for human papillomavirus infection of the anal canal in human immunodeficiency virus (HIV)-positive and HIV-negative homosexual men. J Infect Dis 1998;177(2):361–7.

22. Scholefield JH, Castle MT, Watson NF. Malignant transformation of high-grade anal intraepithelial neoplasia. Br J Surg 2005;92(9):1133–6.

23. Clark MA, Hartley A, Geh JI. Cancer of the anal canal. Lancet Oncol 2004;5(3): 149–57.

24. Abbasakoor F, Boulos PB. Anal intraepithelial neoplasia. Br J Surg 2005;92(3): 277–90.
25. Zbar AP, Fenger C, Efron J, et al. The pathology and molecular biology of anal intraepithelial neoplasia: comparisons with cervical and vulvar intraepithelial carcinoma. Int J Colorectal Dis 2002;17(4):203–15.
26. Dittmer DP. An appraisal of non-AIDS-defining cancers: comment on "spectrum of cancer risk late after AIDS onset in the United States". Arch Intern Med 2010; 170(15):1345–6.
27. Roden R, Wu TC. How will HPV vaccines affect cervical cancer? Nat Rev Cancer 2006;6(10):753–63.
28. Palefsky JM, Giuliano AR, Goldstone S, et al. HPV vaccine against anal HPV infection and anal intraepithelial neoplasia. N Engl J Med 2011;365(17):1576–85.
29. Licitra L, Perrone F, Bossi P, et al. High-risk human papillomavirus affects prognosis in patients with surgically treated oropharyngeal squamous cell carcinoma. J Clin Oncol 2006;24(36):5630–6.
30. Shi W, Kato H, Perez-Ordonez B, et al. Comparative prognostic value of HPV16 E6 mRNA compared with in situ hybridization for human oropharyngeal squamous carcinoma. J Clin Oncol 2009;27(36):6213–21.
31. Mammas IN, Sourvinos G, Giannoudis A, et al. Human papilloma virus (HPV) and host cellular interactions. Pathol Oncol Res 2008;14(4):345–54.
32. Bartelink H, Roelofsen F, Eschwege F, et al. Concomitant radiotherapy and chemotherapy is superior to radiotherapy alone in the treatment of locally advanced anal cancer: results of a phase III randomized trial of the European Organization for Research and Treatment of Cancer Radiotherapy and Gastrointestinal Cooperative Groups. J Clin Oncol 1997;15(5):2040–9.
33. Nilsson PJ, Svensson C, Goldman S, et al. Epidermoid anal cancer: a review of a population-based series of 308 consecutive patients treated according to prospective protocols. Int J Radiat Oncol Biol Phys 2005;61(1):92–102.
34. Renehan AG, Saunders MP, Schofield PF, et al. Patterns of local disease failure and outcome after salvage surgery in patients with anal cancer. Br J Surg 2005; 92:605–14.
35. UKCCCR. Epidermoid anal cancer: results from the UKCCCR randomised trial of radiotherapy alone versus radiotherapy, 5-fluorouracil, and mitomycin. UKCCCR Anal Cancer Trial Working Party. UK Co-ordinating Committee on Cancer Research. Lancet 1996;348(9034):1049–54.
36. Ajani JA, Winter KA, Gunderson LL, et al. Fluorouracil, mitomycin, and radiotherapy vs fluorouracil, cisplatin, and radiotherapy for carcinoma of the anal canal: a randomized controlled trial. JAMA 2008;299(16):1914–21.
37. Das P, Cantor SB, Parker CL, et al. Long-term quality of life after radiotherapy for the treatment of anal cancer. Cancer 2010;116(4):822–9.
38. Klas JV, Rothenberger DA, Wong WD, et al. Malignant tumors of the anal canal: the spectrum of disease, treatment, and outcomes. Cancer 1999;85(8):1686–93.
39. Deniaud-Alexandre E, Touboul E, Tiret E, et al. Results of definitive irradiation in a series of 305 epidermoid carcinomas of the anal canal. Int J Radiat Oncol Biol Phys 2003;56(5):1259–73.
40. Renehan AG, O'Dwyer ST. Initial management through the anal cancer multidisciplinary team meeting. Colorectal Dis 2011;13(Suppl 1):21–8.
41. National Cancer Peer Review Programme. Manual for cancer services 2008; colorectal measures. London: NHS National Cancer Action Team; 2010.
42. National Comprehensive Cancer Network (NCCN) Clinical Practice Guidelines in Oncology. Anal carcinoma version 2.2012. 2011. Available at:

www.nccn.org/professionals/physician_gls/pdf/anal.pdf. Accessed May 16, 2012.

43. Hill J, Meadows H, Haboubi N, et al. Pathological staging of epidermoid anal carcinoma for the new era. Colorectal Dis 2003;5(3):206–13.

44. Wade DS, Herrera L, Castillo NB, et al. Metastases to the lymph nodes in epidermoid carcinoma of the anal canal studied by a clearing technique. Surg Gynecol Obstet 1989;169(3):238–42.

45. Greenall MJ, Quan SH, Urmacher C, et al. Treatment of epidermoid carcinoma of the anal canal. Surg Gynecol Obstet 1985;161(6):509–17.

46. Fenger C, Frisch M, Marti MC, et al. Tumours of the anal canal. In: Hamilton SR, Aaltonen LA, editors. World Health Organization classification of tumours. Pathology and genetics of tumours of the digestive system. Lyon (France): IARC Press; 2000. p. 145–55.

47. Glynne-Jones R, Northover JM, Cervantes A. Anal cancer: ESMO Clinical Practice Guidelines for diagnosis, treatment and follow-up. Ann Oncol 2010; 21(Suppl 5):v87–92.

48. Shepherd NA, Scholefield JH, Love SB, et al. Prognostic factors in anal squamous carcinoma: a multivariate analysis of clinical, pathological and flow cytometric parameters in 235 cases. Histopathology 1990;16(6):545–55.

49. Lampejo T, Kavanagh D, Clark J, et al. Prognostic biomarkers in squamous cell carcinoma of the anus: a systematic review. Br J Cancer 2010;103(12):1858–69.

50. Ogunbiyi OA, Scholefield JH, Smith JH, et al. Immunohistochemical analysis of p53 expression in anal squamous neoplasia. J Clin Pathol 1993;46(6):507–12.

51. Gangopadhyay SA, Lin Y, editors. The tumour suppressor gene p53. Frontiers in molecular biology. New York: Oxford University Press; 1997.

52. Mawdsley S, Meadows H, James R. The role of biological molecular markers in predicting both response to treatment and clinical outcome in squamous cell carcinoma of the anus [abstract 183]. ASCO 2004 Gastrointestinal Cancers Symposium Proceedings, San Francisco, January 2004.

53. Allal AS, Alonso-Pentzke L, Remadi S. Apparent lack of prognostic value of MIB-1 index in anal carcinomas treated by radiotherapy. Br J Cancer 1998;77(8):1333–6.

54. Noffsinger AE, Hui YZ, Suzuk L, et al. The relationship of human papillomavirus to proliferation and ploidy in carcinoma of the anus. Cancer 1995;75(4):958–67.

55. Renehan AG, Yeh HC, Johnson JA, et al. Diabetes and cancer (2): evaluating the impact of diabetes on mortality in patients with cancer. Diabetologia 2012; 55(6):1619–32.

56. Edge SB, Byrd DR, Compton CC, et al. AJCC cancer staging manual. 7th edition. New York: Springer; 2009.

57. Roach SC, Hulse PA, Moulding FJ, et al. Magnetic resonance imaging of anal cancer. Clin Radiol 2005;60(10):1111–9.

58. Salerno G, Daniels IR, Brown G. Magnetic resonance imaging of the low rectum: defining the radiological anatomy. Colorectal Dis 2006;8(Suppl 3):10–3.

59. Koh DM, Dzik-Jurasz A, O'Neill B, et al. Pelvic phased-array MR imaging of anal carcinoma before and after chemoradiation. Br J Radiol 2008;81(962):91–8.

60. Engstrom PF, Arnoletti JP, Benson AB 3rd, et al. NCCN clinical practice guidelines in oncology. Anal carcinoma. J Natl Compr Canc Netw 2010;8(1):106–20.

61. Cotter SE, Grigsby PW, Siegel BA, et al. FDG-PET/CT in the evaluation of anal carcinoma. Int J Radiat Oncol Biol Phys 2006;65(3):720–5.

62. Krengli M, Milia ME, Turri L, et al. FDG-PET/CT imaging for staging and target volume delineation in conformal radiotherapy of anal carcinoma. Radiat Oncol 2010;5:10.

63. Winton E, Heriot AG, Ng M, et al. The impact of 18-fluorodeoxyglucose positron emission tomography on the staging, management and outcome of anal cancer. Br J Cancer 2009;100(5):693–700.

64. Trautmann TG, Zuger JH. Positron emission tomography for pretreatment staging and posttreatment evaluation in cancer of the anal canal. Mol Imaging Biol 2005;7(4):309–13.

65. Bhuva NJ, Glynne-Jones R, Sonoda L, et al. To PET or not to PET? That is the question. Staging in anal cancer. Ann Oncol 2012;23(8):2078–82.

66. De La Rochefordière A, Pontvert D, Asselain B, et al. Radiothérapie des cancers du canal anal. Expérience de l'institut Curie dans le traitement des aires ganglionnaires. Bull Cancer Radiother 1993;80:391–8.

67. Gerard JP, Chapet O, Samiei F, et al. Management of inguinal lymph node metastases in patients with carcinoma of the anal canal: experience in a series of 270 patients treated in Lyon and review of the literature. Cancer 2001;92(1):77–84.

68. Makela PJ, Leminen A, Kaariainen M, et al. Pretreatment sonographic evaluation of inguinal lymph nodes in patients with vulvar malignancy. J Ultrasound Med 1993;12(5):255–8.

69. de Jong JS, Beukema JC, van Dam GM, et al. Limited value of staging squamous cell carcinoma of the anal margin and canal using the sentinel lymph node procedure: a prospective study with long-term follow-up. Ann Surg Oncol 2010;17(10):2656–62.

70. Leichman L, Nigro N, Vaitkevicius VK, et al. Cancer of the anal canal. Model for preoperative adjuvant combined modality therapy. Am J Med 1985;78(2):211–5.

71. Nigro ND, Vaitkevicius VK, Considine B Jr. Combined therapy for cancer of the anal canal: a preliminary report. Dis Colon Rectum 1974;17(3):354–6.

72. Cummings BJ, Keane TJ, O'Sullivan B, et al. Epidermoid anal cancer: treatment by radiation alone or by radiation and 5-fluorouracil with and without mitomycin C [see comments]. Int J Radiat Oncol Biol Phys 1991;21(5):1115–25.

73. Newman G, Calverley DC, Acker BD, et al. The management of carcinoma of the anal canal by external beam radiotherapy, experience in Vancouver 1971-1988. Radiother Oncol 1992;25(3):196–202.

74. Papillon J, Montbarbon JF. Epidermoid carcinoma of the anal canal. A series of 276 cases. Dis Colon Rectum 1987;30(5):324–33.

75. Glimelius B, Pahlman L. Radiation therapy of anal epidermoid carcinoma. Int J Radiat Oncol Biol Phys 1987;13(3):305–12.

76. Eschwege F, Lasser P, Chavy A, et al. Squamous cell carcinoma of the anal canal: treatment by external beam irradiation. Radiother Oncol 1985;3(2):145–50.

77. Cantril ST, Green JP, Schall GL, et al. Primary radiation therapy in the treatment of anal carcinoma. Int J Radiat Oncol Biol Phys 1983;9(9):1271–8.

78. Cummings BJ, Keane TJ, O'Sullivan B, et al. Mitomycin in anal canal carcinoma. Oncology 1993;50(Suppl 1):63–9.

79. Friberg B, Svensson C, Goldman S, et al. The Swedish National Care Programme for Anal Carcinoma—implementation and overall results. Acta Oncol 1998;37(1):25–32.

80. John M, Pajak T, Flam M, et al. Dose escalation in chemoradiation for anal cancer: preliminary results of RTOG 92-08. Cancer J Sci Am 1996;2(4):205–11.

81. Martenson JA, Lipsitz SR, Lefkopoulou M, et al. Results of combined modality therapy for patients with anal cancer (E7283). An Eastern Cooperative Oncology Group study. Cancer 1995;76(10):1731–6.

82. Rich TA, Hughes L, Ajani JA, et al. Low dose, continuous infusion 5-fluorouracil plus radiotherapy for anal cancer. Int J Radiat Oncol Biol Phys 1990;18(3):710.

83. Flam M, John M, Pajak TF, et al. Role of mitomycin in combination with fluorouracil and radiotherapy, and of salvage chemoradiation in the definitive nonsurgical treatment of epidermoid carcinoma of the anal canal: results of a phase III randomized intergroup study. J Clin Oncol 1996;14(9):2527–39.

84. Gunderson LL, Winter KA, Ajani JA, et al. Long-term update of US GI Intergroup RTOG- 98–11 phase III trial for anal carcinoma: comparison of concurrent chemoradiation with 5FU-mitomycin versus 5FU-cisplatin. Gastrointestinal Cancers Symposium. ASCO; San Francisco, January 2012. p. 140. [abstract: 367].

85. Peiffert D, Tournier-Rangeard L, Gerard JP, et al. Induction chemotherapy and dose intensification of the radiation boost in locally advanced anal canal carcinoma: final analysis of the randomized UNICANCER ACCORD 03 Trial. J Clin Oncol 2012;30(16):1941–8.

86. Glynne-Jones R, James R, Meadows H, et al. Optimum time to assess complete clinical response (CR) following chemoradiation (CRT) using mitomycin (MMC) or cisplatin (CisP), with or without maintenance CisP/5FU in squamous cell carcinoma of the anus: Results of ACT II. J Clin Oncol 2012;30(suppl; abstr 4004).

87. Hwang JM, Rao AR, Cosmatos HA, et al. Treatment of T3 and T4 anal carcinoma with combined chemoradiation and interstitial 192Ir implantation: a 10-year experience. Brachytherapy 2004;3(2):95–100.

88. Chong G, Dickson JL, Cunningham D, et al. Capecitabine and mitomycin C as third-line therapy for patients with metastatic colorectal cancer resistant to fluorouracil and irinotecan. Br J Cancer 2005;93(5):510–4.

89. El-Ghazal R, Podoltsev N, Marks P, et al. Mitomycin–C-induced thrombotic thrombocytopenic purpura/hemolytic uremic syndrome: cumulative toxicity of an old drug in a new era. Clin Colorectal Cancer 2011;10(2):142–5.

90. Doci R, Zucali R, Bombelli L, et al. Combined chemoradiation therapy for anal cancer. A report of 56 cases. Ann Surg 1992;215(2):150–6.

91. Gerard JP, Ayzac L, Hun D, et al. Treatment of anal canal carcinoma with high dose radiation therapy and concomitant fluorouracil-cisplatinum. Long-term results in 95 patients. Radiother Oncol 1998;46(3):249–56.

92. Hung A, Crane C, Delclos M, et al. Cisplatin-based combined modality therapy for anal carcinoma: a wider therapeutic index. Cancer 2003;97(5):1195–202.

93. Olivatto LO, Meton F, Bezerra M, et al. Phase I study of cetuximab (CET) in combination with 5-flurouracil (5FU), cisplatin (CP) and radiotherapy (RT) in patients with locally advanced squamous cell anal carcinoma (LAAC) [abstract 4609]. J Clin Oncol 2008;26:15S.

94. Matzinger O, Roelofsen F, Mineur L, et al. Mitomycin C with continuous fluorouracil or with cisplatin in combination with radiotherapy for locally advanced anal cancer (European Organisation for Research and Treatment of Cancer phase II study 22011-40014). Eur J Cancer 2009;45(16):2782–91.

95. Adelstein DJ, Li Y, Adams GL, et al. An intergroup phase III comparison of standard radiation therapy and two schedules of concurrent chemoradiotherapy in patients with unresectable squamous cell head and neck cancer. J Clin Oncol 2003;21(1):92–8.

96. Forastiere AA, Goepfert H, Maor M, et al. Concurrent chemotherapy and radiotherapy for organ preservation in advanced laryngeal cancer. N Engl J Med 2003;349(22):2091–8.

97. Loong HH, Ma BB, Leung SF, et al. Prognostic significance of the total dose of cisplatin administered during concurrent chemoradiotherapy in patients with locoregionally advanced nasopharyngeal carcinoma. Radiother Oncol 2012. [Epub ahead of print].

98. Eng C, Chang GJ, Das P, et al. Phase II study of capecitabine and oxaliplatin with concurrent radiation therapy (XELOX-XRT) for squamous cell carcinoma of the anal canal [abstract 4116]. J Clin Oncol 2009;27:15S.

99. Sadek H, Azli N, Wendling JL, et al. Treatment of advanced squamous cell carcinoma of the skin with cisplatin, 5-fluorouracil, and bleomycin. Cancer 1990; 66(8):1692–6.

100. Meropol NJ, Niedzwiecki D, Shank B, et al. Induction therapy for poor-prognosis anal canal carcinoma: a phase II study of the cancer and Leukemia Group B (CALGB 9281). J Clin Oncol 2008;26(19):3229–34.

101. Peiffert D, Giovannini M, Ducreux M, et al. High-dose radiation therapy and neo-adjuvant plus concomitant chemotherapy with 5-fluorouracil and cisplatin in patients with locally advanced squamous-cell anal canal cancer: final results of a phase II study. Ann Oncol 2001;12(3):397–404.

102. Choi CH, Lee JW, Kim TJ, et al. Phase II study of consolidation chemotherapy after concurrent chemoradiation in cervical cancer: preliminary results. Int J Radiat Oncol Biol Phys 2007;68(3):817–22.

103. Chemoradiotherapy for Cervical Cancer Meta-Analysis Collaboration. Reducing uncertainties about the effects of chemoradiotherapy for cervical cancer: a systematic review and meta-analysis of individual patient data from 18 randomized trials. J Clin Oncol 2008;26(35):5802–12.

104. James R, Meadows H. The second UK phase IIII anal cancer trial of chemoradiation and maintenance therapy (ACT II): preliminary results on toxicity and outcome [abstract]. Proc Am Soc Clin Oncol, J Clin Oncol 2003;22:287.

105. Hatfield P, Cooper R, Sebag-Montefiore D. Involved-field, low-dose chemoradiotherapy for early-stage anal carcinoma. Int J Radiat Oncol Biol Phys 2008;70(2): 419–24.

106. Hu K, Minsky BD, Cohen AM, et al. 30 Gy may be an adequate dose in patients with anal cancer treated with excisional biopsy followed by combined-modality therapy. J Surg Oncol 1999;70(2):71–7.

107. Renehan AG, O'Dwyer ST. Management of local disease relapse. Colorectal Dis 2011;13(s1):44–52.

108. Sebag-Montefiore D, James R, Meadows H, et al. The pattern and timing of disease recurrence in squamous cancer of the anus: Mature results from the NCRI ACT II trial. J Clin Oncol 2012;30(suppl; abstr 4029).

109. Chapet O, Gerard JP, Riche B, et al. Prognostic value of tumor regression evaluated after first course of radiotherapy for anal canal cancer. Int J Radiat Oncol Biol Phys 2005;63(5):1316–24.

110. Tanum G, Holm R. Anal carcinoma: a clinical approach to p53 and RB gene proteins. Oncology 1996;53(5):369–73.

111. Schwarz JK, Siegel BA, Dehdashti F, et al. Tumor response and survival predicted by post-therapy FDG-PET/CT in anal cancer. Int J Radiat Oncol Biol Phys 2008;71(1):180–6.

112. Chauveinc L, Buthaud X, Falcou MC, et al. Anal canal cancer treatment: practical limitations of routine prescription of concurrent chemotherapy and radiotherapy. Br J Cancer 2003;89(11):2057–61.

113. Allal AS, Mermillod B, Roth AD, et al. Impact of clinical and therapeutic factors on major late complications after radiotherapy with or without concomitant chemotherapy for anal carcinoma. Int J Radiat Oncol Biol Phys 1997;39(5):1099–105.

114. Peiffert D, Bey P, Pernot M, et al. Conservative treatment by irradiation of epidermoid cancers of the anal canal: prognostic factors of tumoral control and complications. Int J Radiat Oncol Biol Phys 1997;37(2):313–24.

115. Wagner JP, Mahe MA, Romestaing P, et al. Radiation therapy in the conservative treatment of carcinoma of the anal canal. Int J Radiat Oncol Biol Phys 1994; 29(1):17–23.

116. Glynne-Jones R, Sebag-Montefiore D, Adams R, et al. "Mind the gap"—the impact of variations in the duration of the treatment gap and overall treatment time in the first UK Anal Cancer Trial (ACT I). Int J Radiat Oncol Biol Phys 2011;81(5):1488–94.

117. Cox JD, Stetz J, Pajak TF. Toxicity criteria of the Radiation Therapy Oncology Group (RTOG) and the European Organization for Research and Treatment of Cancer (EORTC). Int J Radiat Oncol Biol Phys 1995;31(5):1341–6.

118. Northover J, Glynne-Jones R, Sebag-Montefiore D, et al. Chemoradiation for the treatment of epidermoid anal cancer: 13-year follow-up of the first randomised UKCCCR Anal Cancer Trial (ACT I). Br J Cancer 2010;102(7):1123–8.

119. Baxter NN, Habermann EB, Tepper JE, et al. Risk of pelvic fractures in older women following pelvic irradiation. JAMA 2005;294(20):2587–93.

120. Tomaszewski JM, Link E, Leong T, et al. Twenty-five-year experience with radical chemoradiation for anal cancer. Int J Radiat Oncol Biol Phys 2012;83(2):552–8.

121. Mai SK, Welzel G, Haegele V, et al. The influence of smoking and other risk factors on the outcome after radiochemotherapy for anal cancer. Radiat Oncol 2007;2:30.

122. Tournier-Rangeard L, Mercier M, Peiffert D, et al. Radiochemotherapy of locally advanced anal canal carcinoma: prospective assessment of early impact on the quality of life (randomized trial ACCORD 03). Radiother Oncol 2008;87(3):391–7.

123. Allal AS, Sprangers MA, Laurencet F, et al. Assessment of long-term quality of life in patients with anal carcinomas treated by radiotherapy with or without chemotherapy. Br J Cancer 1999;80(10):1588–94.

124. Vordermark D, Sailer M, Flentje M, et al. Curative-intent radiation therapy in anal carcinoma: quality of life and sphincter function. Radiother Oncol 1999;52(3):239–43.

125. Vordermark D, Sailer M, Flentje M, et al. Impaired sphincter function and good quality of life in anal carcinoma patients after radiotherapy: a paradox? Front Radiat Ther Oncol 2002;37:132–9.

126. Boman BM, Moertel CG, O'Connell MJ, et al. Carcinoma of the anal canal. A clinical and pathologic study of 188 cases. Cancer 1984;54(1):114–25.

127. Kuehn PG, Eisenberg H, Reed JF. Epidermoid carcinoma of the perianal skin and anal canal. Cancer 1968;22(5):932–8.

128. Wells IT, Fox BM. PET/CT in anal cancer—is it worth doing? Clin Radiol 2012; 67(6):535–40.

129. Evans TR, Lofts FJ, Mansi JL, et al. A phase II study of continuous-infusion 5-fluorouracil with cisplatin and epirubicin in inoperable pancreatic cancer. Br J Cancer 1996;73(10):1260–4.

130. Ajani JA, Carrasco CH, Jackson DE, et al. Combination of cisplatin plus fluoro-pyrimidine chemotherapy effective against liver metastases from carcinoma of the anal canal. Am J Med 1989;87(2):221–4.

131. Faivre C, Rougier P, Ducreux M, et al. 5-fluorouracile and cisplatinum combination chemotherapy for metastatic squamous-cell anal cancer. Bull Cancer 1999; 86(10):861–5 [in French].

132. Fisher WB, Herbst KD, Sims JE, et al. Metastatic cloacogenic carcinoma of the anus: sequential responses to adriamycin and cis-dichlorodiammineplatinum(II). Cancer Treat Rep 1978;62(1):91–7.

133. Gurfinkel R, Walfisch S. Combined treatment of basaloid anal carcinoma using cisplatin, 5-fluorouracil and resection of hepatic metastasis. Tech Coloproctol 2005;9(3):235–6.

134. Jaiyesimi IA, Pazdur R. Cisplatin and 5-fluorouracil as salvage therapy for recurrent metastatic squamous cell carcinoma of the anal canal. Am J Clin Oncol 1993;16(6):536–40.

135. Khater R, Frenay M, Bourry J, et al. Cisplatin plus 5-fluorouracil in the treatment of metastatic anal squamous cell carcinoma: a report of two cases. Cancer Treat Rep 1986;70(11):1345–6.

136. Salem PA, Habboubi N, Anaissie E, et al. Effectiveness of cisplatin in the treatment of anal squamous cell carcinoma. Cancer Treat Rep 1985;69(7–8):891–3.

137. Tanum G, Tveit K, Karlsen KO, et al. Chemotherapy and radiation therapy for anal carcinoma. Survival and late morbidity. Cancer 1991;67(10):2462–6.

138. Hainsworth JD, Burris HA 3rd, Meluch AA, et al. Paclitaxel, carboplatin, and long-term continuous infusion of 5-fluorouracil in the treatment of advanced squamous and other selected carcinomas: results of a Phase II trial. Cancer 2001;92(3):642–9.

139. Jhawer M, Mani S, Lefkopoulou M, et al. Phase II study of mitomycin-C, adriamycin, cisplatin (MAP) and Bleomycin-CCNU in patients with advanced cancer of the anal canal: an Eastern Cooperative Oncology Group study E7282. Invest New Drugs 2006;24(5):447–54.

140. Wilking N, Petrelli N, Herrera L, et al. Phase II study of combination bleomycin, vincristine and high-dose methotrexate (BOM) with leucovorin rescue in advanced squamous cell carcinoma of the anal canal. Cancer Chemother Pharmacol 1985;15(3):300–2.

141. Tanum G. Treatment of relapsing anal carcinoma. Acta Oncol 1993;32(1):33–5.

142. Golub DV, Civelek AC, Sharma VR. A regimen of taxol, Ifosfamide, and platinum for recurrent advanced squamous cell cancer of the anal canal. Chemother Res Pract 2011;2011:163736.

143. Vuong T, Devic S, Belliveau P, et al. Contribution of conformal therapy in the treatment of anal canal carcinoma with combined chemotherapy and radiotherapy: results of a phase II study. Int J Radiat Oncol Biol Phys 2003;56(3):823–31.

144. Moreau-Claeys MV, Peiffert D. Normal tissue tolerance to external beam radiation therapy: anal canal. Cancer Radiother 2010;14(4–5):359–62 [in French].

145. Salama JK, Mell LK, Schomas DA, et al. Concurrent chemotherapy and intensity-modulated radiation therapy for anal canal cancer patients: a multicenter experience. J Clin Oncol 2007;25(29):4581–6.

146. Mell LK, Schomas DA, Salama JK, et al. Association between bone marrow dosimetric parameters and acute hematologic toxicity in anal cancer patients treated with concurrent chemotherapy and intensity-modulated radiotherapy. Int J Radiat Oncol Biol Phys 2008;70(5):1431–7.

147. Alvarez G, Perry A, Tan BR, et al. Expression of epidermal growth factor receptor in squamous cell carcinomas of the anal canal is independent of gene amplification. Mod Pathol 2006;19(7):942–9.

148. Van Damme N, Deron P, Van Roy N, et al. Epidermal growth factor receptor and K-RAS status in two cohorts of squamous cell carcinomas. BMC Cancer 2010;10:189.

149. Bussink J, van der Kogel AJ, Kaanders JH. Activation of the PI3-K/AKT pathway and implications for radioresistance mechanisms in head and neck cancer. Lancet Oncol 2008;9(3):288–96.

150. Miyaguchi M, Olofsson J, Hellquist HB. Expression of epidermal growth factor receptor in glottic carcinoma and its relation to recurrence after radiotherapy. Clin Otolaryngol Allied Sci 1991;16(5):466–9.

151. Bosset JF, Roelofsen F, Morgan DA, et al. Shortened irradiation scheme, continuous infusion of 5-fluorouracil and fractionation of mitomycin C in locally advanced anal carcinomas. Results of a phase II study of the European Organization for Research and Treatment of Cancer. Radiotherapy and Gastrointestinal Cooperative Groups. Eur J Cancer 2003;39(1):45–51.

152. Glynne-Jones R, Meadows H, Wan S, et al. EXTRA—a multicenter phase II study of chemoradiation using a 5 day per week oral regimen of capecitabine and intravenous mitomycin C in anal cancer. Int J Radiat Oncol Biol Phys 2008; 72(1):119–26.

153. Zampino MG, Magni E, Sonzogni A, et al. K-ras status in squamous cell anal carcinoma (SCC): it's time for target-oriented treatment? Cancer Chemother Pharmacol 2009;65(1):197–9.

154. Lukan N, Strobel P, Willer A, et al. Cetuximab-based treatment of metastatic anal cancer: correlation of response with KRAS mutational status. Oncology 2009; 77(5):293–9.

155. Kronfli M, Glynne-Jones R. Chemoradiotherapy in anal cancer. Colorectal Dis 2011;13(Suppl 1):33–8.

156. Sischy B, Doggett RLS, Krall JM, et al. Definitive irradiation and chemotherapy for radiosensitization in management of anal carcinoma: interim report on Radiation Therapy Oncology Group study no 8314. J Natl Cancer Inst 1989;81: 850–6.

157. Martenson JA, Lipsitz SR, Wagner H, et al. Initial results of a phase II trial of high dose radiation therapy, 5-fluorouracil, and cisplatin for patients with anal cancer (E4292). Int J Radiation Oncol Biol Phys 1996;35:745–9.

158. Doci R, Zucali R, La Monica G, et al. Primary chemoradiation therapy with fluorouracil and cisplatin for cancer of the anus: results in 35 consecutive patients. J Clin Oncol 1996;14:3121–5.

159. Konski A, Garcia M, John M, et al. Evaluation of planned treatment breaks during radiation therapy for anal cancer: update of of RTOG 92-08. Int J Radiat Oncol Biol Phys 2008;72(1):114–8.

160. Vaz F, Trindade C, Barata A, et al. Sequential and concomitant chemoradiation (CTR) therapy with flurouracil (5FU) and cisplatin (CDDP) for anal squamous cell carcinoma (ASCC). J Clin Oncol 1998;17:304. [abstract 1173].

161. Gerard JP, Romestaing P, Mornex F, et al. Radiochemotherapy in anal carcinoma (ACC). A randomised trial comparing fluorouracil-cisplatin (5FU-CDDP) and CDDP alone. Eur J Cancer 1999;S143. [abstract 523].

162. Matthews JH, Burmeister BH, Borg M, et al. T1-2 anal carcinoma requires elective inguinal radiation treatment–the results of Trans Tasman Radiation Oncology Group study TROG 99.02. Radiother Oncol 2011;98(1):93–8.

163. Sebag-Montefiore D, Meadows HM, Cunningham D, et al. Three cytotoxic drugs combined with pelvic radiation and as maintenance chemotherapy for patients with squamous cell carcinoma of the anus (SCCA): Long-term follow-up of a phase II pilot study using 5-fluorouracil, mitomycin C and cisplatin. Radiother Oncol 2012 Aug;104(2):155–60.

164. Crehange G, Bosset M, Lorchel F, et al. Combining cisplatin and Mitomycin with radiotherapy in anal carcinoma. Dis Colon Rectum 2006;50:43–9.

165. Kachnic L, Winter K, Myerson R, et al. Early efficacy of RTOG-0529: a phase II evaluation of dose painted IMRT in combination with 5-fluorouracil and Mitomycin-C for the reduction of acute morbidity in carcinoma of the anal canal. Int J Radiation Oncol Biol Phys 2010;78(3S) suppl PROC ASTRO:s55. [abstract 116].

Merkel Cell Carcinoma

Sandra Y. Han, MD[a], Jeffrey P. North, MD[a], Theresa Canavan, BS[a],
Nancy Kim, MD[b], Siegrid S. Yu, MD[a],*

KEYWORDS

- Merkel cell • Skin cancer • Neuroendocrine carcinoma

KEY POINTS

- Merkel cell carcinoma (MCC) is a cutaneous malignancy with an aggressive course.
- MCCs has no specific distinctive features, although many present as an asymptomatic red or pink papule or nodule.
- The recent discovery of the Merkel cell polyomavirus (MCPyV) offers the potential for understanding the basis of the disease and creating targeted therapies.
- The first consensus staging system for MCC was developed in 2010 and emphasizes the importance of sentinel lymph node in staging of disease.
- Currently, there are no standardized guidelines for treatment, although surgery with possible adjuvant radiation is favored for local or locoregional disease. Chemotherapy is reserved for distant metastatic disease.

INTRODUCTION

MCC is a rare neuroendocrine carcinoma of the skin. MCC was originally described by Toker in 1972 in his report of 5 cases of trabecular cell carcinoma of the skin.[1] Subsequently, through electron microscopy, these tumors were found to contain dense core granules.[2] Because Merkel cells were known to be the only cells in the skin containing these granules, it was hypothesized that trabecular carcinoma of the skin originated from Merkel cells. The exact origin of Merkel cells is still a matter of debate, with some investigators hypothesizing that Merkel cells arise from stem cells of neural crest origin. Other investigators suggest that Merkel cells differentiate from epidermal keratinocyte-like cells (reviewed by Boulais and Misery[3]). Currently, the former is the favored viewpoint. Other names for MCC have previously been used, including

Funding Sources: None.
Conflicts of Interest: None.
[a] Department of Dermatology, University of California, San Francisco, 1701 Divisadero Street, 3rd Floor, San Francisco, CA 94115, USA; [b] Spectrum Dermatology, 7425 East Shea Boulevard, Suite 110, Scottsdale, AZ 85260, USA
* Corresponding author.
E-mail address: yus@derm.ucsf.edu

Hematol Oncol Clin N Am 26 (2012) 1351–1374
http://dx.doi.org/10.1016/j.hoc.2012.08.007
0889-8588/12/$ – see front matter © 2012 Elsevier Inc. All rights reserved.

neuroendocrine or primary small cell carcinoma of the skin and anaplastic cancer of the skin.

Although MCC is a rare malignancy, it has an aggressive clinical course. At the time of presentation, 66% of patients have local disease, 27% have nodal involvement, and 7% have distant metastases.[4] The 5-year survival of MCC patients (relative to age-matched and gender-matched controls) is 64% for local, 39% for regional nodal, and 18% for distant metastatic disease.[4] Given the rarity of this malignancy, there is a paucity of prospective trials, and management of MCC remains challenging in the absence of standardized guidelines for treatment. In 2010, the first consensus staging system for MCC was adopted by the American Joint Committee on Cancer (AJCC) (**Table 1**). Unlike other previously proposed guidelines, a distinction was made between clinical versus pathologic examination of regional lymph nodes. The

Table 1
2010 American Joint Committee on Cancer staging system for Merkel cell carcinoma

T	N	M
Tx, primary tumor cannot be assessed	Nx, regional nodes cannot be assessed	Mx, distant metastasis cannot be assessed
T0, no primary tumor	N0, no regional node metastasis[a]	M0, no distant metastasis
Tis, in situ primary tumor	cN0, nodes not clinically detectable[a]	M1, distant metastasis[b]
T1, primary tumor ≤2 cm	cN1, nodes clinically detectable[a]	M1a, distant skin, distant subcutaneous tissues, or distant lymph nodes
T2, primary tumor >2 but ≤5 cm	N1a, micrometastasis[c]	M1b, lung
T3, primary tumor >5 cm	N1b, macrometastasis[d]	M1c, metastasis to all other visceral sites
T4, primary tumor invades	N2, in-transit metastasis[e]	

Stage			
0	Tis	N0	M0
IA	T1	pN0	M0
IB	T1	cN0	M0
IIA	T2/T3	pN0	M0
IIB	T2/T3	cN0	M0
IIC	T4	N0	M0
IIIA	Any T	N1a	M0
IIIB	Any T	N1b/N2	M0
IV	Any T	Any N	M1

[a] N0 denotes negative nodes by clinical, pathologic, or both types of examination. Clinical detection of nodal disease may be via inspection, palpation, and/or imaging; cN0 is used only for patients who did not undergo pathologic node staging.
[b] Because there are no data to suggest significant effect of M categories on survival in MCC, M1a–c are included in same stage grouping.
[c] Micrometastasis are diagnosed after sentinel or elective lymphadenectomy.
[d] Macrometastasis are defined as clinically detectable nodal metastases confirmed pathologically by biopsy or therapeutic lymphadenectomy.
[e] In-transit metastasis is tumor distinct from primary lesion and located either (1) between primary lesion and draining regional lymph nodes or (2) distal to primary lesion.

mainstay of treatment remains surgical, and there is support for the use of adjuvant radiation for localized and regional disease whereas chemotherapy is often reserved for palliative therapy in cases of distant metastases.

EPIDEMIOLOGY

The epidemiology and survival of MCC patients have been studied by several groups using data from the Surveillance, Epidemiology and End Result (SEER) Program of the National Cancer Institute, which included 10% to 14% of the US population observed starting in 1973 and continuing onward as a prospective cohort.[5–8] The incidence of MCC among the SEER population was reported sporadically before the mid-1980s. Between the years 1986 and 2006, however, the incidence of primary MCC grew significantly, from 0.15 cases per 100,000[8] to 0.6 cases per 100,000.[5] Similar to the findings from the SEER database, Reichgelt and Visser[9] reported that the incidence of MCC in the Netherlands increased between 1993 and 2007, albeit at a slower rate, from 0.17 to 0.35 cases per 100,000. The increased incidence during this time is at least in part due to improvements in the methods used to accurately diagnose MCC as the immunologic profile specific for MCC has been better elucidated.

Not all groups have found such a dramatic rise in MCC incidence during this same time period; some researchers found a stable incidence since the mid-1990s. In Denmark, Kaae and colleagues[10] used the Danish national health and population registers to assess MCC incidence, and they found that the incidence remained stable between 1995 and 2006 at 0.22 cases per 100,000 person-years. Likewise, the incidence of MCC in Western Australia between 1993 and 2007 increased only slightly for men and did not increase at all for women.[11]

Although the incidence for this population in Western Australia has remained stable, it remains the group with the highest incidence reported worldwide. Girschik and colleagues[11] analyzed histologically confirmed cases of MCC from the Western Australia Cancer Registry from 1993 to 2007 and found an age-standardized incidence over this time frame of 0.82 cases per 100,000. This high incidence corresponds to a high level of UV exposure in this location. The geographic association for MCC development has been studied for the United States as well. The highest age-adjusted incidence in white patients from the SEER database was in Hawaii, which is the geographic location from the SEER database with the highest UV index. Further supporting the causative role of UV in development of MCC is the finding that patients with psoriasis who underwent oral methoxsalen (psoralen) and UVA photochemotherapy have an MCC incidence 100-times greater than the general population.[12]

The majority of patients (71.6%) with MCC are first diagnosed at age 70 or older,[5] and it is infrequently found in patients under age 50. The incidence of primary MCC is higher in men than in women when all ethnic groups are examined, with a ratio of 2:1 in whites and 1.5:1 in other ethnic groups.[7] Men tend to have an initial diagnosis at a slightly younger age than women, with a mean age of 73.6 for men and 76.2 for women at diagnosis.[7] Nearly 95% of the cases reported in the SEER population between 1973 and 2006 occurred in white patients, and only 1.0% and 4.1% were in black and other races (Asian Pacific Islander, American Indian, other), respectively.[7]

ETIOLOGY

The groundbreaking discovery by Feng and colleagues[13] in 2008 of a novel polyomavirus associated with the development of MCC has led to several investigative efforts in viral tumorigenesis. In their study, the MCPyV genome was detected in 8 of 10 MCC tumors but only 16% (4/25) of normal skin and non-MCC tumor tissue. The presence of MCPyV in 80% of MCC cases has been substantiated in several studies (reviewed by Kuwamoto[14]).

Members of the *Polyomaviridae* family are small, nonencapsulated, circular, double-stranded DNA viruses with the potential to cause transformation in experimental animal models and cultured cells. To date, 17 members of the family have been identified, and 9 are known to infect humans (BK, JC, KI, WU, MCPyV, Human polyomavirus 6, Human polyomavirus 7, Trichodysplasia spinulosa-associated polyomavirus, and Human polyomavirus 9). The first 2 members, BK virus and JC virus, were discovered in 1971. BK virus causes nephropathy in immunosuppressed kidney transplant patients,[15] and JC virus is responsible for progressive multifocal leukoencephelopathy in patients with profound immunosuppression.[16] KI, WU, and TS are not as yet known to cause disease in humans. Simian virus 40 is the most well-known polyomavirus, although its role in human disease and tumorigenesis remains controversial.[17]

The genome of MCPyV is comprised of early and late regions. The former consists of large T-antigen (LT) and small T-antigen regions, which encode proteins necessary for viral replication. The late region encodes viral proteins (VPs) responsible for capsid assembly. LT antigen contains 3 different domains: a binding site for retinoblastoma tumor suppressor protein, a binding site for heat shock protein, and a helicase domain. In Feng and colleagues'[13] initial study, MCPyV was observed as integrated into MCC tumor genome in a monoclonal pattern, implying viral infection and genome integration occurred before clonal expansion of tumor cells. A follow-up study by Shuda and colleagues[18] identified mutations within the LT antigen in the MCPyV present in MCC tumors. These mutations did not affect the retinoblastoma and heat shock protein binding domains but did result in loss of the helicase domain. As a result, the viral replication capacity of DNA was lost, and the investigators suggested that MCPyV-positive MCC tumor cells underwent selection for LT mutations to prevent autoactivation of integrated virus replication that would be detrimental to cell survival.

MCPyV is ubiquitous in its infection of humans. The seroprevalence of MCPyV antibodies against viral capsid proteins 1 and 2 (VP1 and VP2) ranges from 42% to 88% in healthy adult subjects.[19–22] In children, the prevalence is 9% under the age of 4, but this increases to 35% by age 13.[23] Although the seroprevalence of antibodies to VP1 and VP2 has been shown higher among MCC subjects, the titers have not been shown to correlate with tumor characteristics or viral load. The presence of a high titer did correspond with a better progression-free survival,[24] although the mechanism of immunoprotection is unclear because MCC tumors do not express VP1 or VP2 proteins.[25] In contrast, another study demonstrated a greater specificity of antibodies directed at MCPyV large and small tumor-associated antigens (T-Ag) among MCC patients.[26] The importance of T-Ag was demonstrated by Houben et al[27] in that its expression is necessary for the maintenance of MCPyV-positive MCC. The seroprevalence of these antibodies was 0.9% among healthy control subjects, while it was 40.5% among MCC patients. Moreover, antibody levels were found to be predictive of clinical course, and therefore Paulson and colleagues[26] concluded that antibodies recognizing T-Ag are specifically associated with MCC, do not effectively protect against disease progression, and may serve as a clinically useful indicator of disease status.

Studies have also been conducted on the cellular immune response to MCPyV. Intratumoral infiltration of CD8+ lymphocytes has been demonstrated as an independent predictor of improved survival among MCC patients. Of 156 cases, patients with robust CD8+ intratumoral infiltration had 100% MCC-specific survival compared with 60% survival among patients with sparse or no CD8+ intratumoral infiltration.[28] This improved prognosis with tumor-infiltrating lymphocytes was recently confirmed by Sihto and colleagues.[29]

The role immunology plays in MCC development is highlighted by the fact that patients with immunosuppression at higher risk for development of MCC. Moreover, immunosuppressed patients with MCC are younger and have more advanced disease at the time of diagnosis.[30–32] MCC is associated with a diverse number of autoimmune diseases as well as with organ transplantation.[33–39] A cohort of 309,365 individuals with AIDS was assessed for the development of MCC between −60 to +27 months relative to AIDS onset. Six individuals from this cohort developed MCC, which corresponds to a relative risk of 13.4 (95% CI, 4.9–29.1) compared with the general population, suggesting that a weakened immune system increases the risk of MCC.[31] In Heath and colleagues[40] analysis, 7.8% of MCC patients were found to have some form of immunosuppression, including HIV, chronic lymphocytic leukemia (CLL), and solid organ transplants. A 2009 study examining the Finnish Cancer Registry demonstrated a standardized incidence ratio of 17.9 for developing CLL after a diagnosis of MCC and a standardized incidence ratio of 15.7 for developing MCC among patients already diagnosed with CLL.[41] Another recent study showed that among MCC patients, the standardized incidence ratio was 3.67 for men and 3.62 for women in developing a hematological malignancy. In this study, CLL was the most common at 45%.[42]

Among transplant patients, renal transplant patients most commonly acquire MCC, with the average time span of 7 years between organ transplantation and development of MCC.[30] Thirty-six cases of MCC have been reported to the Cincinnati Transplant Tumor Registry, which translates to an incidence of approximately 3 cases per 1000 transplant patients.[43] The MCPyV may explain the increased incidence of MCC in immunosuppressed patients, but its pathogenesis has not been fully elucidated. The importance of immune status is further highlighted by cases in which MCC tumors have temporarily regressed in transplant patients upon the cessation of immunosuppressive medications.[44,45]

PRESENTATION

MCC can be a difficult tumor to clinically diagnose, because it tends to be asymptomatic and does not have pathognomonic clinical features. Ultimately, the diagnosis is made by biopsy and histopathologic examination. Typically, lesions present as firm, red-to-purple, nontender papules or nodules (**Figs. 1** and **2**). In Heath and colleagues[40] study, 56% of patients presented with a tumor having a red or pink hue, whereas 26% had blue/violaceous lesions (**Fig. 3**). Moreover, 63% of patients in the study reported rapid growth in the size of their tumor over a period of 3 months. Only 11% of patients did not notice any changes in size of primary lesions.

As discussed previously, UV exposure is believed to play a role in the development of MCC. Accordingly, MCC is most commonly located on UV-exposed areas, such as the head and neck, which account for 48% of all MCC diagnoses.[5,40] Incidence of MCC of the upper limb is 19%, followed by a 16% incidence of MCC of the lower limb and 11% incidence of MCC of the trunk.[6] UV-protected locations, such as the trunk, back, and buttocks, are less commonly affected than UV-exposed sites. The MCC site with the best prognosis is presentation on the limbs, which generally correlates with less advanced disease. MCC presentation on the trunk is associated with distant metastasis at the time of diagnosis.[6]

Some unusual primary sites for MCC to occur include mucosal sites, including the lacrimal gland[46] and the parotid gland.[47] Approximately 5% of all cases of first primary MCC present in mucosal sites. From 1992 to 2001, the total number of cases of first primary MCC was 1027 and of these cases, 50 had an initial presentation in a mucosal anatomic site.[6] The most common sites affected by mucosal MCC are the larynx,

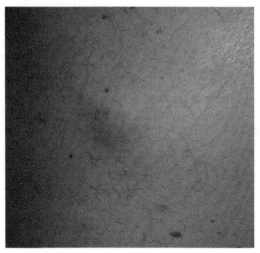

Fig. 1. A less common presentation of MCC is a subcutaneous nodule with minimal overlying surface change. This highlights the importance of maintaining a high index of suspicion for diagnosing and treating this entity.

followed by the nasal cavity, pharynx, and mouth.[6] There have also been rare reports of vulvar[48] and penile MCC.[49] Mucosal MCC is associated with a worse prognosis than primary cutaneous MCC at other anatomic sites. Part of the reason for the worse prognosis may lie in the difficulty of detection and delayed diagnosis.

Subcutaneous primary tumor is a less common presentation of MCC (see **Fig. 4**). Reports in the literature describe a subcutaneous nodule or mass with minimal to no overlying epidermal change as the initial presentation.[50–54] The sites of these nodules have included the cheek[50] and the arm.[51] Differential diagnoses for these

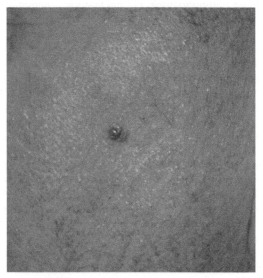

Fig. 2. This small, asymptomatic, red papule on the cheek of an elderly patient was diagnosed as MCC on histopathology. This is a typical presentation of MCC.

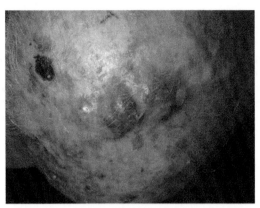

Fig. 3. These erythematous, firm scalp nodules presented in a patient with known renal cell carcinoma. Initial clinical suspicion was that of metastatic renal cell carcinoma. Biopsy, however, revealed in-transit MCC, which can mimic other carcinomas.

nodules and masses have included lipoma, carcinoid, epidermal cyst, and cutaneous metastases until pathologic examination rendered the diagnosis of MCC.

Another less common presentation of MCC is an enlarged lymph node without any findings of primary cutaneous disease.[55–65] In Heath and colleagues'[45] series, nodal MCC with an unknown primary was reported as the initial presentation in 14% of MCCs. Of reported cases, the most common site of MCC presenting in the lymph node was inguinal, although axillary,[55,57] submandibular,[55,56,62] and retroperitoneal[63] sites also were reported. The prognosis of these primary nodal presentations of MCC

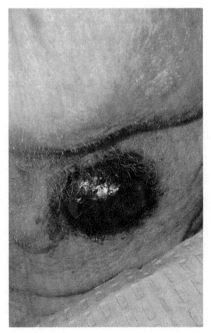

Fig. 4. Some MCCs have a more violaceous hue and can expand rapidly. This nodule grew 4 cm within 1 month.

is speculated as being similar to those of primary cutaneous MCCs with nodal metastasis.[65] The origin of these nodal MCCs is not entirely understood. The general prevailing viewpoint is that these nodal MCCs represent nodal metastasis from a regressed primary cutaneous MCC. An alternative theory is that lymph nodal MCCs are primary sites of tumor formation,[55] but given that Merkel cells have never been localized as primary cells of lymph nodes, this theory is less favorable. Because distinction from other poorly differentiated small cell or neuroendocrine tumors may be difficult, stringent pathologic techniques must be used to diagnose MCC presenting in a lymph node without a known corresponding cutaneous lesion.

DIAGNOSTIC EVALUATION
Pathology

Histopathologic features
All neuroendocrine tumors (eg, MCC, small cell lung carcinoma, and carcinoid tumors) share similar histopathologic features, featuring small to medium-sized cells with round nuclei and scant cytoplasm. The nuclei have finely granular or stippled chromatin, sometimes exhibiting a smudged appearance with inconspicuous nucleoli (**Fig. 5**). The high nucleus:cytoplasm ratio imparts a blue or basaloid appearance at scanning magnification. Some MCCs have cells with more vesicular chromatin with multiple small nucleoli, irregular nuclear contours, and more abundant cytoplasm. The latter two features were associated with a lack of detectable MCPyV infection in one small study.[66] Nuclear pleomorphism is typically mild, whereas mitotic figures and apoptotic cells abound (see **Fig. 5**).

MCC is divided into subtypes based on growth pattern and cell size. Most MCCs have a nodular architecture with multiple, interconnecting aggregations of cells forming a tumor centered in the dermis with infiltrative strands of cells at the tumor periphery. The presence or absence of these infiltrative strands is used to classify MCCs into infiltrative or nodular patterns.[67] The so-called diffuse pattern consists of large collections of neoplastic cells coalescing into sheet-like aggregations of cells. The trabecular pattern, for which MCC was originally named trabecular carcinoma by Toker in 1972,[1] consists of interconnecting strands of cells (**Fig. 6**). Epidermal involvement can be seen in any of these subtypes and occurs in approximately 10% of all cases.[68] Purely intraepidermal MCC, also called MCC in situ, is rare.

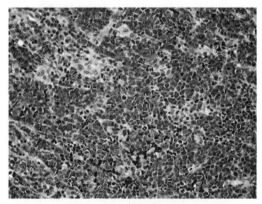

Fig. 5. The cells of MCC have round nuclei with finely granular chromatin, inconspicuous nucleoli, and scant cytoplasm. Mitotic figures are numerous. The neoplastic cells are significantly larger than interspersed lymphocytes. H&E ×400.

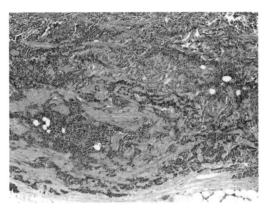

Fig. 6. Aggregations of tumor cells form interanastamosing cords in the dermis in a trabecular pattern with some infiltrate strands of cells in the deep reticular dermis. H&E ×100.

Combinations of these patterns frequently occur in the same tumor and, with the exception of improved survival associated with cases lacking an infiltrative pattern,[67] separation based on growth pattern does not seem to have clinical significance.

In addition to architectural subclassification, MCC is classified according to cell size. The majority of MCCs are the intermediate cell type, with medium-sized nuclei (10–15 microns), which are significantly larger than nearby lymphocytes (see **Fig. 5**). Some degree of nuclear molding is present, often manifesting as the ball-in-mitt pattern with compression of some nuclei into crescent shapes around adjacent circular nuclei. The small cell variant of MCC features cells approximately the size of lymphocytes, which can lead to misclassification of the tumor as a lymphocytic process. An uncommon large cell variant with greater nuclear pleomorphism is also described.

Immunohistochemical and ultrastructural features

Due to histopathologic overlap with neuroendocrine tumors, hematologic malignancies, poorly differentiated carcinomas, and various other neoplasms, confirmatory studies are used in the vast majority of suspected MCCs. Electron microscopy played a critical role in identifying MCC as a neuroendocrine carcinoma and can be used as an ancillary test to confirm the diagnosis. The presence of paranuclear and/or cytoplasmic bundles of tonofilaments (keratin intermediate filaments), cytoplasmic dense-core granules, and desmosomal attachments is characteristic of MCC. Currently, widespread access to immunostains, which offer rapid results with good sensitivity and specificity, has made immunostaining the confirmatory test of choice for MCC.

Although many immunostains have been studied in MCC, cytokeratin 20, low-molecular-weight cytokeratins (eg, CAM5.2), and neurofilaments have a high sensitivity for MCC and are the most frequently used immunostains in this differential diagnosis. A paranuclear dot staining pattern is characteristic of MCC (**Fig. 7**). Diffuse cytoplasmic staining is less specific. Negative staining with thyroid transcription factor 1 and cytokeratin 7 can be used to increase specificity, especially when differentiating from small cell lung carcinoma. Neuroendocrine markers, such as synaptophysin, chromogranin, and neuron-specific enolase, are frequently used, but these are nonspecific and of limited diagnostic value. In exceptionally challenging cases, chromosomal analysis with array-based comparative genomic hybridization can be helpful.

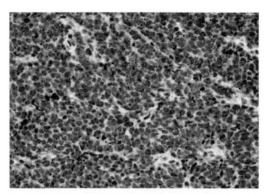

Fig. 7. Paranuclear dot pattern in MCC. Cytokeratin 20 ×400.

Prognostic features

Tumor size and thickness, along with lymphovascular invasion, have prognostic significance in MCC.[67] Intravascular invasion occurs in 56% to 93% of cases and sometimes requires a vascular immunostain (eg, D2-40) for identification.[69,70] Promising data have shown positive p63 staining correlates with a remarkably worse prognosis,[71] but most prognostic studies of immunostains, including MCPyV large T antigen, Ki-67, p53, and Rb, are small and have inconsistent results.

Staging

Several staging guidelines for MCC had been developed before 2010.[72–75] Because of the overall paucity of cases of MCC, however, none of these cohorts included more than 251 cases. In 2010, the first consensus staging system was published based on 5823 cases registered in the National Cancer Data Base (a US-based registry founded by the American Cancer Society and the American College of Surgeons) (**Table 1**).[4] The staging system has subsequently been adopted by the AJCC and the International Union Against Cancer.

The new consensus staging system has 4 stages determined by tumor size (T), the presence or absence of metastases to regional lymph nodes (N), and the presence or absence of distant metastases (M). For local disease, a distinction was made between those primary tumors less than or equal to 2 cm in size (T1) at the time of presentation, which showed a 66% 5-year survival. In contrast, those tumors between 2 cm and 5 cm in size (T2) carried a 51% 5-year survival. The T3 designation was given to those tumors that exceeded 5 cm in size. Although the prognoses of these patients were similar to those of those having T2 disease, this format was chosen so that the T4 designation could be assigned to those tumors invading deeper underlying structures so as to maintain congruence with other AJCC staging systems.

The staging system also takes into consideration whether examination of regional lymph nodes has occurred clinically or pathologically. Data in the cohort demonstrate a worse prognosis for those with undetectable lymph nodes on clinical examination alone compared with those who have pathologically proven negative lymph nodes. Accordingly, those with pathologically negative lymph nodes are categorized as having either stage IA or stage IIA disease. In contrast, those with negative lymph nodes based on clinical examination alone are regarded as having either stage IB or stage IIB disease. Sentinel lymph node biopsy (SLNB), therefore, should be considered for all patients presenting with clinically localized disease.

For distant metastases, staging criteria are similar to that of melanoma. Distinctions are made between having no metastatic disease, metastases to distant skin, subcutaneous tissue, or lymph nodes, metastases to lung, or metastases to any other visceral site.

Prognosis

The prognosis of MCC is generally poor. Stage at time of presentation is the most important prognostic indicator. Under the revised staging guidelines (discussed previously), patients with local disease have a 5-year survival of 66% if the primary tumor is less than or equal to 2 cm in diameter, whereas those who present with tumors greater than 2 cm have a 5-year survival of 51%. Patients who have local disease confirmed with pathologically negative lymph nodes have a better prognosis (76% at 5 years) compared with those who have negative lymph nodes based on clinical examination alone (59% at 5 years). Among those patients with metastases to regional lymph nodes, the 5-year survival ranges from 26% to 42%. Patients with distant metastases have a prognosis of 18% survival at 5 years.

In addition to stage at the time of diagnosis, clinical features have been evaluated as potential prognostic factors. Smith and colleagues[76] reported that in a review of 2104 MCCs in head and neck locations, the lip had a significantly worse prognosis with a higher rate of invasion into deeper underlying structures and a higher rate of nodal metastasis. For MCCs of any location, a primary tumor presenting on the trunk is associated with a worse prognosis.[77] Men have been found to have a worse prognosis compared with women. Older patients (>70 years old) have a worse prognosis compared with their younger counterparts.[6] A recent review of a database of 500 MCC cases demonstrated a strong association between lymphovascular invasion by MCC and disease-specific death.[69]

Imaging

Currently, there are no consensus guidelines regarding which patients should be imaged after an initial diagnosis of MCC. Although SLNB is useful for detection of microscopic locoregional metastasis, imaging may be useful as an adjunct to determine the presence of distant metastasis. In general, those patients with clinically localized disease and no clinical evidence of metastatic nodal disease should be assessed first for candidacy for SLNB with possible adjunctive imaging for evaluation and staging. Those with evidence of nodal or metastatic disease on initial history and physical examination are recommended to have preoperative imaging to evaluate for distant metastasis and facilitate staging at the time of MCC diagnosis.

The preferred modality for imaging MCC has yet to be established. Conventional imaging has primarily been with CT, ultrasound, and MRI.[78–81] More recently, the role of (18)F–fluorodeoxyglucose positron emission tomography (FDG PET) alone or in combination with CT (FDG PET–CT) has been investigated. Yao and colleagues[82] reported 2 cases in which FDG PET detected metastatic disease in subcentimeter nodes that were not detected on initial CT scans. The investigators argue that FDG PET has increased sensitivity compared with conventional CT in identifying these small foci of metastases. Similarly, Lin and colleagues[83] reported the increased sensitivity of FDG PET to detect recurrent MCC compared with conventional CT. A retrospective review of 18 patients demonstrated that all proven sites of MCC greater than 5 mm were visualized on FDG PET–CT, and these findings led to changes in management of 9 patients.[84] In a study of head and neck cancers, Shintani and colleagues[85] determined that 2 of 5 MCC patients had their postsurgical adjuvant treatment plan change as a result of findings on PET CT. Two recent case series, however, comparing the utility of FDG PET–CT to traditional imaging modalities showed no demonstrable difference in sensitivity or specificity between the two.[86,87] However, FDG PET–CT has greater sensitivity in detecting bony metastases for more common tumors, such as lung and colorectal carcinoma. This may be applicable to neuroendocrine tumors over traditional imaging for MCC.[88]

The frequency of imaging is also a matter of controversy. Given that the median time to recurrence of MCC is 9 months and that 90% of MCC recurrences occur within the first 2 years of diagnosis of the primary tumor, more frequent surveillance when clinically indicated during this period is advocated.[72,89] Currently there is no standardized algorithm for the role of imaging in monitoring for recurrence. At the authors' institution, the preferred imaging modality is FDG PET–CT, which is used to screen high-risk patients or those with clinical evidence of metastasis at the time of primary MCC diagnosis. The frequency of follow-up is handled on an individual basis using FDG PET–CT, although patients are typically reimaged every 6 months for the first 2 years.

TREATMENT
Surgery

Surgery is the primary therapy for MCC. Given the absence of prospective studies comparing optimal margins for wide local excision, guidelines on ideal surgical management have not been established. Historically, excision of 2 cm to 3 cm to investing fascia has been the margin used. There have been no prospective studies that directly compare ideal margins and guide standards for treatment. In a retrospective review at a single institution, however, an average surgical margin of 1.1 cm yielded negative margins in 94% of cases (185/196),[72] prompting some physicians to favor narrower margins, particularly for smaller tumors. Current National Comprehensive Cancer Network (NCCN) guidelines recommend 1-cm to 2-cm margin for wide local excision or, alternatively, treatment with Mohs surgery to ensure clear margins with a central debulk for permanent fixation for microstaging.[89]

Mohs surgery for MCC has been evaluated as a favorable approach for MCC. In a small, retrospective study comparing outcomes of patients who underwent Mohs surgery to those patients receiving standard excision, 92% (11/12) of those who had Mohs surgery were free from recurrence at 36 months versus 32% (13/41) of those with wide local excision alone.[90] Mohs surgery for MCC is demonstrated as having even greater efficacy with adjuvant radiation therapy. Boyer and colleagues[91] described 4 of 25 recurrent or in-transit metastases developing after Mohs surgery in patients with stage I MCC treated with surgery alone compared with 0 of 20 in those receiving adjuvant radiation. This difference failed to reach statistical significance, although the limitation of its small sample size must be taken into account. The recurrence rate of 4% to 16% with Mohs surgery is similar to that of published reports of wide local excision of 4% to 14%.

The most important aspect of surgical treatment through wide local excision or Mohs surgery is to establish clear surgical margins. In addition, all MCC patients who are surgical candidates for SLNB are advised to undergo the procedure (described later). For patients who are undergoing wide local excision, SLNB is performed intraoperatively. Those patients treated with Mohs surgery for MCC should have SLNB performed before Mohs surgery because lymphatic drainage may be altered through the Mohs procedure leading to alterations in lymphoscintigraphy.

Sentinel Lymph Node Biopsy

Although prophylactic lymphadenectomy has previously been recommended for the management of MCC,[74,92] this is no longer advised; rather, with few exceptions, those patients who are surgical candidates should undergo SLNB at the time of wide local excision, because it is the most consistent prognosticator. As originally described by Messina and colleagues[93] for MCC in 1997, this method allows detection of local nodal metastasis not evident on clinical examination. Further studies have substantiated that approximately 20% to 32% of clinically negative nodes display microscopic metastasis on SLNB, supporting the rationale for wide use of this practice in diagnostic evaluation.[72,94,95] As discussed previously, the prognosis is favorable (76% survival at 5 years) for those patients with localized disease and negative SLNB. Moreover, Gupta and colleagues[94] observed that 60% of patients with a positive SLNB recurred within 3 years in contrast to 20% with a negative SLNB. A meta-analysis by Mehrany and colleagues[96] showed the odds of recurrent MCC were 19-fold greater in those patients with a positive SLNB compared with those with a negative result. The status of sentinel lymph node on prognosis has, however, been recently disputed by Fields and colleagues.[95] In their analysis of 146 patients undergoing SLNB, there was no significant difference in recurrence ($P = .86$) or death ($P = .84$) from MCC.

In cases of small, localized primary MCC tumors less than 1 cm and no clinical evidence of regional nodal involvement, Stokes and colleagues[97] have advocated that SLNB may be avoided. This conclusion is based on their study that only 4% (2/54) of patients with subcentimeter tumors had lymph nodes metastases, and their metastases were clinically evident even before SLNB. Conversely, other investigators, including Sarnaik and colleagues,[98] Schwartz and colleagues,[99] and Tai and colleagues[100] indicate that SLNB should be performed for all MCC regardless of tumor size, given their data that even small tumors may harbor micrometastases and reveal positive results with SLNB. In Schwartz and colleagues'[99] study, of 42 tumors less than 1 cm, 23.8% demonstrated a positive SLNB (28.5 months vs 11.8 months).[101] It is important to perform immunostains on all SLNB histologic specimens because micrometastatic disease may be missed on routine hematoxylin-eosin (H&E) stain. In one study, cytokeratin 20 detected MCC in 22% of lymph node sections that were missed on routine staining.[102]

Radiation Therapy

For those patients with positive SLNB, the traditional treatment approach has been complete lymph node dissection alone, lymph node dissection with adjuvant radiation, or radiation therapy (RT) alone. Given the rarity of this disease, no prospective, randomized controlled trials exist to support one of these approaches over the other. The decision of which option to pursue is often dependent on comorbidities and consideration of adverse events as well as institutional protocol. At the authors' institution, patients with positive SLNB are treated with either complete lymphadenectomy or radiation monotherapy but typically not a combination of both, due to the morbidity of dual treatment of draining lymphatics. In instances of grossly positive disease at the time of dissection or evidence of extracapsular extension of MCC on pathology, however, adjuvant RT to the nodal bed is considered.

Radiation as monotherapy for definitive treatment

MCC is a radiosensitive malignancy, and RT has been used for monotherapy of primary tumors and to obtain locoregional control, although its role as the primary therapeutic agent is generally reserved for patients who are not surgical candidates for resection of MCC. Data supporting the use of RT as definitive monotherapy of primary tumors have emerged with a recent study. In a retrospective analysis of patients with more localized disease (stage IB to IIB under current AJCC criteria) by

Pape and colleagues,[103] 25 patients who were treated with RT alone to the primary tumor site were compared with 25 patients who underwent surgery with adjuvant RT to the primary tumor site. Most patients in both groups received RT to the nodal basin. The investigators found no significant difference in clinical outcome between these 2 groups.

The use of RT as monotherapy for patients with more advanced disease has also been evaluated. In a case series by Koh and Veness,[104] of 8 patients treated with RT to the primary tumor and regional lymph nodes, 6 patients eventually succumbed to distant metastases at the time of follow-up. The median time to relapse was 3.5 months. The same group reported a 60% rate of relapse among a cohort of 43 patients treated with RT alone.[105] In this group of patients with poor prognosis, 77% were known to have nodal metastases. Patients received a median of 51 Gy in fractionated doses to the primary tumor and a median of 50 Gy to the regional nodal bed. Of the relapses, only 25% were within the irradiated field, and thus the investigators conclude RT monotherapy may be beneficial to those with nodal disease who are not surgical candidates, although most die of distant disease.

In contrast, a recent study by Fang and colleagues[106] supports the use of RT as definitive treatment of regional disease. This is the largest study to date of RT monotherapy used to treat known regional disease based on clinical examination (24 patients) or a positive SLNB (26 patients). The authors compared RT treatment of known metastatic regional lymph nodes with RT monotherapy versus *completion lymph node dissection*(CLND) ± RT. The investigators found those with microscopic disease to have 100% regional recurrence-free survival regardless of treatment modality at 18 months. For those patients with clinically palpable disease at presentation, similar regional recurrence-free survival was found between the RT monotherapy group (78%) and CLND ± RT group (73%) at 2 years ($P = .8$). Patients in the Veness study had their primary tumor treated with RT and not surgery whereas most of the patients in Fang and colleagues' study had surgical resection of their primary tumor.

Radiation as adjuvant therapy

RT as adjuvant therapy to surgical treatment of primary MCC has also been evaluated in limited studies. A meta-analysis of 1254 patients by Lewis and colleagues[107] compared outcomes between those who received a combination of surgery and adjuvant radiation and those who underwent surgery alone. This analysis included study types of all sample sizes in which MCC was treated primarily with surgery with or without adjuvant RT. The investigators found decreases in both local (88% vs 61%) and regional (77% vs 44%) recurrences at 5 years with combination therapy. With the inclusion of all cases for the analysis, there was no difference in overall or disease-specific mortality. One major limitation of this study, however, is that it did not distinguish between the treatment fields for RT because it included those who received RT to the primary tumor bed, to local in-transit disease, and to regional lymph nodes.

A retrospective analysis by Gillenwater and colleagues[108] was conducted of 66 patients with MCC who received either surgical treatment alone or combination therapy with surgery and RT to the primary tumor bed and draining lymphatics. Most of the patients in both groups had localized MCC and were staged at N_0. Like Lewis and colleagues,[107] the investigators found a decrease in both local and regional recurrence rates for those with combination therapy compared with surgery alone (44% vs 12% for local and 85% vs 27% for regional recurrence). Similar to Lewis and colleagues' study, there was no difference in disease-specific survival. Further supporting the use of adjuvant RT, Mojica and colleagues[109] reported data from the

SEER database showing a median survival of 63 months for patients treated with adjuvant RT compared with 45 months survival for those who did not receive RT (P = .0002). Further the use of adjuvant RT, Jabbour and colleagues reviewed the records of 82 patients with MCC and found that its use was associated with prolonged time to first recurrence (P = 0.04) and survival (P = .013).[102]

Based on the available data, the NCCN Clinical Practice Guidelines in Oncology for MCC recommend consideration of adjuvant local RT for most patients with MCC and regional RT as either primary or adjuvant therapy after CLND in patients with lymph node metastases. In addition, for patients with micrometastatic disease on SLNB, the NCCN indicates RT monotherapy may be a suitable treatment without CLND.[89]

In contrast, some investigators found no benefit to adjuvant RT to regional lymph nodes and dispute this recommendation. In a study of a prospective database of MCC patients, Fields and colleagues[110] found no significant difference in the cumulative incidence of local recurrence at 2 years between patients who were selected to receive adjuvant local RT (1.7%) compared with those who were not selected (3.8%; P = .77). Similarly, there was no significant difference in the lymph node recurrence rate at 2 years between patients who were selected to receive lymph node RT (5.2%) compared with those who were not selected (13.8%; P = .15). Although most patients undergo local RT to the primary tumor bed, the NCCN identifies a group for which clinical observation may also be appropriate. For those patients with small tumors who have undergone successful wide local excision and without any other adverse factors, clinical observation alone may be sufficient.[89]

Chemotherapy

In patients with locoregional MCC, the use of chemotherapy has been evaluated in limited studies. In a multivariate reanalysis of a study of MCC patients with high-risk features treated with adjuvant etoposide and carboplatin, Poulsen and colleagues[111] found no survival benefit to the use of chemotherapy. Similarly, a retrospective review by Kokoska and colleagues[112] led to the same conclusion. Given the significant morbidity conferred by treatment toxicities, adjuvant chemotherapy currently has a minimal role in locoregional MCC therapy.[113] Given the increased incidence of MCC among immunocompromised patients as well as the implications of its viral etiology, having an intact immune system is speculated as being important for preventing further progression of MCC. With the effect of traditional chemotherapeutic agents on reducing immune function, it has been advised that these medications be limited in its use for patients with locoregional disease for which surgery and RT are treatment alternatives.

Patients with distant disease at the time of diagnosis have few treatment options, and chemotherapy is generally the mainstay of therapy with palliative intent. Based on the similarity of MCC to small cell lung cancer in biologic behavior, chemotherapeutic regimens for the latter have guided MCC regimens.[114] The most common regimen is etoposide/carboplatin whereas cyclophosphamide/doxorubicin/vincristine ± prednisone has also been used.[115] MCC has been shown a chemosensitive malignancy,[116] but it has a high recurrence rate and overall poor prognosis. In a study by Pectasides and colleagues,[117] among 11 patients with locally advanced or metastatic MCC, there was a response rate of 73% to combination chemotherapy. Two patients achieved complete remission with adjuvant RT. All of the others experienced disease recurrence, with a median progression-free survival of 10 months and overall survival of 14 months. A retrospective study by Voog and colleagues[118] demonstrated a similarly favorable response rate of 61% to first-line chemotherapy, but overall survival was poor, especially for those with metastatic disease. Median overall survival was 9 months for those with metastatic disease and 24 months for those with locally advanced disease at the time of treatment initiation.

Given that many MCC patients are elderly with significant comorbidities, the decision to pursue chemotherapy must take treatment-related toxicities into account. In the review by Tai and colleagues,[119] there was a 3.5% mortality rate for patients who received chemotherapy. Voog and colleagues'[118] study reported an even higher rate of 7.7%. Among those patients receiving combination RT and chemotherapy with etoposide/carboplatin, neutropenia was found to be the most significant toxicity, with the greatest risk occurring during the second cycle of chemotherapy.[120]

FUTURE DEVELOPMENTS

Given the few results of treatment with traditional chemotherapeutic agents, one avenue of future MCC therapy is the development of treatments directed at molecular targets. At this time, no specific pathway for tumorigenesis has been elucidated although various targets have been investigated. MCC has been demonstrated to over-express the KIT receptor tyrosine kinase protein as detected by CD117 staining,[121,122] prompting the clinical trial of imatinib mesylate as a potential treatment of MCC.[123] The trial was discontinued because it was not found efficacious in treating MCC. Studies subsequent to enrollment of the trial demonstrated the lack of activating mutations in c-KIT, which provides explanation as to the outcome seen with imatinib.[124,125]

More recently CD56, a neural cell adhesion molecule expressed by a variety of human cells, including Merkel cells, has been the focus of pharmacologic targeting. Lorvotuzumab mertansine is a humanized monoclonal antibody that selectively binds CD56. This medication has received Orphan Drug Designation from the US Food and Drug Administration and is currently in clinical trials.[126]

A study by Nardi and colleagues[127] demonstrated activating mutations of PIK3CA in 6 of 60 MCC tumors. With the exception of one case, these mutations were present only in MCPyV-negative tumors. These PIK3CA mutations result in downstream activation of AKT and, ultimately, antiapoptotic and cell proliferative pathways.[128] This opens up the potential for therapy with PIK3 inhibitors, such as ZSTK474[129] and NVP-BEZ235.[130] Similar findings were demonstrated by Hafner and colleagues.[131]

The increasing state of knowledge of MCPyV in MCC pathogenesis may lead to the development immunologic therapies. Given the antiviral property of interferons, several studies have been conducted to evaluate their efficacy against MCC. In experimental models, type I interferon (IFN), which includes IFN-α and IFN-β, was shown to strongly inhibit the viability of MCPyV cell lines.[132,133] Although attempts at treatment in vivo of two patients with IFN-α were unsuccessful,[134] the IFNs remain a potential treatment under further study.

Given the effect of cellular immunity on MCC, an area of potential therapy is the development of a vaccine against MCPyV. One potential target is LT, because this protein has been shown to be necessary for maintenance of MCC in MCPyV-infected cells.[27] Iyer and colleagues[135] identified MCPyV-specific epitopes immunogenic to CD8+ and CD4+ T cells that opened the possibility of producing epitope-specific vaccines. Zeng and colleagues[136] identified an LT-specific CD4+ T helper epitope at MCPyV LT aa136-160. As demonstrated in a mouse model, mice innoculated with the vaccine construct demonstrated significantly smaller tumor volume and a significantly higher survival rate than mice vaccinated with control vectors.

As another potential way to stimulate the cytotoxic response of the host immune system, the therapeutic role of interleukin (IL)-12 is being evaluated. A phase II trial using intratumoral delivery of IL-12 plasmid DNA followed by in vivo electroporation of MCC tumors is currently enrolling participants.[137] Subjects will receive delivery of the plasmid on three occasions and will be followed for expression of IL-12 and clinical response.

SUMMARY

MCC is a rare and aggressive neuroendocrine carcinoma of the skin with an increased incidence over the past 2 decades. The malignancy is most commonly seen in elderly white and immunosuppressed populations, such as HIV positive patients or solid organ transplant recipients.

The etiology of MCC has yet to be fully elucidated, although the recent discovery of the MCPyV, which is present in 80% of MCCs, has sparked immense interest in understanding its tumorigenesis. Clinical manifestations are varied, although most MCCs start as asymptomatic growths on sun-exposed sites. MCC can be definitively diagnosed through using a combination of routine histology and immunohistochemical stains on tumor biopsy specimens with a cytokeratin 20 paranuclear dot staining pattern virtually pathognomonic for MCC.

The 2010 AJCC staging system classifies MCC by tumor size, presence or absence of nodal disease, and distant metastasis at time of presentation. Accurately staging MCC is important because it influences treatment and provides the most accurate prognostic data. To prevent the understaging of patients with subclinical nodal disease or distant metastases, SLNBs and advanced imaging are often incorporated into the staging process.

At this time, there is no consensus on how to optimally treat this disease, and, therefore, a multidisciplinary approach is advised to optimize patient outcomes. Surgical excision of the primary tumor, either via wide local excision or Mohs surgery, is the cornerstone of treatment with adjuvant RT in cases of high-risk patients or tumor characteristics providing improved locoregional control compared with surgery alone. Chemotherapy is reserved for patients with distant metastatic disease, but unfortunately, it has not been found to induce prolonged remission. The discovery of the novel MCPyV offers exciting opportunities for the development of oncologic therapies by capitalizing on immunologic mechanisms.

REFERENCES

1. Toker C. Trabecular carcinoma of the skin. Arch Dermatol 1972;105(1):107–10.
2. Tang CK, Toker C. Trabecular carcinoma of the skin: an ultrastructural study. Cancer 1978;42(5):2311–21.
3. Boulais N, Misery L. Merkel cells. J Am Acad Dermatol 2007;57(1):147–65.
4. Lemos BD, Storer BE, Iyer JG, et al. Pathologic nodal evaluation improves prognostic accuracy in Merkel cell carcinoma: analysis of 5823 cases as the basis of the first consensus staging system. J Am Acad Dermatol 2010;63(5):751–61.
5. Albores-Saavedra J, Batich K, Chable-Montero F, et al. Merkel cell carcinoma demographics, morphology, and survival based on 3870 cases: a population based study. J Cutan Pathol 2010;37(1):20–7.
6. Agelli M, Clegg LX. Epidemiology of primary Merkel cell carcinoma in the United States. J Am Acad Dermatol 2003;49(5):832–41.
7. Agelli M, Clegg LX, Becker JC, et al. The etiology and epidemiology of Merkel cell carcinoma. Curr Probl Cancer 2010;34(1):14–37.
8. Hodgson NC. Merkel cell carcinoma: changing incidence trends. J Surg Oncol 2005;89(1):1–4.

9. Reichgelt BA, Visser O. Epidemiology and survival of Merkel cell carcinoma in the Netherlands. A population-based study of 808 cases in 1993-2007. Eur J Cancer 2011;47(4):579–85.

10. Kaae J, Hansen AV, Biggar RJ, et al. Merkel cell carcinoma: incidence, mortality, and risk of other cancers. J Natl Cancer Inst 2010;102(11):793–801.

11. Girschik J, Thorn K, Beer TW, et al. Merkel cell carcinoma in Western Australia: a population-based study of incidence and survival. Br J Dermatol 2011;165(5): 1051–7.

12. Lunder EJ, Stern RS. Merkel-cell carcinomas in patients treated with methoxsalen and ultraviolet A radiation. N Engl J Med 1998;339(17):1247–8.

13. Feng H, Shuda M, Chang Y, et al. Clonal integration of a polyomavirus in human Merkel cell carcinoma. Science 2008;319(5866):1096–100.

14. Kuwamoto S. Recent advances in the biology of Merkel cell carcinoma. Hum Pathol 2011;42(8):1063–77.

15. Gardner SD, Field AM, Coleman DV, et al. New human papovavirus (B.K.) isolated from urine after renal transplantation. Lancet 1971;1(7712):1253–7.

16. Padgett BL, Walker DL, ZuRhein GM, et al. Cultivation of papova-like virus from human brain with progressive multifocal leucoencephalopathy. Lancet 1971; 1(7712):1257–60.

17. Poulin DL, DeCaprio JA. Is there a role for SV40 in human cancer? J Clin Oncol 2006;24(26):4356–65.

18. Shuda M, Feng H, Kwun HJ, et al. T antigen mutations are a human tumor-specific signature for Merkel cell polyomavirus. Proc Natl Acad Sci U S A 2008;105(42):16272–7.

19. Viscidi RP, Rollison DE, Sondak VK, et al. Age-specific seroprevalence of Merkel cell polyomavirus, BK virus, and JC virus. Clin Vaccine Immunol 2011;18(10): 1737–43.

20. Kean JM, Rao S, Wang M, et al. Seroepidemiology of human polyomaviruses. PLoS Pathog 2009;5(3):e1000363.

21. Tolstov YL, Pastrana DV, Feng H, et al. Human Merkel cell polyomavirus infection II. MCV is a common human infection that can be detected by conformational capsid epitope immunoassays. Int J Cancer 2009;125(6):1250–6.

22. Carter JJ, Paulson KG, Wipf GC, et al. Association of Merkel cell polyomavirus-specific antibodies with Merkel cell carcinoma. J Natl Cancer Inst 2009;101(21): 1510–22.

23. Chen T, Hedman L, Mattila PS, et al. Serological evidence of Merkel cell polyomavirus primary infections in childhood. J Clin Virol 2011;50(2):125–9.

24. Touze A, Le Bidre E, Laude H, et al. High levels of antibodies against merkel cell polyomavirus identify a subset of patients with merkel cell carcinoma with better clinical outcome. J Clin Oncol 2011;29(12):1612–9.

25. Pastrana DV, Tolstov YL, Becker JC, et al. Quantitation of human serorespon-siveness to Merkel cell polyomavirus. PLoS Pathog 2009;5(9):e1000578.

26. Paulson KG, Carter JJ, Johnson LG, et al. Antibodies to merkel cell polyomavirus T antigen oncoproteins reflect tumor burden in merkel cell carcinoma patients. Cancer Res 2010;70(21):8388–97.

27. Houben R, Shuda M, Weinkam R, et al. Merkel cell polyomavirus-infected Merkel cell carcinoma cells require expression of viral T antigens. J Virol 2010;84(14):7064–72.

28. Paulson KG, Iyer JG, Tegeder AR, et al. Transcriptome-wide studies of merkel cell carcinoma and validation of intratumoral CD8+ lymphocyte invasion as an independent predictor of survival. J Clin Oncol 2011;29(12):1539–46.

29. Sihto H, Bohling T, Kavola H, et al. Tumor Infiltrating immune cells and outcome of merkel cell carcinoma: a population-based study. Clin Cancer Res 2012; 18(10):2872–81.

30. Buell JF, Trofe J, Hanaway MJ, et al. Immunosuppression and Merkel cell cancer. Transplant Proc 2002;34(5):1780–1.

31. Engels EA, Frisch M, Goedert JJ, et al. Merkel cell carcinoma and HIV infection. Lancet 2002;359(9305):497–8.

32. Penn I, First MR. Merkel's cell carcinoma in organ recipients: report of 41 cases. Transplantation 1999;68(11):1717–21.

33. Gooptu C, Woollons A, Ross J, et al. Merkel cell carcinoma arising after therapeutic immunosuppression. Br J Dermatol 1997;137(4):637–41.

34. Lentz SR, Krewson L, Zutter MM. Recurrent neuroendocrine (Merkel cell) carcinoma of the skin presenting as marrow failure in a man with systemic lupus erythematosus. Med Pediatr Oncol 1993;21(2):137–41.

35. Nemoto I, Sato-Matsumura KC, Fujita Y, et al. Leukaemic dissemination of Merkel cell carcinoma in a patient with systemic lupus erythematosus. Clin Exp Dermatol 2008;33(3):270–2.

36. McLoone NM, McKenna K, Edgar D, et al. Merkel cell carcinoma in a patient with chronic sarcoidosis. Clin Exp Dermatol 2005;30(5):580–2.

37. Lillis J, Ceilley RI, Nelson P. Merkel cell carcinoma in a patient with autoimmune hepatitis. J Drugs Dermatol 2005;4(3):357–9.

38. Satolli F, Venturi C, Vescovi V, et al. Merkel-cell carcinoma in Behcet's disease. Acta Derm Venereol 2005;85(1):79.

39. Gianfreda M, Caiffi S, De Franceschi T, et al. Merkel cell carcinoma of the skin in a patient with myasthenia gravis. Minerva Med 2002;93(3):219–22 [in Italian].

40. Heath M, Jaimes N, Lemos B, et al. Clinical characteristics of Merkel cell carcinoma at diagnosis in 195 patients: the AEIOU features. J Am Acad Dermatol 2008;58(3):375–81.

41. Koljonen V, Kukko H, Pukkala E, et al. Chronic lymphocytic leukaemia patients have a high risk of Merkel-cell polyomavirus DNA-positive Merkel-cell carcinoma. Br J Cancer 2009;101(8):1444–7.

42. Tadmor T, Liphshitz I, Aviv A, et al. Increased incidence of chronic lymphocytic leukaemia and lymphomas in patients with Merkel cell carcinoma—a population based study of 335 cases with neuroendocrine skin tumour. Br J Haematol 2012; 157(4):457–62.

43. Miller RW, Rabkin CS. Merkel cell carcinoma and melanoma: etiological similarities and differences. Cancer Epidemiol Biomarkers Prev 1999;8(2): 153–8.

44. Friedlaender MM, Rubinger D, Rosenbaum E, et al. Temporary regression of Merkel cell carcinoma metastases after cessation of cyclosporine. Transplantation 2002;73(11):1849–50.

45. Muirhead R, Ritchie DM. Partial regression of Merkel cell carcinoma in response to withdrawal of azathioprine in an immunosuppression-induced case of metastatic Merkel cell carcinoma. Clin Oncol 2007;19(1):96.

46. Gess AJ, Silkiss RZ. A merkel cell carcinoma of the lacrimal gland. Ophthal Plast Reconstr Surg 2012;28(1):e11–3.

47. Ghaderi M, Coury J, Oxenberg J, et al. Primary Merkel cell carcinoma of the parotid gland. Dermatol Surg 2010;89(7):E24–7.

48. Iavazzo C, Terzi M, Arapantoni-Dadioti P, et al. Vulvar merkel carcinoma: a case report. Case Report Med 2011;2011:546972.

49. Tomic S, Warner TF, Messing E, et al. Penile Merkel cell carcinoma. Urology 1995;45(6):1062–5.

50. Sarma DP, Heagley DE, Chalupa J, et al. An unusual clinical presentation of merkel cell carcinoma: a case report. Case Report Med 2010;2010:905414.

51. Huang GS, Chang WC, Lee HS, et al. Merkel cell carcinoma arising from the subcutaneous fat of the arm with intact skin. Dermatol Surg 2005;31(6): 717–9.

52. Balaton AJ, Capron F, Baviera EE, et al. Neuroendocrine carcinoma (Merkel cell tumor?) presenting as a subcutaneous tumor. An ultrastructural and immunohistochemical study of three cases. Pathol Res Pract 1989;184(2):211–6.

53. Tsai YY, Hsiao CH, Chiu HC, et al. CK7+/CK20- Merkel cell carcinoma presenting as inguinal subcutaneous nodules with subsequent epidermotropic metastasis. Acta Derm Venereol 2010;90(4):438–9.

54. Gambichler T, Kobus S, Kreuter A, et al. Primary merkel cell carcinoma clinically presenting as deep oedematous mass of the groin. Eur J Med Res 2010;15(6): 274–6.

55. Eusebi V, Capella C, Cossu A, et al. Neuroendocrine carcinoma within lymph nodes in the absence of a primary tumor, with special reference to Merkel cell carcinoma. Am J Surg Pathol 1992;16(7):658–66.

56. Straka JA, Straka MB. A review of Merkel cell carcinoma with emphasis on lymph node disease in the absence of a primary site. Am J Otol 1997;18(1): 55–65.

57. Ferrara G, Ianniello GP, Di Vizio D, et al. Lymph node Merkel cell carcinoma with no evidence of cutaneous tumor–report of two cases. Tumori 1997;83(5):868–72.

58. Samarendra P, Berkowitz L, Kumari S, et al. Primary nodal neuroendocrine (Merkel cell) tumor in a patient with HIV infection. South Med J 2000;93(9):920–2.

59. Fotia G, Barni R, Bellan C, et al. Lymph nodal Merkel cell carcinoma: primary or metastatic disease? a clinical case. Tumori 2002;88(5):424–6.

60. Silberstein E, Koretz M, Cagnano E, et al. Neuroendocrine (Merkel cell) carcinoma in regional lymph nodes without primary site. Isr Med Assoc J 2003;5(6):450–1.

61. Kuwabara H, Mori H, Uda H, et al. Nodal neuroendocrine (Merkel cell) carcinoma without an identifiable primary tumor. Acta Cytol 2003;47(3):515–7.

62. Nazarian Y, Shalmon B, Horowitz Z, et al. Merkel cell carcinoma of unknown primary site. J Laryngol Otol 2007;121(4):e1.

63. Boghossian V, Owen ID, Nuli B, et al. Neuroendocrine (Merkel cell) carcinoma of the retroperitoneum with no identifiable primary site. World J Surg Oncol 2007;5:117.

64. Kim EJ, Kim HS, Kim HO, et al. Merkel cell carcinoma of the inguinal lymph node with an unknown primary site. J Dermatol 2009;36(3):170–3.

65. De Cicco L, Vavassori A, Jereczek-Fossa BA, et al. Lymph node metastases of Merkel cell carcinoma from unknown primary site: report of three cases. Tumori 2008;94(5):758–61.

66. Kuwamoto S, Higaki H, Kanai K, et al. Association of Merkel cell polyomavirus infection with morphologic differences in Merkel cell carcinoma. Hum Pathol 2011;42(5):632–40.

67. Andea AA, Coit DG, Amin B, et al. Merkel cell carcinoma: histologic features and prognosis. Cancer 2008;113(9):2549–58.

68. Skelton HG, Smith KJ, Hitchcock CL, et al. Merkel cell carcinoma: analysis of clinical, histologic, and immunohistologic features of 132 cases with relation to survival. J Am Acad Dermatol 1997;37(5 Pt 1):734–9.

69. Fields RC, Busam KJ, Chou JF, et al. Five hundred patients with Merkel cell carcinoma evaluated at a single institution. Ann Surg 2011;254(3):465–73 [discussion: 473–5].

70. Kukko HM, Koljonen VS, Tukiainen EJ, et al. Vascular invasion is an early event in pathogenesis of Merkel cell carcinoma. Mod Pathol 2010;23(8):1151–6.

71. Asioli S, Righi A, Volante M, et al. p63 expression as a new prognostic marker in Merkel cell carcinoma. Cancer 2007;110(3):640–7.

72. Allen PJ, Bowne WB, Jaques DP, et al. Merkel cell carcinoma: prognosis and treatment of patients from a single institution. J Clin Oncol 2005;23(10):2300–9.

73. Allen PJ, Zhang ZF, Coit DG. Surgical management of Merkel cell carcinoma. Ann Surg 1999;229(1):97–105.

74. Yiengpruksawan A, Coit DG, Thaler HT, et al. Merkel cell carcinoma. Prognosis and management. Arch Surg 1991;126(12):1514–9.

75. Clark JR, Veness MJ, Gilbert R, et al. Merkel cell carcinoma of the head and neck: is adjuvant radiotherapy necessary? Head Neck 2007;29(3):249–57.

76. Smith VA, Madan OP, Lentsch EJ. Tumor location is an independent prognostic factor in head and neck Merkel cell carcinoma. Otolaryngol Head Neck Surg 2012;146(3):403–8.

77. Ott MJ, Tanabe KK, Gadd MA, et al. Multimodality management of Merkel cell carcinoma. Arch Surg 1999;134(4):388–92 [discussion: 392–3].

78. Eftekhari F, Wallace S, Silva EG, et al. Merkel cell carcinoma of the skin: imaging and clinical features in 93 cases. Br J Radiol 1996;69(819):226–33.

79. Gollub MJ, Gruen DR, Dershaw DD. Merkel cell carcinoma: CT findings in 12 patients. AJR Am J Roentgenol 1996;167(3):617–20.

80. Nguyen BD, McCullough AE. Imaging of Merkel cell carcinoma. Radiographics 2002;22(2):367–76.

81. Anderson SE, Beer KT, Banic A, et al. MRI of merkel cell carcinoma: histologic correlation and review of the literature. AJR Am J Roentgenol 2005;185(6):1441–8.

82. Yao M, Smith RB, Hoffman HT, et al. Merkel cell carcinoma: two case reports focusing on the role of fluorodeoxyglucose positron emission tomography imaging in staging and surveillance. Am J Clin Oncol 2005;28(2):205–10.

83. Lin O, Thomas A, Singh A, et al. Complementary role of positron emission tomography in merkel cell carcinoma. South Med J 2004;97(11):1110–2.

84. Concannon R, Larcos GS, Veness M. The impact of (18)F-FDG PET-CT scanning for staging and management of Merkel cell carcinoma: results from Westmead Hospital, Sydney, Australia. J Am Acad Dermatol 2010;62(1):76–84.

85. Shintani SA, Foote RL, Lowe VJ, et al. Utility of PET/CT imaging performed early after surgical resection in the adjuvant treatment planning for head and neck cancer. Int J Radiat Oncol Biol Phys 2008;70(2):322–9.

86. Peloschek P, Novotny C, Mueller-Mang C, et al. Diagnostic imaging in Merkel cell carcinoma: lessons to learn from 16 cases with correlation of sonography, CT, MRI and PET. Eur J Radiol 2010;73(2):317–23.

87. Maury G, Dereure O, Du-Thanh A, et al. Interest of (18)F-FDG PET-CT scanning for staging and management of merkel cell carcinoma: a retrospective study of 15 patients. J Eur Acad Dermatol Venereol 2011;25(12):1420–7.

88. Werner MK, Aschoff P, Reimold M, et al. FDG-PET/CT-guided biopsy of bone metastases sets a new course in patient management after extensive imaging and multiple futile biopsies. Br J Radiol 2011;84(999):e65–7.

89. National Comprehensive Cancer Network. NCCN Clinical Practice Guidlines in Oncology—Merkel cell carcinoma. 2012(Version 1.2012).

90. O'Connor WJ, Roenigk RK, Brodland DG. Merkel cell carcinoma. Comparison of Mohs micrographic surgery and wide excision in eighty-six patients. Dermatol Surg 1997;23(10):929–33.
91. Boyer JD, Zitelli JA, Brodland DG, et al. Local control of primary Merkel cell carcinoma: review of 45 cases treated with Mohs micrographic surgery with and without adjuvant radiation. J Am Acad Dermatol 2002;47(6):885–92.
92. Hitchcock CL, Bland KI, Laney RG 3rd, et al. Neuroendocrine (Merkel cell) carcinoma of the skin. Its natural history, diagnosis, and treatment. Ann Surg 1988;207(2):201–7.
93. Messina JL, Reintgen DS, Cruse CW, et al. Selective lymphadenectomy in patients with Merkel cell (cutaneous neuroendocrine) carcinoma. Ann Surg Oncol 1997;4(5):389–95.
94. Gupta SG, Wang LC, Penas PF, et al. Sentinel lymph node biopsy for evaluation and treatment of patients with Merkel cell carcinoma: the Dana-Farber experience and meta-analysis of the literature. Arch Dermatol 2006;142(6):685–90.
95. Fields RC, Busam KJ, Chou JF, et al. Recurrence and survival in patients undergoing sentinel lymph node biopsy for merkel cell carcinoma: analysis of 153 patients from a single institution. Ann Surg Oncol 2011;18(9):2529–37.
96. Mehrany K, Otley CC, Weenig RH, et al. A meta-analysis of the prognostic significance of sentinel lymph node status in Merkel cell carcinoma. Dermatol Surg 2002;28(2):113–7 [discussion: 117].
97. Stokes JB, Graw KS, Dengel LT, et al. Patients with Merkel cell carcinoma tumors < or = 1.0 cm in diameter are unlikely to harbor regional lymph node metastasis. J Clin Oncol 2009;27(23):3772–7.
98. Sarnaik AA, Zager JS, Cox LE, et al. Routine omission of sentinel lymph node biopsy for merkel cell carcinoma <= 1 cm is not justified. J Clin Oncol 2010;28(1):e7.
99. Schwartz JL, Griffith KA, Lowe L, et al. Features predicting sentinel lymph node positivity in Merkel cell carcinoma. J Clin Oncol 2011;29(8):1036–41.
100. Tai P, Yu E, Assouline A, et al. Management of Merkel cell carcinoma with emphasis on small primary tumors–a case series and review of the current literature. J Drugs Dermatol 2010;9(2):105–10.
101. Jabbour J, Cumming R, Scolyer RA, et al. Merkel cell carcinoma: assessing the effect of wide local excision, lymph node dissection, and radiotherapy on recurrence and survival in early-stage disease—results from a review of 82 consecutive cases diagnosed between 1992 and 2004. Ann Surg Oncol 2007;14(6):1943–52.
102. Su LD, Lowe L, Bradford CR, et al. Immunostaining for cytokeratin 20 improves detection of micrometastatic Merkel cell carcinoma in sentinel lymph nodes. J Am Acad Dermatol 2002;46(5):661–6.
103. Pape E, Rezvoy N, Penel N, et al. Radiotherapy alone for Merkel cell carcinoma: a comparative and retrospective study of 25 patients. J Am Acad Dermatol 2011;65(5):983–90.
104. Koh CS, Veness MJ. Role of definitive radiotherapy in treating patients with inoperable Merkel cell carcinoma: the Westmead Hospital experience and a review of the literature. Australas J Dermatol 2009;50(4):249–56.
105. Veness M, Foote M, Gebski V, et al. The role of radiotherapy alone in patients with merkel cell carcinoma: reporting the Australian experience of 43 patients. Int J Radiat Oncol Biol Phys 2010;78(3):703–9.
106. Fang LC, Lemos B, Douglas J, et al. Radiation monotherapy as regional treatment for lymph node-positive Merkel cell carcinoma. Cancer 2010;116(7):1783–90.

107. Lewis KG, Weinstock MA, Weaver AL, et al. Adjuvant local irradiation for Merkel cell carcinoma. Arch Dermatol 2006;142(6):693–700.
108. Gillenwater AM, Hessel AC, Morrison WH, et al. Merkel cell carcinoma of the head and neck: effect of surgical excision and radiation on recurrence and survival. Arch Otolaryngol Head Neck Surg 2001;127(2):149–54.
109. Mojica P, Smith D, Ellenhorn JD. Adjuvant radiation therapy is associated with improved survival in Merkel cell carcinoma of the skin. J Clin Oncol 2007; 25(9):1043–7.
110. Fields RC, Busam KJ, Chou JF, et al. Recurrence after complete resection and selective use of adjuvant therapy for stage I through III Merkel cell carcinoma. Cancer 2012;118(13):3311–20.
111. Poulsen MG, Rischin D, Porter I, et al. Does chemotherapy improve survival in high-risk stage I and II Merkel cell carcinoma of the skin? Int J Radiat Oncol Biol Phys 2006;64(1):114–9.
112. Kokoska ER, Kokoska MS, Collins BT, et al. Early aggressive treatment for Merkel cell carcinoma improves outcome. Am J Surg 1997;174(6):688–93.
113. Garneski KM, Nghiem P. Merkel cell carcinoma adjuvant therapy: current data support radiation but not chemotherapy. J Am Acad Dermatol 2007;57(1):166–9.
114. Sharma D, Flora G, Grunberg SM. Chemotherapy of metastatic Merkel cell carcinoma: case report and review of the literature. Am J Clin Oncol 1991; 14(2):166–9.
115. Henness S, Vereecken P. Management of Merkel tumours: an evidence-based review. Curr Opin Oncol 2008;20(3):280–6.
116. Wynne CJ, Kearsley JH. Merkel cell tumor. A chemosensitive skin cancer. Cancer 1988;62(1):28–31.
117. Pectasides D, Papaxoinis G, Pectasides E, et al. Merkel cell carcinoma of the skin: a retrospective study of 24 cases by the Hellenic Cooperative Oncology Group. Oncology 2007;72(3–4):211–8.
118. Voog E, Biron P, Martin JP, et al. Chemotherapy for patients with locally advanced or metastatic Merkel cell carcinoma. Cancer 1999;85(12):2589–95.
119. Tai PT, Yu E, Winquist E, et al. Chemotherapy in neuroendocrine/Merkel cell carcinoma of the skin: case series and review of 204 cases. J Clin Oncol 2000;18(12):2493–9.
120. Poulsen M, Rischin D, Walpole E, et al. Analysis of toxicity of Merkel cell carcinoma of the skin treated with synchronous carboplatin/etoposide and radiation: a Trans-Tasman Radiation Oncology Group study. Int J Radiat Oncol Biol Phys 2001;51(1):156–63.
121. Su LD, Fullen DR, Lowe L, et al. CD117 (KIT receptor) expression in Merkel cell carcinoma. Am J Dermatopathol 2002;24(4):289–93.
122. Feinmesser M, Halpern M, Kaganovsky E, et al. c-kit expression in primary and metastatic merkel cell carcinoma. Am J Dermatopathol 2004;26(6):458–62.
123. Samlowski WE, Moon J, Tuthill RJ, et al. A phase II trial of imatinib mesylate in merkel cell carcinoma (neuroendocrine carcinoma of the skin): a Southwest Oncology Group study (S0331). Am J Clin Oncol 2010;33(5):495–9.
124. Swick BL, Ravdel L, Fitzpatrick JE, et al. Merkel cell carcinoma: evaluation of KIT (CD117) expression and failure to demonstrate activating mutations in the C-KIT proto-oncogene - implications for treatment with imatinib mesylate. J Cutan Pathol 2007;34(4):324–9.
125. Kartha RV, Sundram UN. Silent mutations in KIT and PDGFRA and coexpression of receptors with SCF and PDGFA in Merkel cell carcinoma: implications for tyrosine kinase-based tumorigenesis. Mod Pathol 2008;21(2):96–104.

126. Woll PJ, Moore KN, Bhatia S, et al. Efficacy results from a phase I study of lorvotuzumab mertansine (IMGN901) in patients with CD56-positive solid tumors [abstract]. J Clin Oncol 2011;29(Suppl):e.13582.

127. Nardi V, Song Y, Santamaria-Barria JA, et al. Activation of PI3K signaling in Merkel cell carcinoma. Clin Cancer Res 2012;18(5):1227–36.

128. Cully M, You H, Levine AJ, et al. Beyond PTEN mutations: the PI3K pathway as an integrator of multiple inputs during tumorigenesis. Nat Rev Cancer 2006;6(3): 184–92.

129. Kong D, Yaguchi S, Yamori T. Effect of ZSTK474, a novel phosphatidylinositol 3-kinase inhibitor, on DNA-dependent protein kinase. Biol Pharm Bull 2009; 32(2):297–300.

130. Maira SM, Stauffer F, Brueggen J, et al. Identification and characterization of NVP-BEZ235, a new orally available dual phosphatidylinositol 3-kinase/mammalian target of rapamycin inhibitor with potent in vivo antitumor activity. Mol Cancer Ther 2008;7(7):1851–63.

131. Hafner C, Houben R, Baeurle A, et al. Activation of the PI3K/AKT pathway in Merkel cell carcinoma. PLoS One 2012;7(2):e31255.

132. Willmes C, Adam C, Alb M, et al. Type I and II IFNs inhibit merkel cell carcinoma via modulation of the merkel cell polyomavirus T antigens. Cancer Res 2012; 72(8):2120–8.

133. Krasagakis K, Kruger-Krasagakis S, Tzanakakis GN, et al. Interferon-alpha inhibits proliferation and induces apoptosis of merkel cell carcinoma in vitro. Cancer Invest 2008;26(6):562–8.

134. Biver-Dalle C, Nguyen T, Touze A, et al. Use of interferon-alpha in two patients with Merkel cell carcinoma positive for Merkel cell polyomavirus. Acta Oncol 2011;50(3):479–80.

135. Iyer JG, Afanasiev OK, McClurkan C, et al. Merkel cell polyomavirus-specific CD8 and CD4 T-cell responses identified in Merkel cell carcinomas and blood. Clin Cancer Res 2011;17(21):6671–80.

136. Zeng Q, Gomez BP, Viscidi RP, et al. Development of a DNA vaccine targeting Merkel cell polyomavirus. Vaccine 2012;30(7):1322–9.

137. National Institutes of Health. Interleukin-12 gene and in vivo electroporation-mediated plasmid DNA vaccine therapy in treating patients with Merkel cell cancer. Available at: http://clinicaltrials.gov/ct2/show/NCT01440816?term=merkel+cell&rank=3. Accessed June 22, 2012.

Index

Note: Page numbers of article titles are in **boldface** type.

Hematol Oncol Clin N Am 26 (2012) 1375–1384
http://dx.doi.org/10.1016/S0889-8588(12)00189-X
0889-8588/12/$ – see front matter © 2012 Elsevier Inc. All rights reserved.

Moving?

Make sure your subscription moves with you!

To notify us of your new address, find your **Clinics Account Number** (located on your mailing label above your name), and contact customer service at:

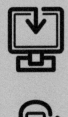

Email: journalscustomerservice-usa@elsevier.com

800-654-2452 (subscribers in the U.S. & Canada)
314-447-8871 (subscribers outside of the U.S. & Canada)

Fax number: 314-447-8029

Elsevier Health Sciences Division
Subscription Customer Service
3251 Riverport Lane
Maryland Heights, MO 63043

*To ensure uninterrupted delivery of your subscription, please notify us at least 4 weeks in advance of move.

Printed and bound by CPI Group (UK) Ltd, Croydon, CR0 4YY

03/10/2024

01040446-0010